THE MEDICAL CLINICS OF NORTH AMERICA

VOLUME 55 / NUMBER 2
MARCH 1971

SYMPOSIUM ON
TREATMENT OF COMMON MEDICAL DISORDERS

José Bocles, M.D., and
Roger F. Palmer, M.D., *Guest Editors*

W. B. SAUNDERS COMPANY – Philadelphia · London · Toronto

W. B. Saunders Company: West Washington Square
Philadelphia, Pa.   19105

12 Dyott Street
London, WC1A   1DB

1835 Yonge Street
Toronto 7, Ontario

Soon after publication in English, the Medical Clinics
appear in translated editions, published by the following:

Spanish   Editorial Interamericana, S.A., Cedro 512,
               Apartado 26370, Mexico 4, D.F., Mexico

Italian   Piccin Editore, Via Porciglia, 10,
               35100 Padua, Italy

Portuguese   Editora Guanabara Koogan, S.A., Rua do Ouvidor,
               132 ZC 21, Rio de Janeiro, Brazil

Greek   John Mihalopoulos and Son,
               Thessaloniki, Greece

THE MEDICAL CLINICS OF NORTH AMERICA
March, 1971   Volume 55 — Number 2

The Medical Clinics of North America is published every other month by W. B. Saunders Company,
West Washington Square, Philadelphia, Pennsylvania 19105, at Hampton Road, Cherry Hill, New Jersey
08034. Subscription price is $21.00 per year. Second class postage paid at Cherry Hill, New Jersey 08034.
This issue is Volume 55, Number 2.
The editor of this publication is Albert E. Meier, W. B. Saunders Company, West Washington Square,
Philadelphia, Pennsylvania 19105.

Library of Congress catalog card number 17-28505

Contributors

ROY D. ALTMAN, M.D., Research Associate, University of Miami School of Medicine; Attending Physician, Jackson Memorial Hospital and Miami Veterans Administration Hospital

AZUCENA G. ARCEBAL, M.D., Senior Fellow in Cardiology, University of Miami School of Medicine and Jackson Memorial Hospital

JOSÉ S. BOCLES, M.D., Clinical Assistant Professor of Medicine, University of Miami School of Medicine

JONATHAN J. BRAUNSTEIN, M.D., Assistant Professor of Medicine, University of Miami School of Medicine

BENJAMIN BRAUZER, M.D., Assistant Professor of Psychiatry, University of Miami School of Medicine

LEE A. BRICKER, M.D., Assistant Professor of Medicine, University of Miami School of Medicine; Attending Physician, Jackson Memorial Hospital and University of Miami Hospital

HARVEY E. BROWN, JR., M.D., Associate Professor of Medicine, University of Miami School of Medicine; Attending Physician, Jackson Memorial Hospital and Miami Veterans Administration Hospital

AUGUSTIN CASTELLANOS, JR., M.D., Assistant Professor of Medicine, University of Miami School of Medicine; Cardiologist, Miami Veterans Administration Hospital

NOBLE J. DAVID, M.D., Professor of Neurology, University of Miami School of Medicine; Chief, Neurology Service, Miami Veterans Administration Hospital

HUGH R. GILMORE, III, M.D., Clinical Associate Professor of Medicine, Division of Cardiology, Department of Medicine, University of Miami School of Medicine

CARL GOLDSMITH, M.D., F.A.C.P., Associate Professor of Medicine, University of Miami School of Medicine; Chief, Renal Section, Jackson Memorial Hospital

BURTON J. GOLDSTEIN, M.D., Associate Professor, and Assistant Chairman, Department of Psychiatry, University of Miami School of Medicine

NORMAN L. GOTTLIEB, M.D., Instructor in Medicine, University of Miami School of Medicine; Attending Physician, Jackson Memorial Hospital and Miami Veterans Administration Hospital

DAVID S. HOWELL, M.D., Professor of Medicine, University of Miami School of Medicine; Director, Arthritis Training and Research Program, Jackson Memorial Hospital and Miami Veterans Administration Hospital

RAMANUJA N. V. IYENGAR, M.D., Senior Fellow in Cardiology, University of Miami School of Medicine and Jackson Memorial Hospital

HARVEY S. KANTOR, M.D., Instructor in Medicine, University of Miami School of Medicine; Research and Education Associate, Infectious Disease Section, Miami Veterans Administration Hospital

JAMES L. KATSIKAS, M.D., Senior Fellow in Nephrology, University of Miami School of Medicine

KURT LANGE, M.D., F.A.C.P., Professor of Medicine, Professor of Clinical Pediatrics, and Chief, Renal Service and Laboratory, New York Medical College; Attending Physician, Flower and Fifth Avenue Hospitals, Metropolitan Hospital, and Bird S. Coler Hospital; Consultant, Horton Memorial Hospital, Middletown, New York, and Chenango Hospital, Norwich, New York

KENNETH C. LASSETER, M.D., Postdoctoral Fellow, Department of Pharmacology, University of Miami School of Medicine

LOUIS LEMBERG, M.D., Professor of Clinical Cardiology, and Chief, Division of Electrophysiology, University of Miami School of Medicine; Director, Coronary Care Unit, Jackson Memorial Hospital

ROBERTO LLAMAS, M.D., Clinical Assistant Professor of Medicine, University of Miami School of Medicine; Associate Director, Cardiopulmonary Laboratory, Miami Heart Institute, Miami Beach, Florida

BARRY J. MATERSON, M.D., Instructor, Department of Medicine, University of Miami School of Medicine; Research Associate, Miami Veterans Administration Hospital

DANIEL H. MINTZ, M.D., Professor of Medicine, and Chief, Division of Endocrinology and Metabolism, University of Miami School of Medicine; Attending Physician, Jackson Memorial Hospital and University of Miami Hospital

ROBERT J. MYERBURG, M.D., Assistant Professor of Medicine and Physiology, University of Miami School of Medicine; Chief, Cardiology Section, Miami Veterans Administration Hospital

ROGER F. PALMER, M.D., Professor and Chairman, Department of Pharmacology, and Professor of Medicine, University of Miami School of Medicine

SOLOMON PAPPER, M.D., Professor and Co-Chairman, Department of Medicine, University of Miami School of Medicine; Chief, Medical Service, Miami Veterans Administration Hospital

ELISEO C. PEREZ-STABLE, M.D., Professor, Department of Medicine, University of Miami School of Medicine; Assistant Chief, Medical Service, Miami Veterans Administration Hospital

ARVEY I. ROGERS, M.D., Associate Professor of Medicine, University of Miami School of Medicine; Chief, Gastroenterology, Miami Veterans Administration Hospital

EUGENE R. SCHIFF, M.D., Assistant Professor of Medicine, University of Miami School of Medicine; Staff Physician, Gastroenterology, Miami Veterans Administration Hospital and Jackson Memorial Hospital

WILLIAM V. SHAW, M.D., Associate Professor of Medicine, University of Miami School of Medicine; Chief, Infectious Disease Section, Miami Veterans Administration Hospital

CARLOS A. VAAMONDE, M.D., Associate Professor of Medicine, University of Miami School of Medicine; Chief, Nephrology Section, Miami Veterans Administration Hospital

RECENT SYMPOSIA

May 1970
NEW DEVELOPMENTS IN MEDICINE

July 1970
SOPHISTICATED DIAGNOSTIC PROCEDURES

September 1970
EFFICACY OF ANTIMICROBIAL AND ANTIFUNGAL AGENTS

November 1970
CURRENT CONCEPTS IN CLINICAL NUTRITION

January 1971
DISEASES OF THE KIDNEY

FORTHCOMING SYMPOSIA

May 1971
MEDICAL ADVANCES IN CANCER
IRWIN H. KRAKOFF, M.D., *Guest Editor*

July 1971
DIABETES MELLITUS
PHILIP FELIG, M.D.,
PHILIP K. BONDY, M.D., *Guest Editors*

September 1971
ATHEROSCLEROSIS
MARK D. ALTSCHULE, M.D., *Guest Editor*

November 1971
INTENSIVE CARE UNITS
JAMES S. TODD, M.D., *Guest Editor*

January 1972
DIAGNOSIS AND TREATMENT OF HEMORRHAGIC DISORDERS
ENNIO C. ROSSI, M.D., *Guest Editor*

Contents

The Treatment of Arrhythmias Following Acute Myocardial
Infarction 273

*Louis Lemberg, Augustin Castellanos, Jr., Azucena G. Arcebal,
and Ramanuja N. V. Iyengar*

Minor disturbances in rhythm associated with myocardial infarction frequently precede primary electrical death due to ventricular fibrillation or cardiac
standstill. Early and aggressive therapy, based on an
understanding of the mechanisms and clinical signs
of these arrhythmias, results in significant reduction
in mortality.

Insulin-Independent Diabetes Mellitus 295

Lee A. Bricker, and Daniel H. Mintz

A discussion of some major controversies: diagnostic
criteria, the degree to which hyperglycemia should be
corrected, the effectiveness of various therapies in
retarding subsequent development of complications.

Treatment of Uncomplicated Peptic Ulcer Disease............................ 305

Eugene R. Schiff

What constitutes "adequate medical therapy" for
peptic ulcer disease? An understanding of the normal
control of gastric acid secretion provides a more
rational basis for currently advocated medical and
surgical techniques for reduction of gastric acidity to
a level at which pepsin activity is insignificant.

The Treatment of Chronic Hypertension.. 317
Hugh R. Gilmore, III

Environmental control and current drug therapy in a
comprehensive regimen for carefully reducing blood
pressure. Consideration of possible harmful effects.

Hypertensive Emergencies.. 325
Carlos A. Vaamonde, Noble J. David, and Roger F. Palmer

A nephrologist, a neurologist, and a clinical pharmacologist discuss malignant hypertension and hypertensive encephalopathy.

Renal Failure 335
Solomon Papper

A comprehensive discussion of pathophysiology, clinical manifestations, and therapy of acute and chronic
kidney dysfunction.

Diuretic Drug Therapy of Edema....................................... 359
Eliseo C. Perez-Stable, and Barry J. Materson

An empirical approach to the management of a variety
of diseases characterized by renal salt and water retention and the formation of edema, based on an
understanding of the mechanisms of action of diuretic
drugs, and the physiologic effects of diuresis.

Therapeutic Considerations in Selected Forms of Acute and
Chronic Liver Disease 373
Arvey I. Rogers

Recent therapeutic advances in acute uncomplicated
viral hepatitis, fulminant hepatic failure, alcoholic
hepatitis, and chronic hepatitis.

Management of the Obese Patient....................................... 391
Jonathan J. Braunstein

Obesity as a nutritional disorder. Diagnosis, underlying causes, complications, and therapeutic programs
for weight reduction.

A Clinical Approach to the Hyperlipidemias...................................... 403

Lee A. Bricker

While primary hypercholesterolemia remains discouraging to treat, the hyperlipemias quite often lend
themselves to successful therapy. Rational diagnostic
decisions can be made in the physician's office using
chemical determinations of plasma cholesterol and
fasting triglyceride, and simple inspection of the fasting plasma, as well as history and physical examination.

Diagnostic and Therapeutic Aspects of Stable Angina Pectoris 421

Robert J. Myerburg

A brief overview of the clinical, metabolic, and patho-
physiologic knowledge accumulated over the past 10
to 15 years: toward a modern approach to management.

Treatment of Arrhythmias: Basic Considerations 435

Kenneth C. Lasseter

Mechanisms by which pharmacologic agents produce
beneficial effects, and the mediation of these effects
in the intact organism through indirect mechanisms
such as the autonomic nervous system.

Airway Obstruction.. 445

José S. Bocles, and Roberto Llamas

Chronic obstruction and acute respiratory failure in
emphysema, chronic bronchitis, and asthma. Precipitating causes and treatment of reversible factors.
The artificial airway. Mechanical ventilatory aids.

A Comprehensive Regimen for Osteoarthritis 457

David S. Howell, Roy D. Altman, Harvey E. Brown, Jr.,
and Norman L. Gottlieb

Recent information on the biochemistry of inflammation and connective tissues, and orthopedic materials
science have opened new vistas for future therapeutic
approaches. A review of current trends in therapy,
with special emphasis on methods employed by the
authors.

Microbial Suprainfection 471

> Harvey S. Kantor, and William V. Shaw

> Antimicrobial agents as a major cause of suprainfection
> in man: a review of selected aspects, including patho-
> genesis and factors influencing colonization and
> suprainfection.

Pharmacologic Considerations in the Treatment of Anxiety and
Depression in Medical Practice 485

> Burton J. Goldstein, and Benjamin Brauzer

> Minor tranquilizers, and antianxiety and antidepres-
> sant drugs in treatment of the anxious-depressed pa-
> tient. Symptom cues, and a frame of reference for
> rational drug therapy.

Drug Interactions 495

> Roger F. Palmer

> Propensity for adverse reactions in patients receiving
> multiple drugs: clinical implementation of pharma-
> cologic data. The effects of drugs on each other in such
> areas as drug metabolism, interference with renal or
> biliary elimination, and alteration of adrenergic
> mechanisms.

Disorders of Potassium Metabolism 503

> James L. Katsikas, and Carl Goldsmith

> Normal potassium metabolism and maintenance of
> cellular function. Evaluating the status of body potas-
> sium: relationship of intracellular to extracellular
> concentrations.

ADDITIONAL ARTICLE

Nutritional Management of Kidney Disorders 513

> Kurt Lange

> Protein metabolism and the maintenance of positive
> nitrogen balance. Dietary considerations in the treat-
> ment of acute and chronic glomerulonephritis, uremia,
> the nephrotic syndrome, and acute renal failure.

Index 521

Foreword

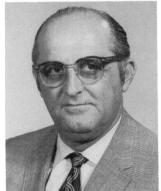 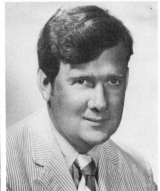

JOSÉ S. BOCLES, M.D.   ROGER F. PALMER, M.D.

Many approaches to the treatment of common medical disorders have changed little in the last decade; others have changed considerably even in the last 2 or 3 years. New modes of therapy are being recognized and with their recognition come new therapeutic pitfalls. Such is the case for example in the problem of drug interactions. In his article Dr. Palmer has outlined serious problems associated with the administration of multiple drugs. Many new interactions of drugs appear weekly in the medical literature, confounding the practitioner, and a synthesis of these mechanisms is presented as a guide to future therapy when multiple drugs are present. The availability of more potent agents has created problems due to overextensions of pharmacologic activity. The newer diuretics present such an example and are discussed in perspective by Drs. Perez-Stable and Materson.

Significant and rapid advances are being made in the understanding of disease. New understandings of the pathophysiology of angina have altered the therapeutic approach to this disease. Dr. Myerburg brings us up to date with recent therapeutic advances in this field. In the area of antiarrhythmic agents much new knowledge has been forthcoming through a better understanding of intracellular events of the cardiac action potential and how they relate to the clinical management of arrhythmias. Accordingly, a section by Dr. Kenneth C. Lasseter on these basic concepts, and an article by Dr. Lewis Lemberg and co-authors on the management of arrhythmias have been included. These seem particularly pertinent since more and more of our population is suffering from various forms of heart disease and there is intensive investigation into the development of new drugs for these purposes.

271

Recent developments in the field of the hyperlipidemias and their potential modification by drugs have been taking place at a rapid rate. Dr. Bricker describes many of the problems involved and some of the newer drugs available for therapy of the hyperlipidemias.

Other areas which have been chronic problems in medicine have received new insights by the various authors that contributed to this issue, and it is hoped that most of the material covered will enable the practicing physician to deal with recent developments in therapy, and their problems.

JOSÉ S. BOCLES, M.D.,
ROGER F. PALMER, M.D.
Guest Editors

University of Miami
School of Medicine
P. O. Box 875, Biscayne Annex
Miami, Florida 33153

The Treatment of Arrhythmias Following Acute Myocardial Infarction

Louis Lemberg, M.D.,* Augustin Castellanos, Jr., M.D.,†
Azucena G. Arcebal, M.D.,‡
and Ramanuja N. V. Iyengar, M.D.§

The introduction of electronic monitoring systems in coronary care units (CCU), coupled with the recent advances in electrophysiology, has resulted in a better understanding of the mechanisms and clinical significance of arrhythmias following myocardial infarction.

Hemodynamic alterations usually result when heart rates fall below 40 per minute or exceed 160 per minute. At these extremes, compensatory mechanisms are brought into play in order to maintain adequate cardiac output or normal blood pressure. In disease states, on the other hand, the reserves may be insufficient to compensate for these extremes in heart rate. A fall in cardiac output may result, with a fall in blood pressure accompanied by diminished blood flow to vital organs. In patients with acute myocardial infarction, therefore, excessively rapid or slow heart rates that occur in the presence of arrhythmias may precipitate or aggravate hypotension or left ventricular failure, or extend the area of injury.

Furthermore, although atrial contribution to cardiac output has been shown to be of little clinical significance in normal hearts, its loss (i.e., during atrial fibrillation of atrioventricular dissociation) in patients with acute myocardial infarction, who already have a compromised circulatory state by virtue of the myocardial damage, may lead to progressive deterioration. Studies have shown that atrial contraction may contribute 20 to 30 per cent of the cardiac output in diseased hearts.

From the Division of Cardiology, Department of Medicine, University of Miami School of Medicine, and the Coronary Care Unit, Jackson Memorial Hospital, Miami, Florida

*Professor of Clinical Cardiology, and Chief, Division of Electrophysiology, University of Miami School of Medicine; Director, Coronary Care Unit, Jackson Memorial Hospital
†Assistant Professor of Medicine, University of Miami School of Medicine; Cardiologist, Veterans Administration Hospital
‡Senior Fellow in Cardiology, University of Miami School of Medicine and Jackson Memorial Hospital
§Senior Fellow in Cardiology, University of Miami School of Medicine and Jackson Memorial Hospital

Thus, in the coronary care unit, early aggressive and prophylactic therapy of arrhythmias is the keynote by which the rapid clinical degradation that is a constant threat during the early days of an acute myocardial infarction is frequently averted or modified.

Following acute myocardial infarction, particularly during the first 48 hours after onset of chest pain, some form of irregularity of the heart beat is exhibited by nearly 95 per cent of patients. An essential and consistent observation is that minor disturbances in rhythm frequently precede primary electrical death due to ventricular fibrillation or cardiac standstill.[18, 22-24] Early and aggressive therapy of these seemingly insignificant arrhythmias in order to prevent the more lethal forms has reduced mortality from acute myocardial infarction by 50 per cent.[24]

MANAGEMENT IN THE CORONARY CARE UNIT

Table 1 illustrates a physiologic classification of arrhythmias occurring in acute myocardial infarction and provides guidelines to therapy. The incidence of the various arrhythmias was obtained from computerized data obtained from the coronary care unit of the University of Miami at the Jackson Memorial Hospital. There were a total of 400 patients with proven acute myocardial infarction.

The ventricular premature beat, by virtue of its frequency (present in 80 per cent of cases) and potentiality for predisposing to ventricular fibrillation, is the most important arrhythmia following an acute myocardial infarction. Since electrical death is primarily due to ventricular

Table 1. *Clinical Classification of Arrhythmias*

ARRHYTHMIAS	INCIDENCE	TREATMENT
Electrical instability		*Drug*
Premature ventricular contraction	80%	Lidocaine
Paroxysmal ventricular tachycardia	28%	Quinidine
		Procainamide
		Propranolol
		Diphenylhydantoin
		Electrical
		Cardioversion
Bradyarrhythmias		*Drug*
Sinus bradycardia	30%	Atropine
Junctional rhythms	8%	Isoproterenol
Slow ventricular tachycardia	16%	*Electrical*
Atrioventricular block	8%	Pacemaker
		Atrial
		Ventriculo-inhibited
Pump failure		*Drug*
Atrial arrhythmias	27.3%	Digitalis
Premature atrial contractions		Propranolol
Paroxysmal atrial tachycardia		*Electrical*
Atrial fibrillation		Cardioversion

fibrillation, the suppression of the ventricular premature beat has significantly reduced the incidence of this lethal complication to less than 5 per cent.

Electrical instability is manifested clinically by a high frequency of ventricular premature beats (more than 6 per minute), salvos of repetitive ventricular beats or ventricular tachycardia with ectopic rates over 100 per minute, ventricular premature beats that are multiform, or even a single ventricular premature beat interrupting the T wave of a preceding sinus or ectopic beat.[23] The latter instance favors ventricular fibrillation because the ventricular premature beat falls during the vulnerable period of the ventricular excitability cycle or ascending limb of the T wave.[34] The threshold of excitability to ventricular fibrillation is reduced following ischemia or injury.

Lidocaine is currently the most useful cardiodepressant drug for the immediate suppression of ventricular premature beats or ventricular tachycardia.[37] It has a rapid onset of action (15 to 30 seconds) and a duration of effect of 20 minutes. Single bolus injections of 50 to 75 mg. of lidocaine are given intravenously for arrhythmias of electrical instability, and are well tolerated without untoward reactions. The dose may be repeated every 15 to 30 minutes, or when necessary.

Persistent or recurrent episodes of the arrhythmia indicate the use of slow intravenous infusion of 1 to 2 gm. of lidocaine in 500 ml. of 5 per cent dextrose in water given at a rate of 1 to 2 mg. per minute, depending on the need. Arrhythmias of electrical instability are suppressed in 88 per cent of cases.[23] With recurrence of the rhythm disturbances, and if continued anti-arrhythmic effect is desired beyond 24 hours, quinidine orally in doses of 200 to 400 mg. four times daily or procainamide 500 mg. every 6 hours is added to the regimen.

Transient hypotension may follow administration of lidocaine rarely, primarily because of its short duration of action. Other side-effects which disappear promptly after cessation of the drug are drowsiness, dryness of the mouth, and slight mental confusion. Rarely, convulsions or respiratory depression may be seen in the elderly patient.

Propranolol, a beta-adrenergic blocking agent, is useful when rapid control of ventricular arrhythmia is desired and when there is intolerance or sensitivity to lidocaine. Small doses, of 0.5 mg. every 2 minutes given intravenously up to a total dose of 3 to 4 mg., have resulted in sinus rhythm in almost all cases (Fig. 1).[20] The presence of concomittant left ventricular failure is not a deterring factor in the management of these patients, as will be shown later.

Electrical cardioversion is indicated when ventricular tachycardia does not respond to drug therapy and a rapidly deteriorating clinical state accompanies the tachyarrhythmia.

During the very early phases following an acute myocardial infarction, bradyarrhythmias complicate the clinical picture in 20 to 30 per cent of patients. Slow ventricular rates may be seen in any one of three mechanisms: sinus bradycardia, atrioventricular dissociation with junctional rhythm, or atrioventricular block (Table 1). Bradyarrhythmias occur more frequently following inferior or diaphragmatic infarctions

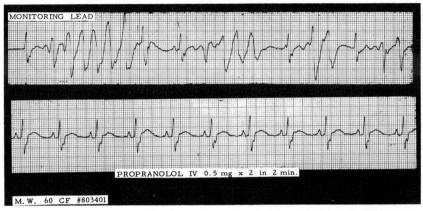

Figure 1. The upper strip shows multifocal ventricular premature beats and runs of ventricular tachycardia occurring in a 60 year old patient with acute myocardial infarction. The second strip shows suppression of the arrhythmias following 1 mg. of propranolol given intravenously in 2 divided doses.

(44 per cent), as compared to anterior wall infarctions (13 per cent). This has been partly attributed to the blood supply. The sinoatrial nodal artery arises from the right coronary artery in 60 per cent of cases, and acute right coronary artery occlusion results in inferior wall or diaphragmatic infarction. However, this alone does not explain the increased incidence of bradyarrhythmias in recent inferior infarctions, since the arrhythmias are usually promptly abolished by vagolytic drugs, such as atropine. Another explanation is the impairment of circulation to the parasympathetic nerve terminals along the lower portions of the interatrial septum. The blood supply to this area comes from the right coronary system.

Sinus bradycardia, the most frequent disorder, occurs alone in 30 per cent of cases of acute myocardial infarction. In 24 per cent, atrioventricular dissociation was present, with either a junctional rhythm or, more commonly, a slow or non-paroxysmal type (ectopic ventricular beats at below 100 per minute with or without exit block) of ventricular tachycardia[2] dominating, and usually making its appearance as an escape mechanism. Although atrioventricular block has a more grave pathogenesis, it is included in this category because the slow ventricular response that occurs with it produces similar hemodynamic and electrophysiologic alterations. The main therapeutic objective in atrioventricular block, as well as in the other bradyarrhythmias, is cardio-acceleration.

Normally, when the heart rate falls below 60 per minute, normal vasomotor control mechanisms and adequate cardiac function produce an increase in stroke volume to maintain cardiac output. In patients with acute myocardial infarction the damaged heart is unable to compensate, and increases in stroke volume do not occur even when rates fall below normal. As a result, systemic blood pressure falls, with consequent reduction in regional blood flow to the heart, brain, and kidneys. Clinically, this is manifested by hypotension, dizziness or syncope, low urine output, left ventricular failure, and arrhythmias due to the resulting acidosis.

One of the essential observations in the coronary care unit is the enhanced frequency of ventricular premature beats and other ventricular arrhythmias in the presence of sinus bradycardia (Fig. 2).[14, 23, 36] Through animal experiments it has been demonstrated that with the longer ventricular cycles that occur in sinus bradycardia, great disparity in the rate of recovery of excitability develops between neighboring groups of fibers.[15] This may be further enhanced by repetitive ventricular ectopic beats, sympathetic stimulation, digitalis toxication, and myocardial ischemia.[6] Therefore, in the clinical setting of acute myocardial injury, cardiac rates below 60 per minute will favor multiform ventricular premature beats, ventricular tachycardia, and even ventricular fibrillation. Although bradyarrhythmias are potentially serious, the prognosis is excellent,[23] provided that prompt therapy is directed toward accelerating the heart to a "critical" rate. The critical rate is considered to be that rate below which hypotension, poor cardiac output, or ventricular premature beats appear. There is no fixed optimal rate, because it varies from patient to patient and may even vary in the same patient from time to time.

Cardio-acceleration can be attained pharmacologically with atropine or isoproterenol, or by electrical pacing. Transvenous endocardial pacing may be done by atrial pacing, ventricular pacing, or both. The latter can be accompanied by the newer technique of sequential atrioventricular pacing (Fig. 3).[10]

Since heightened vagal tone frequently accompanies acute infarctions of the inferior or diaphragmatic wall,[14, 37] sinus slowing is treated initially with 0.4 to 1 mg. of atropine administered intravenously. At times, doses up to 2 mg. may be required. This may be repeated every 1 to 2 hours as needed in order to prevent the untoward effects of the bradyarrhythmia. When undesirable reactions to atropine occur (hallucinations or mental confusion in elderly patients, urinary retention) or when an "optimal" rate is not obtained, isoproterenol is given as a slow intravenous infusion beginning with doses of 0.5 mg. in 500 ml. of 5 per cent dextrose in water. The mixture is carefully titrated to maintain the

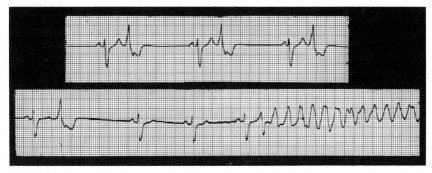

Figure 2.   Ventricular premature beats and ventricular flutter associated with sinus bradycardia in a patient with recent inferior wall myocardial infarction.

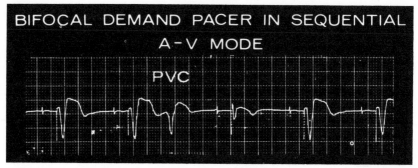

Figure 3. Demand pacemaker which can be dormant or pace the atria or atria and ventricles with sequential delay.

desired rate while preventing increased ventricular automaticity which may occur.

The persistence of ventricular ectopic beats or the occurrence of angina with isoproterenol dictates cessation of therapy. When normal atrioventricular conduction exists, atrial pacing reverses the adverse effects of the bradyarrhythmia while maintaining a fixed, clinically desirable rate. A disadvantage of the latter procedure is the difficulty in maintaining an adequate electrode catheter position for effective atrial pacing, in which case, ventricular pacing is substituted. Figures 4 through 6 show bradyarrhythmias treated with atropine, isoproterenol, and atrial pacing respectively.

There are special features and special therapeutic problems associated with heart block complicating acute myocardial infarction. Although heart block is an infrequent complication (7 to 10 per cent)[27, 33] it has generated more controversy than any of the other arrhythmias occurring in the coronary care unit. The differences in opinion relate to the indications for the use of pacemakers and to the judgment as to their beneficial effects.

The incidence and mortality figures for the varying degrees of atrioventricular block are shown in Table 2. Of interest is that no death was noted among those with first degree atrioventricular block and second degree atrioventricular block of the Wenckebach type that did not progress to third degree atrioventricular block. The overall mortality of complete atrioventricular block in the coronary care unit at the Jackson Memorial Hospital is 43 per cent, which is only slightly higher than the figure for second degree atrioventricular block of the Mobitz II variety, indicating the malignant nature of the latter.[31]

Knowledge of the site of the infarction is a critical factor in determining the prognosis as well as the management of atrioventricular block complicating acute myocardial infarction.[23, 27, 32, 33] In Table 3 it is apparent that although atrioventricular block follows inferior or diaphragmatic infarctions more than twice as often as it follows anterior wall infarctions, the mortality rate is three times greater in the latter than in the former.

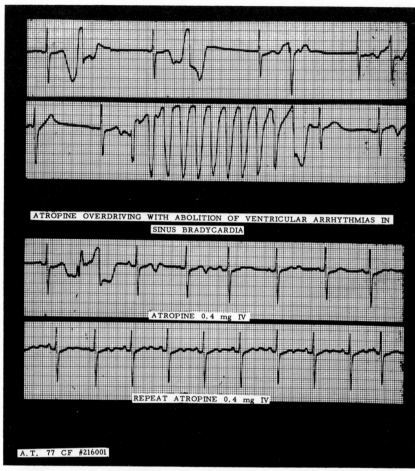

ATROPINE OVERDRIVING WITH ABOLITION OF VENTRICULAR ARRHYTHMIAS IN
SINUS BRADYCARDIA

ATROPINE 0.4 mg IV

REPEAT ATROPINE 0.4 mg IV

A.T. 77 CF #216001

Figure 4. The upper two strips show multifocal premature ventricular contractions and a run of ventricular tachycardia in a patient with sinus bradycardia and transient atrioventricular dissociation. Overdriving with 0.8 mg. of atropine intravenously accelerated sinus node discharge with abolition of the arrhythmia.

The pathogenesis of acute atrioventricular conduction disturbances helps to explain these differences. Heart block in acute infarction of the inferior wall is located high in the atrioventricular node (above the bundle of His) and consists pathologically of edema or inflammation due to transient ischemia, or infarction of contiguous myocardium rather than involvement of the conduction tissue proper. The block is usually transient, and seldom is there a residual conduction defect. In anterior wall infarctions, heart block is secondary to destruction and necrosis of the bundle branches and distal parts of the conducting tissues, so that permanent damage results with residual block of one or both bundles. With the use of His bundle electrocardiography, studies of patients with acute atrioventricular block following acute myocardial infarction have

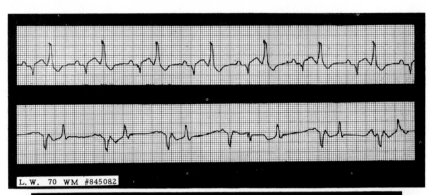

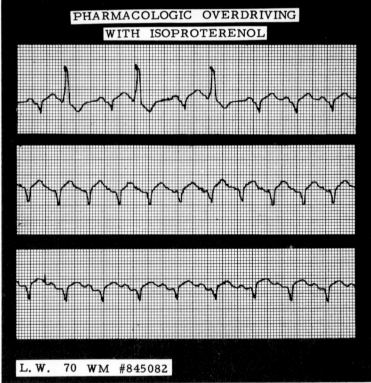

Figure 5. *Above,* Seventy year old white man with acute anterolateral myocardial infarction with ventricular bigeminy. Intravenous administration of 50 mg. of lidocaine, transient atrioventricular dissociation with multifocal premature ventricular contractions as seen in the second strip, resulted.

Below, With persistence of ventricular bigeminy, isoproterenol was used for overdrive. With an increase in sinus rates to 125 to 150 per minute, the arrhythmia was completely eliminated.

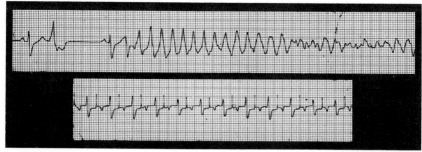

Figure 6.   Recurrent ventricular irritability with ventricular fibrillation in a setting of sinus bradycardia prevented by overdriving, using atrial pacing at a rate of 125 per minute.

localized the area of conduction disturbance to be above the bundle of His in inferior wall infarction and below the bundle of His in atrioventricular block complicating anterior wall infarctions.[4] Table 4 shows the other differences that characterize these two forms of atrioventricular block.

In general, first degree atrioventricular block alone, irrespective of the site of infarction, requires no treatment. In the presence of higher degrees of block complicating inferior wall infarctions, initial drug therapy is indicated if the existing ventricular rate is inadequate and undesirable effects of bradyarrhythmia develop. In the clinical setting, therefore, the critical factor is the heart rate and not the degree of block.

In inferior wall infarctions, early acute atrioventricular block of any degree may result from excessive vagal discharge, and in these situations, sinus bradycardia is also present. Atropine, in doses mentioned earlier, has been shown to improve atrioventricular conduction in more than half of these patients (Fig. 7). Intravenous infusion of isoproterenol may improve atrioventricular conduction when atropine is ineffective. One mg. of isoproterenol in 500 ml. of 5 per cent dextrose in water is titrated for the desired clinical rate and rhythm.

The clinical course and prognosis of atrioventricular block in inferior wall infarction are not significantly altered by endocardial pacing. The following are the indications for pacing in atrioventricular block due to acute inferior wall infarction: (1) when the ventricular rate cannot be effectively maintained at optimal levels by drug therapy; (2) second degree atrioventricular block, Mobitz type II (very rare); (3) third degree

Table 2.   *Incidence and Mortality Rates in Various Types of Atrioventricular Block*

TYPE	INCIDENCE	MORTALITY
First degree	10.7%	0
Second degree, Wenckebach type	2.3%	0
Second degree, Mobitz type II	2.0% } 4.3%	33%
Third degree	7.2%	43%

Table 3. *Incidence of Third Degree Atrioventricular Block Complicating Myocardial Infarction and Associated Mortality Rates*

SITE	INCIDENCE	MORTALITY
Diaphragmatic infarction	69%	27.1%
Anterior infarction	31%	80.0%

atrioventricular block with wide QRS complexes and a ventricular rate below 60 per minute.

Earlier experiences in the coronary care unit have shown that most patients who develop acute atrioventricular block following anterior wall infarctions have a poor prognosis even with electrical pacing. This is attributed to the extensive myocardial damage and has frequently been complicated by cardiogenic shock, pump failure, or myocardial rupture.

With more advances in electrophysiology, and following retrospective reviews of particular clinical situations, it has been noted that atrioventricular block with anterior wall infarctions was frequently ushered in by the appearances of block in any of the bundle branches.[28] Specific ECG patterns are produced by interruption of any one or any combination of the right bundle and the two divisions (anterosuperior and posteroinferior) of the left bundle.[3, 5, 28] With this knowledge, prophylactic insertion of a pacing catheter when any two of these branches are blocked improve prognosis.

The approach to therapy for atrioventricular block complicating anterior wall myocardial infarction is quite different. Here atropine is ineffective and isoproterenol may be transiently helpful if advanced

Table 4. *Atrioventricular Block Complicating Myocardial Infarction*

	ATRIOVENTRICULAR BLOCK COMPLICATING ANTERIOR WALL INFARCTION	ATRIOVENTRICULAR BLOCK COMPLICATING INFERIOR WALL INFARCTION
Pathogenesis	Destruction due to infarction of the bundle branches	Edema or inflammation due to transient ischemia of atrioventricular node and contiguous myocardium
Location of block	Below the bundle of His	Above the bundle of His
Premonitory signs	Sudden asystole or appearance of bundle branch block	Sinus bradycardia often; first degree atrioventricular or second degree Wenckebach often precedes atrioventricular block
Adam-Stokes attacks	Almost always present	Rare (7 to 10 per cent)
QRS complexes	Usually wide (idioventricular)	Usually narrow, maintaining supraventricular pattern
Subsidiary pacemaker	Ventricular	Probably junctional
Mobitz II	Usual	Rare
Residual block	Bundle branch block (any form)	Almost always none
Treatment	Pacemaker	Drugs usually effective
Prognosis	Poor	Good

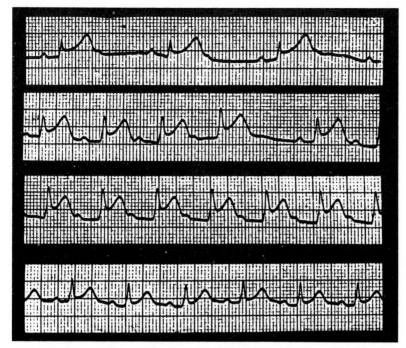

Figure 7.   Sinus rhythm with normal PR interval followed the intravenous adminis-tration of 0.6 mg. of atropine to a 70 year old patient with a recent inferior wall myocardial infarction complicated by third degree atrioventricular block.

atrioventricular block or asystole occurs before a pacing catheter can be introduced (Fig. 8). Therefore, in the following acute situations, a pace-maker catheter should be inserted prophylactically for standby pacing:

1. Complete right bundle branch block and block of the superior division of the left bundle.

2. Complete right bundle branch block and block of the inferior division of the left bundle.

3. Complete right bundle branch block and first degree atrioventric-ular block.

4. Complete left bundle branch block and first or second degree atrioventricular block.

5. Complete left bundle branch block alternating with complete right bundle branch block.

6. Any type of bundle branch block with shock or progressive heart failure.

The above includes the different degrees of bifascicular or incom-plete trifascicular block.[28] Active pacing is initiated in the presence of complete atrioventricular block, second degree block, Mobitz type II, commonly seen in anterior wall infarction, or progressive first degree block with a P-R interval longer than 0.30 seconds.

Atrioventricular conduction disturbances that follow myocardial infarction are transient in nature and seldom require permanent pacing. Because regular sinus rhythm may return at anytime during the course

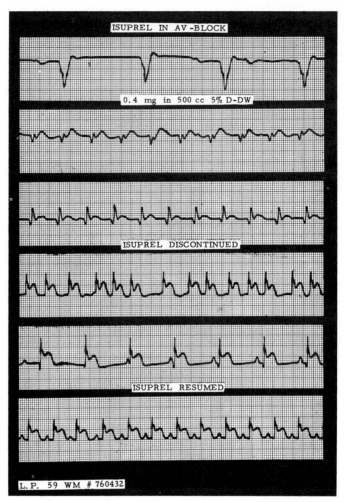

Figure 8. Restoration of sinus rhythm with normal atrioventricular conduction with isoproterenol (Isuprel) in a case of complete atrioventricular block. Initially, isoproterenol caused an increase in rate of a ventricular rhythm (strip 2). When atrial fibrillation with a ventricular response of +120 per minute occurred (strip 4), isoproterenol was discontinued. The drip had to be restarted when sinus bradycardia with transient atrioventricular dissociation resulted (strip 5), and sinus rhythm with normal atrioventricular conduction was maintained at rates of 125 to 130 per minute.

of an acute myocardial infarction, the pacemaker of choice is the ventriculo-inhibited or demand pacemaker.[1, 21] This type of pacemaker reduces the risk of repetitive ventricular beats or ventricular fibrillation. Figure 9 shows an episode of ventricular fibrillation initiated by a pacemaker impulse occurring in a patient with acute myocardial infarction prior to the use of demand pacemaker.

 In spite of the transient character of atrioventricular blocks in patients with myocardial infarction, a review of the second week postinfarction arrhythmias[27] have revealed a 15 per cent incidence of either

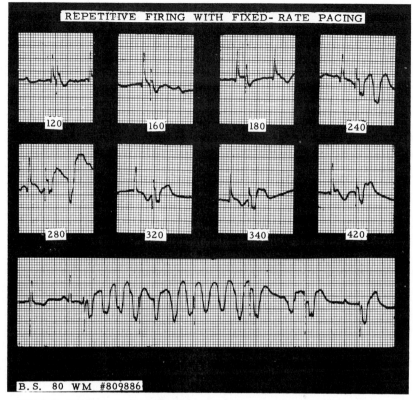

Figure 9. Episodes of repetitive firing and ventricular fibrillation initiated by a pace-maker inpulse occurring in a patient with acute myocardial infarction when the spikes fell, 240 to 280 msec following the onset of the QRS.

a return of atrioventricular abnormalities or deaths due to cardiac arrest. Whether re-infarction or recurrent ischemia contributed to this incidence or whether it resulted from drug usage,[19] the question is ever present as to how long a pacing catheter for standby pacing should be retained in the ventricular cavity. The use of continued monitoring by telemetry in an intermediate coronary care unit would help answer this question in addition to improving the prognosis during this period.[35]

Supraventricular arrhythmias occurring during an acute myocardial infarction are generally considered to be benign and transient.[30] Excluding sinus tachycardia, atrial fibrillation is the most common and occurs in 10 to 15 per cent of cases of myocardial infarction. Most episodes of atrial fibrillation are preceded by premature atrial beats and occasionally by short runs of atrial tachycardia.[17] It is not unusual to see spurts of atrial tachycardia, flutter, and fibrillation in the same patient within short periods of time. These arrhythmias are usually associated with anterior or lateral wall infarctions resulting from involvement of the left coronary system. Their occurrence in these situations has been attributed either to elevated left atrial pressures secondary to left ventricular failure[23] or to atrial infarction.[29] Although atrial fibrillation was more commonly seen after the first 24 hours following an acute myocardial infarction when the degree of left ventricular failure is expected to be greater, it also occurred with inferior or true posterior wall infarctions within the first few hours after the onset of chest pain. In this instance, involvement of the right coronary artery, which supplies the sinoatrial node in 60 per cent of cases, has been implicated as a factor contributing to the etiology of atrial fibrillation.

Short paroxysms of supraventricular arrhythmias may be tolerated during an acute myocardial infarction provided that the ventricular rate is not rapid. In most instances, however, particularly following the acute onset of atrial fibrillation and flutter, the ventricular response to the rapid atrial ectopic beats exceeds 150 per minute and may aggravate existing left ventricular failure and cause hypotension, thus widening the area of damage or injury. In this setting, the patient's intolerance to the rapid rates with potential deterioration of the clinical state dictate rapid control of the arrhythmia.

A special consideration in acute atrial fibrillation other than the rapid ventricular response is the loss of atrial transport, which may be critical in the presence of a damaged myocardium; therefore, there is an urgent need not only to slow the heart rate immediately, but also to restore atrial contribution to cardiac output by establishing sinus rhythm.

Although electrical cardioversion has been highly successful in terminating atrial flutter, its effects in atrial fibrillation are transient, and the arrhythmia returns after a brief period of sinus rhythm (Fig. 10).

Digitalis has been the drug of choice for atrial arrhythmias, particularly in left ventricular failure. Oral digoxin, 0.25 mg. two or three times daily, plus diuretics may help abolish ectopic atrial contractions, and may prevent progression to atrial flutter or fibrillation. When a more rapid atrial arrhythmia occurs in spite of digitalization, adequate control of ventricular response may require added increments of digitalis, parenterally or orally, depending upon the urgency of the situation.

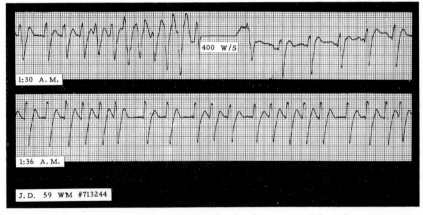

Figure 10. Recurrent atrial fibrillation shortly after successful cardioversion; sinus rhythm was maintained only for 6 minutes.

Patients with acute myocardial infarction have been shown to be more sensitive to digitalis, tolerating only 70 per cent of the usual digitalizing dose.[8] However, in the presence of atrial arrhythmias, particularly atrial fibrillation, the use of large amounts of the drug to slow the ventricular rate by more effective atrioventricular blocking of rapid atrial impulses may be required.

The rapidity of obtaining an optimal slow ventricular response to atrial fibrillation with the use of digitalis alone is unpredictable. Furthermore, the possibility of digitalis overdosage in acute myocardial infarction dictates caution and prevents its use in amounts needed to achieve the end point of desired ventricular rate control. Beta blocking agents can be successfully employed in this clinical setting. They are effective alone or combined with the glycosides to enhance the atrioventricular effect.[25]

Supraventricular and ventricular arrhythmias accompanied by varying degrees of heart failure not responding to conventional measures were successfully treated with propranolol (Table 5).[20] The clinical state required urgent and immediate therapy. Propranolol, 0.5 mg. given intravenously every 2 minutes up to an average amount of 4.5 mg., is effective within 5 to 15 minutes in controlling the rapid ventricular rate, and frequently may convert the rhythm to sinus (Fig. 11). As a result, prompt objective and subjective improvement may occur. The heart failure may also respond more easily to the usual anticongestive heart failure therapy.

In digitalized patients, less propranolol is needed to slow atrioventricular conduction or achieve sinus rhythm because of the synergistic effect of the drugs on delaying atrioventricular transmission. Likewise, in the presence of propranolol, smaller doses of digitalis are required to obtain the therapeutic effect on atrioventricular conduction, thus minimizing the risk of digitalis intoxication.

Following resumption of sinus rhythm and control of left ventricular failure, there is usually no need for long-term administration of propranolol. Maintenance doses of digitalis and intermittent diuretic therapy frequently suffice to keep these patients compensated and free from arrhythmias. Quinidine sulfate, 200 to 400 mg. every 4 hours 4

Table 5.   *Treatment of Arrhythmias in Acute Myocardial Infarction with Propranolol*

ARRHYTHMIAS	NO. OF EPISODES	HEART FAILURE		
		Mild	Moderate	Severe
Atrial flutter	18	6	8	4
Atrial fibrillation	6	4	2	0
Supraventricular tachycardia	8	3	3	2
Ventricular tachycardia	11	4	4	3
Total		16	18	9

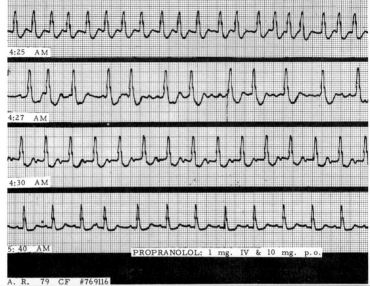

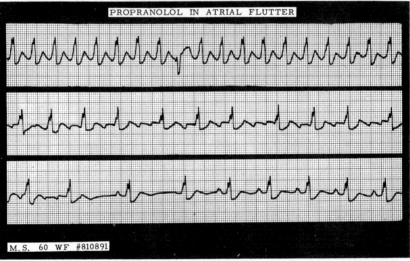

Figure 11. *Above,* Conversion of atrial fibrillation with rapid ventricular response (+ 160 per minute) to sinus rhythm with intravenous propranolol. Following the initial doses of propranolol, the ventricular rate dropped to +90 per minute. Atrial tachycardia at 125 per minute is shown in the third strip, before sinus rhythm with one premature atrial contraction occurring in the fourth strip.

Below, Top strip shows atrial flutter with a ventricular rate of 150 per minute. Propranolol at increments of 0.5 mg. intravenously every 2 minutes resulted in increasing degrees of atrioventricular block and slower ventricular rates with conversion to sinus rhythm after a total dose of 4 mg.

times daily, or diphenylhydantoin, 100 mg. every 4 hours 4 times daily, given orally, will be required when, on occasion, premature atrial contractions or atrial fibrillation persist or recur in spite of adequate control of heart failure and no evidence of new injury.

The known negative inotropic properties of the beta blocking agents[33] are frequently referred to when discussing contraindications to their use in clinical states complicated by heart failure. Hence, there is very little information about its use in the treatment of arrhythmias that follow an acute myocardial infarction. In our experience, the negative chronotropic property of propranolol, producing prompt ventricular slowing in settings where the rapid rates were judged to significantly enhance the hemodynamic abnormalities, plus its quinidine-like property, resulting in conversion to sinus rhythm, were important factors in reducing the oxygen demands of the heart and improving the clinical state. Thus, the benefit obtained with the use of beta blocking agents far outweighed its adverse effects on myocardial contractility.

Few side effects were observed. Sinus bradycardia with atrioventricular dissociation can be promptly counteracted by intravenous administration of 1.0 mg. of atropine. Rarely when atropine is ineffective, isoproterenol IV will be effective. Occasionally, respiratory wheezing due to bronchial constriction occurs with propranolol therapy. This responds promptly to intravenous aminophylline or isoproterenol inhalation.

At all times when using propranolol intravenously, continuous ECG monitoring is mandatory. There should also be available for immediate use a syringe containing 1 mg. of atropine sulfate and 0.2 mg. isoproterenol in 250 ml. of 5 per cent dextrose in water. These are necessary to counteract any excessive slowing of the heart rate resulting from excessive beta blocking effect.

With the introduction of a new beta blocking agent, alprenolol (Aptine), the incidence of slowing of the sinus nodal discharge, or excessive reduction in the ventricular rate has been much less. This is due to the mild beta stimulating property of this new drug, along with its beta blocking effect.

The occurrence of ventricular arrhythmias during the later stages of an acute myocardial infarction (beyond the seventh day) in the absence of clinical or ECG evidence of recurrent ischemic episodes or reinfarction is not unusual. Electrical instability is probably not the cause, and the following factors may be contributory: left ventricular failure, drugs (specifically digitalis), electrolyte imbalance, and hypoxia or blood gas abnormalities. In these clinical settings, therapy is directed towards the underlying etiologic factor. Antiarrhythmic therapy, as with the ventricular arrhythmias of electrical instability, may be given. Patients who have had serious electrical disturbances during the first 5 days in the coronary care unit require maintenance antiarrhythmic therapy to prevent the 5 to 10 per cent incidence of sudden death during the second week. An ideal situation would be the establishment of a "second week" coronary care unit or intermediate unit for continued monitoring on a semi-ambulatory basis.

THE INTERMEDIATE CORONARY CARE UNIT

Statistics indicate that a significant number of deaths occur in hospitalized patients, after discharge from the coronary care unit. Lown et al. reported 22 hospital deaths among 120 patients, 7 (33 per cent) of which occurred after the first week.[22] In a series reported by Day,[25] 4 out of 85 deaths occurred outside the coronary care unit, among a total of 411 patients. The mortality rate in patients discharged from the coronary care unit was 10 per cent in the first 100 patients followed by Killip and Kimball.[18] These patients had either cardiac arrest or life-threatening arrhythmias during their stay in the coronary care unit. However, in the next 150 patients studied by Killip and Kimball, only 2 per cent died after the first week.[18] These authors attributed the reduction in mortality to the fact that, in the second group, all patients with complications were kept in the coronary care unit for a longer period of time. MacMillan et al. reported that 74 late deaths (of a total of 235 demises) occurred in 787 patients with acute myocardial infarction.

Grace et al., who have done the most extensive studies on this aspect of acute myocardial infarctions, followed 305 patients and observed 39 late deaths, half of which were sudden and were thought to be related to ventricular fibrillation, complete atrioventricular block, or asystole.[12] Although these late deaths continued to occur, there have been very few reports dealing with the mechanisms of death and their prevention. At Jackson Memorial Hospital, the mortality rate in patients who had been discharged from the coronary care unit was 11.8 per cent when the patients had been kept only 3 or 4 days in the unit, but was reduced to 6.5 per cent when their stay in the unit had been 1 week. Thirteen of the last 200 patients discharged from the coronary care unit died while still in the hospital. Pump failure could be incriminated in two patients, but arrhythmias were probably responsible in the remaining ones. "Reinfarction" was diagnosed in only two of the four in which post-mortem studies were performed.

In general, it appears that patients having acute transmural infarction complicated by severe arrhythmias have a greater chance of dying suddenly in the post-coronary care period. One obvious solution of this problem would be to keep the patients in the coronary care unit for the entire 3 week period. This is impractical from both the economic viewpoint and bed availability. For this reason, Grace and co-workers at St. Vincent's Hospital in New York elaborated the concept of the Intermediate Coronary Care Unit.[11, 13]

Structure of an Intermediate Coronary Care Unit

Patients with transmural acute myocardial infarction who develop life-threatening arrhythmias or congestive heart failure in the first week are the best candidates for the intermediate coronary care unit. However, if beds are available, all patients should be monitored. The intermediate coronary care unit, which should ideally be located in an area close to the coronary care unit, consists of a single four-bed room designed to provide an additional 12 to 14 days of observation. At St. Vincent's Hospital, tracings are taken every 4 hours by special nurses' aides and are analyzed immediately by a staff or resident physician.[13] This unit is equipped for resuscitation and defibrillation. If the patient's condition deteriorates he is transferred back to the coronary care unit.

At Jackson Memorial Hospital, we are currently evaluating a telemetry system by means of which the electrical signals from the patient are displayed at the nurses' console. The Multichannel RKG Monitor Biomedical Telemetry System* may be used to observe both bedridden and ambulatory patients. The patient's signal is transmitted to the receiver console at the nursing station. The transmitter is a miniature frequency-modulated radiotransmitter circuit housed in a rugged aluminum case. It is connected to the patient by a short cable which, in turn, is attached to the adhesive electrodes applied to the patient's chest. Each transmitter is factory-tuned to one of the receiver channels.

The console is composed of four receiving units: an oscilloscope monitor to display the signals, an electrocardiographic receiver, and a mode selector unit housed in a metal cabinet. This system is equipped with both a high and low frequency alarm system. Tracings are obtained every 4 hours by trained registered nurses. A cardiologist is called if any abnormality is noted. Although data are displayed visually on a monitoring screen, the nurse does not watch the monitor constantly. In contrast to the coronary care unit, where the patient/nurse ratio is 2 to 1, in the intermediate coronary care unit the patient/nurse ratio is 10 to 1. One possible solution to this problem is the use of trained paramedical personnel capable of identifying arrhythmias. Another solution is the addition of an ectopic beat detector. The extrasystole detector is connected to the receiver console to identify arrhythmias appearing in the periods between the recording of the tracings when the monitor is not watched closely.

The Ectopic Beat Detector† is presented in a compact 7×15 module placed close to the nurse's console. It is designed to detect, display, and count ectopic beats of both atrial and ventricular origin. Included is a standard electrocardiographic recorder which writes out 3 second chart segments containing the programed ectopic event, approximately 2 seconds of recording preceding the beat under consideration, and 1 second afterward. This instrument also includes another recorder which plots the heart rate and trend of ectopic activity on a slow moving paper.

The efficacy of the Ectopic Beat Detector or telemetry in general depends on an adequate electrocardiographic signal. This is fundamental, since the patients are not confined to the bed. Therefore, proper electrode placement and optimal care of the electrodes are essential.

Gains Obtained with the Use of an Intermediate Coronary Care Unit

Since our unit has been operating for only 2 months, it is too early to arrive at any conclusions regarding its usefulness. However, Dr. Grace's

---

*Hamilton Standard, Farmington, Connecticut.
†American Optical Company, Framingham Center, Massachussets

experience at St. Vincent's Hospital is impressive.[11] For instance, 117 patients were admitted to the intermediate coronary care unit during its first year of operation. One hundred were discharged directly from the unit and the hospital; 14 were transferred back to the coronary care unit; one died after transfer, and 3 died in the unit.

A dividend of the intermediate coronary care unit is the knowledge gained from following the natural history of patients with acute myocardial infarction after their discharge from the coronary care unit. It should be emphasized again that 10 per cent have life-threatening arrhythmias and about 5 per cent have recurrent chest pain, suggesting recurrent injury or infarction or extension of the previous infarction.[24] The number of patients (6) who returned to the coronary care unit because of severe chest pain was surprisingly high, since no patients were returned to the coronary care unit for recurrence of chest pain prior to the establishment of the intermediate coronary care unit. Of the 9 patients who were returned to the coronary care unit because of arrhythmias, 6 had been in congestive heart failure in the coronary care unit and the other 3 had no complications.

REFERENCES

1. Castellanos, A. Jr., Iyengar, R., Arcebal, A. G., et al.: Intermediate coronary care unit. (In press)
2. Castellanos, A. Jr., Lemberg, L., and Arcebal, A. G.: Mechanisms of slow ventricular tachycardias in acute myocardial infarction. Dis. Chest, 56:470–476, 1969.
3. Castellanos, A. Jr., Lemberg, L., Arcebal, A. G., et al.: Pacing in acute myocardial infarction: A programmed introduction. Chest, 58:152, 1970.
4. Castellanos, A. Jr., Lemberg, L., Arcebal, A. G., et al.: Post-infarction conduction disturbances: A self-teaching program. Dis. Chest, 56:421, 1969.
5. Castellanos, A. Jr., Maytin, O. Arcebal, A. G., et al.: Alternating and coexisting block in the divisions of the left bundle branch. Dis. Chest, 56:103–109, 1969.
6. Castillo, C., Berkovits, B. V., Castellanos, A. Jr., et al.: Bifocal demand pacing. Chest, (In Press).
7. Day, H. W.: Acute coronary care: A five year report. Amer. J. Cardiol., 21:252, 1967.
8. Dreifus, L., Watanabe, Y., Cardenas, N., et al.: Newer anti-arrhythmic drugs. Cardiovascular Clinics, Vol. 1, No. 3. Philadelphia, F. A. Davis Co., 1969.
9. Fluck, D. C., Olsen, E., Pentecost, B., et al.: Natural history and clinical significance of arrhythmias after cardiac infarction. Brit. Heart J., 29:170, 1967.
10. Friedberg, C., Cohen, H., and Donoso, E.: Advanced heart block as a complication of acute myocardial infarction. Role of pacemaker therapy. Prog. Cardiovasc. Dis., 10:466, 1968.
11. Grace, W. J.: Coronary's "half-way stop." Med. World News, 11:25, 1970.
12. Grace, W. J., and Sossia, J. L.: Reducing mortality from acute myocardial infarction—current ideas. Cardiol. Digest, 4:29, 1969.
13. Grace, W. J., and Yarvote, P. M.: The intermediate coronary care unit—preliminary observations. Presented at the Regional Meeting of the American College of Physicians, New York, 1969.
14. Han, J.: Mechanisms of ventricular arrhythmias associated with myocardial infarction. Amer. J. Cardiol., 24:800, 1969.
15. Han, J.: Ventricular vulnerability during acute coronary occlusion. Amer. J. Cardiol., 24:857, 1969.
16. Hurst, J. W., and Logue, B.: The Heart. New York, McGraw-Hill, 2nd ed., 1970.
17. James, T. N.: Myocardial infarction and atrial arrhythmias. Circulation, 24:761, 1961.
18. Killip, T., and Kimball, J.: Treatment of myocardial infarction in a coronary care unit: A two-year experience with 250 patients. Amer. J. Cardiol., 20:457, 1967.
19. Klass, H. J.: Atrial fibrillation associated with acute myocardial infarction. A study of 34 cases. Amer. Heart J., 79:752, 1970.

20. Lemberg, L., Castellanos, A. Jr., and Arcebal, A. G.: The use of propranolol in arrhythmias complicating acute myocardial infarction. Amer. Heart J., 4:479–487, 1970.
21. Lemberg, L., Castellanos, A. Jr., Berkovits, B. V.: Pacemaking on demand in A-V block. J.A.M.A., 191:12–14, 1965.
22. Lown, B., Fakhro, A., Hosdi, W., et al.: The coronary care unit: New perspectives and directions. J.A.M.A., 199:188, 1967.
23. Lown, B., and Klein, M.: Coronary and pre-coronary care. Amer. J. Med., 46:705, 1969.
24. Lown, B., Kosowsky, B., and Klein, M.: Pathogenesis, prevention and treatment of arrhythmias in myocardial infarction. Circulation, 29(Suppl. 4):261, 1969.
25. Lucchesi, B., and Whitsitt, L.: The pharmacology of beta-adrenergic blocking agents. Prog. Cardiovasc. Dis., 11:410, 1969.
26. MacMillan, R. L., Brown, K. W. G., Peckham, G. B., Kahn, O., Hutchinson, D. B., and Paton, M.: Changing perspectives in coronary care. Amer. J. Cardiol., 20:451, 1967.
27. McNally, E., and Benchimol, A.: Medical and physiological considerations in the use of artificial cardiac pacing (Part I). Amer. Heart J., 75:380, 1968.
28. Maytin, O., Castellanos, A. Jr., Arcebal, A. G., et al.: Significance of complete right bundle branch block with right axis deviation in the absence of right ventricular hypertrophy. Brit. Heart J., 1:85–92, 1970.
29. Morris, J., Taft, C., Whalen, R., et al.: Digitalis and experimental myocardial infarction. Amer. Heart J., 77:342, 1969.
30. Mounsey, P.: Intensive coronary care. Amer. J. Cardiol., 20:475, 1967.
31. Norris, R. M.: Heart block in posterior and anterior myocardial infarction. Brit. Heart J., 31:352, 1969.
32. Rosen, K., Loeb, H., Rahimtoola, S., et al.: Site of heart block in acute myocardial infarction. Abst. Clinical Res., 18:326, 1970.
33. Scott, M., Geddes, J., Patterson, G., et al.: Management of complete heart block complicating acute myocardial infarction. Lancet, 2:1382, 1970.
34. Smirk, F. H.: R waves interrupting T waves. Brit. Heart J., 11:23, 1949.
35. Spraklen, F., Bisterman, E., Everest, M., et al.: Late ventricular dysrhythmias after myocardial infarction. Brit. Med. J., 4:364, 1968.
36. Zipes, D.: The clinical significance of bradycardia rhythms in acute myocardial infarction. Amer. J. Cardiol., 24:814, 1969.
37. Zipes, D.: Treatment of arrhythmias in myocardial infarction. Arch. Intern. Med., 124:101, 1969.

Department of Medicine
University of Miami School of Medicine
P.O. Box 875, Biscayne Annex
Miami, Florida 33152

Insulin-Independent Diabetes Mellitus

Lee A. Bricker, M.D.,* and Daniel H. Mintz, M.D.**

Major controversies over the criteria for the diagnosis of diabetes mellitus, the degree to which its hyperglycemia should be corrected, and the effects of various therapies on retarding the subsequent development of complications, remain far from settled.[4] Nonetheless, by examining the several schools of thought and the results obtained in various clinics, one can arrive at a set of workable definitions and practices which will serve the great majority of patients quite well.

DIAGNOSIS

A number of approaches to the diagnosis of diabetes mellitus can be taken. Certainly the adult individual who presents with complaints of the sudden or gradual onset of severe thirst and nocturia, who has a family history of diabetes mellitus, and who may manifest such diverse findings as microaneurysms in the optic fundi, proteinuria, and peripheral neuropathy, presents no diagnostic problem. Perhaps more typical, however, is the patient who may be overweight, whose family history is vague, and who may be noted on routine examination to have an elevated postprandial blood glucose concentration. A decision about whether or not such a patient actually has diabetes mellitus may be difficult.

Glucose Tolerance Test

Perhaps the commonest way of establishing a diagnosis of diabetes mellitus is with the oral glucose tolerance test.[17, 22] In our clinic, the standard method of performing this study consists of obtaining a blood specimen prior to, and 30, 60, 90, 120, and 180 minutes following, the oral administration of 1.75 gm. of glucose per kg. of body weight. The patterns of plasma glucose disappearance following oral glucose ingestion characterize either a normal individual or one with diabetes mellitus.

---

*Assistant Professor of Medicine, University of Miami School of Medicine; Attending Physician, Jackson Memorial Hospital and University of Miami Hospital

**Professor of Medicine, and Chief, Division of Endocrinology and Metabolism, University of Miami School of Medicine; Attending Physician, Jackson Memorial Hospital and University of Miami Hospital

A wide variety of disease states and metabolic derangements influence the rate of glucose disappearance from the blood after its oral administration. Acromegaly, hyperthyroidism, Cushing's syndrome, pheochromocytoma, insulin-secreting tumors, certain central nervous system diseases, chronic liver disease, chronic renal failure, potassium depletion, and other states can significantly reduce glucose tolerance. Moreover, drugs, particularly benzothiadiazine diuretics and oral contraceptive agents, can impair glucose metabolism and chemically produce changes which mimic diabetes mellitus. It should be borne in mind, moreover, that diabetes mellitus and a secondary cause for hyperglycemia may co-exist in a single patient.

Four circumstances deserve special clinical emphasis in the interpretation of the oral glucose tolerance test.

AGE. Table 1 shows a set of normal values for 2-hour postprandial blood sugars, and the increases in these values with increasing age.[10] Accordingly, one must be very circumspect in making a diagnosis of diabetes mellitus, being certain that the appropriate age considerations are applied to the patient's blood sugar values. Failure to consider the patient's age is especially likely to lead to error in diagnosis in the elderly patient.

OBESITY. Many obese patients manifest carbohydrate intolerance.[14] Such "chemical" diabetes may be resistant to virtually any form of control except large doses of medications or weight reduction itself. In instances in which weight loss is successfully accomplished, carbohydrate metabolism often reverses to normal. Figure 1 shows the effects of weight loss alone on the oral glucose tolerance curve. The question in this patient remains whether obesity alone was a cause for the postprandial hyperglycemia or whether it constituted a sufficient stress to unmask a latent diabetes mellitus. It is perhaps in these patients that the actual definition of diabetes mellitus becomes most obscure.

CARBOHYDRATE-INDUCED HYPERLIPIDEMIA. This entity is a familial, primary hyperlipidemic state. It tends to become manifest in middle age, and is generally seen in the mildly to moderately obese individual. Such individuals show distinct carbohydrate intolerance, and are often diagnosed as having diabetes mellitus. Furthermore, such individuals appear to have an accelerated rate of development of atherosclerosis and coronary artery disease. Examination of the patient's fasting plasma reveals it to be lactescent. These patients, however, do not seem prone

Table 1. *Upper Limits of Normal for Plasma Glucose Values in the Oral Tolerance Tests in Older Patients**

	AGE			
	Under 50	50–60	60–70	70–80
1 hour	185	195	210	220
2 hours	140	150	160	175

*Criteria of Fajans et al.[10]

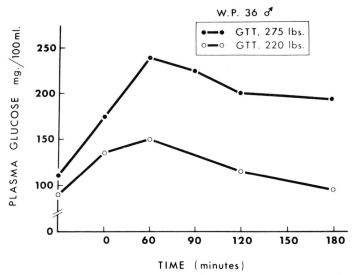

Figure 1. The effect of weight loss on the oral glucose tolerance test.

to develop the vascular complications of diabetes mellitus. This mimicker of diabetes mellitus is effectively treated not by rigid control of the carbohydrate intolerance, but rather by a diet which is relatively restricted in carbohydrates and high in polyunsaturated fats.[6] This dietary regimen alone is usually sufficient to return both plasma glucose and triglyceride levels to normal or near normal levels. The disorder is discussed more fully in a separate section.

PROLONGED BED REST. Bed rest,[16] particularly when associated with carbohydrate restriction, can lead to carbohydrate intolerance. This hyperglycemic response to bed rest is often encountered in hospitalized patients, many of whom maintain the supine position much of the time. Omission of meals between diagnostic tests further contributes to the setting, such that after 3 or 4 days of stressful testing, dietary deprivation, and bed rest, an abnormal oral or intravenous glucose tolerance curve may well be observed.

We have observed that this physiologic response to hospitalization is a frequent cause for an inappropriate diagnosis of diabetes mellitus.

Siperstein et al.[23] have described a technique depending solely on morphologic criteria which we have found useful in the diagnosis of diabetes mellitus. In particular, a sample of quadriceps muscle obtained by needle biopsy is submitted for electron microscopy, and the average thickness of the capillary basement membrane is measured. At present, this test should probably be restricted to adults, where it will more likely offer definitive information. Data for many juvenile patients and for prediabetics remain somewhat indecisive at the present time. Table 2 illustrates the differences in the thickness of muscle capillary basement membranes in a group of adult onset diabetic patients as compared to normal controls. While this test is not widely available, the technique is easy to perform and is inexpensive and safe.

Table 2. *Capillary Basement Membrane Thickness in Thigh Muscle
in Patients with Diabetes Mellitus and in Normal Controls*

	SUBJECTS	NUMBER	WIDTH (Å ± SEM)
Normal	Men	28	1144 ± 35
	Women	22	998 ± 35
Diabetes	Men	23	2217 ± 152
	Women	28	2557 ± 174

*Data of Siperstein, et al.[23]

WHAT IS "GOOD CONTROL"?

Our goal for adequate management of this disease is the maintenance of the patient's general good health and feeling of well-being in a
setting of freedom from symptoms of either hyperglycemia or hypoglycemia. While it is probably logical to suppose that the range of blood
sugar nearest that found in the comparable normal individual might be
least detrimental to the health of the patient with diabetes, such ideal
conditions are, for the most part, unobtainable throughout the day in
most patients. Attempts at such close regulation in insulin-dependent
patients, furthermore, may seriously enhance the risk of hypoglycemia.
Accordingly, we frequently consider it necessary and prudent to accept
postprandial levels of blood sugar higher than this ideal. It is our practice
in patients treated with oral hypoglycemic agents to attempt to obtain
a blood glucose concentration no higher than 160 mg. per 100 ml. before
each meal. In special cases, some patients are able to detect less severe
degrees of hyperglycemia through noting vague feelings of malaise,
inability to think clearly, and other individualized reactions, particularly
early in the disease. The evidence, however, is inconclusive that such
non-euglycemic regulation in any way augments or accelerates the
occurrence of complications.[13]

In our view, then, "good control" represents that state of regulation
in the diabetic patient in which the patient himself feels well and functions at a maximal level. His blood sugar is maintained as close to "normal" as is feasible without risking hypoglycemia. His diet is planned,
palatable, eaten regularly, and is designed to maintain a normal weight.
His therapy is as simple as it can be and encumbers his life to an absolutely minimal degree.

Every effort should be made to keep the patient's morale high and to
encourage him in every possible way. The patient with diabetes is often
terrified at the disclosure that he has the disease. Absolutely paramount
in proper treatment is a thorough, friendly, and enthusiastic dispelling
of these fears, as far as is realistic, and the firm accentuation of that
which is possible. Successful therapy is most likely to occur with continuing physician-patient interaction, in which both parties are prepared
to give time and effort over a long period. There is little room for the
cultivation of guilt or for the intrusion of a reward-and-punishment

philosophy. We avoid, therefore, promulgating a rigid concept of "good" or "bad" control. There is no sound basis for fostering a belief that the patient can somehow dictate the long-range course of his disease simply by religiously following instructions.

PRINCIPLES OF MANAGEMENT

Of paramount importance in total therapy for the diabetic patient is the maintenance of his weight in a normal or near-normal range. A large proportion of adult patients are overweight, and obesity and its complications remain one of the most frustrating problems for the diabetologist and his patient as well. A diet should be individually chosen for the patient, with three goals in mind: (1) palatability, (2) maintenance of normal weight, and (3) a reduction in the content of concentrated or refined carbohydrate. It is beyond the scope of this review to deal with specific diets,[13] but detailed recommendations of some utility have been widely circulated by the American Diabetes Association and the American Dietetic Association.

There is, in addition, increasing evidence to support the contention that diets containing an excess of saturated fat are atherogenic.[12, 24] This, coupled with the well-known tendency of many patients with diabetes to accelerated atherosclerosis,[2, 3, 7, 15] should probably be sufficient grounds for the limitation of saturated fats in the patient's diet. On the other hand, polyunsaturated fats are well known antihypercholesterolemic agents[1] and may have a salutary effect in preventing this type of vascular disease.

In general, caloric allowances should conform to the standards recommended by the Food and Nutrition Board of the National Research Council with individual adjustments for growth, activity, pregnancy, and age.[20] The protein content should approximate 1.2 to 1.5 gm. per kg. per day. Fat should constitute approximately 40 per cent of caloric value of the diet, with 40 per cent represented as polyunsaturated fats, 40 per cent monounsaturated fats, and the remainder saturated fats. These restrictions virtually eliminate dairy fats and restrict meats to those with minimal fat content, with fish and fowl serving as the primary protein source. Fats derived from polyunsaturated vegetable oils (corn, safflower, and soybean) should be emphasized. The carbohydrate content of the diet approximates 40 per cent of its caloric value, the major limitation being placed on restricting rapidly absorbed simple sugars, while emphasizing the more slowly digested and absorbed complex starches.

Diabetic patients should, when possible, be encouraged to exercise regularly. In addition to helping to maintain the patient's sense of well-being, regular and planned exercise may augment peripheral glucose utilization and thereby diminish the dose of insulin or oral hypoglycemic agent required for regulation.

General measures in regulation of the diabetic patient should also include a good state of hygiene. Every effort should be made to avoid infection and unnecessary exposure to colds. In particular, the feet, which are subject to unusually severe complications in diabetes, should be kept scrupulously clean, and in well-fitted, appropriate shoes.

Drug Therapy

Two classes of oral agents are currently in use. One of these is the sulfonylureas. Although we have little insight into the mechanism of their action, the concept that sulfonylurea agents act by enhancing pancreatic beta cell function enjoys considerable support.[11] Table 3 lists the more commonly used sulfonylurea agents and their dosages.

These agents are of value in lowering the blood glucose levels in adult-onset diabetes mellitus, although strict diet may be equally effective. Any of the sulfonylurea compounds may be used initially; the starting dose should be the smallest effective dose. They should not, however, be used in individuals who manifest any major degree of insulin dependence. This, of course, would include most juvenile patients with diabetes mellitus. In this respect, a history of diabetic ketoacidosis at any point in the patient's life would represent contraindication to the use of these agents. While such patients may be easily managed on a small dose of insulin, the substitution of oral agents in their therapy, when they may have virtually no capacity to secrete endogenous insulin, can be quite dangerous. Similarly, patients who have chronic pancreatitis or who have had extensive pancreatic surgery are also not candidates for this type of therapy.

In theory, moreover, these drugs should not be used in obese patients with carbohydrate intolerance until they have successfully undergone weight loss. In practice, this principle is usually difficult to realize, with the obesity proving intractable and the hyperglycemia remaining troublesome. The difficulty may be compounded by the sulfonylureas themselves, since their blood glucose-lowering effects tend to be active in stimulating appetite. The use of sulfonylureas vs. insulin in such diet-resistant patients is currently controversial.

A second classification of orally active agents is the biguanides. These agents may be used alone, or in combination with sulfonylureas.

Table 3. *Commonly Used Oral Agents in Treatment of Diabetes Mellitus*

		TOTAL DAILY DOSES (GM.)		DOSES PER DAY	HALF LIFE (Hr.)
GENERIC NAME	TRADE NAME	Common	Range		
Tolbutamide	Orinase	1.5	0.5 –3.0	2–3	5–7
Acetohexamide	Dymelor	0.75	0.25–1.25	1–2	5–7
Tolazamide	Tolinase	0.25	0.10–0.75	1	7
Chlorpropamide	Diabinese	0.25	0.10–0.50	1	32
Phenformin (phenethylbiguanide)	DBI-TD	0.10	0.05–0.15	2	8

Evidence presently available suggests that, in contrast to the sulfonylureas, they directly stimulate peripheral glucose uptake[18, 25] as a primary mode of action. As with sulfonylureas, biguanides are similarly not used in our clinic in individuals who are insulin-dependent.

Although insulin-biguanide therapy has some advocates, we believe that the major gain of the regimen is merely the reduction in insulin dosage which frequently accompanies it. In our experience, this combination of therapies has generally been successful in patients who have been overinsulinized and are demonstrating the Somogyi phenomenon.[5] The major currently used biguanide agent in the United States is phenethylbiguanide (DBI); the preparation is also formulated in a timed-disintegration capsule (DBI-TD) (see Table 3). The latter preparation is preferred, since there seem to be fewer side-effects with its use. The drug is generally given in doses of 50 to 150 mg. daily. Unlike the sulfonylureas, the biguanide agents seem to function as anorectic agents.[19] Weight reduction with these drugs is easier to achieve than with the sulfonylureas,[26] and the drug may have unique benefit, therefore, in the obese individual with diabetes mellitus.

Some patients not controlled by a sulfonylurea or phenformin alone may be controlled by the combination of phenformin with one of the sulfonylureas. This is due to an apparent[26] synergistic effect. In our clinic, a trial of combined therapy has frequently eliminated the need to resort to insulin.

Toxicity of Oral Hypoglycemic Agents

Undesirable side-effects of the various sulfonylureas are not frequently encountered. Cholestatic jaundice, leukopenia, gastrointestinal upset, a curious intolerance to alcohol, and, most commonly, toxic erythema have been reported, but the combined incidence of these in our clinic appears to be less than 1 per cent. While uncommon, hypoglycemia can occur with any of the sulfonylureas. The persistent nature of the hypoglycemia, particularly that associated with chlorpropamide, frequently necessitates prolonged intravenous glucose therapy. A number of other drugs such as salicylates and phenylbutazone, can interfere with the metabolism or excretion of the active forms of sulfonylureas, and we are therefore especially watchful for hypoglycemia when sulfonylureas are combined with these agents.

Side-effects from phenformin therapy occur more commonly than do those from the sulfonylureas. Anorexia, nausea, vomiting, and diarrhea are frequent. An unpleasant metallic or bitter taste occasionally occurs and serves as a warning sign of impending gastrointestinal intolerance.

Reports of the association of phenformin with lactic acidosis suggest a causal relationship, although the evidence that the drug can actually cause lactic acidosis is inconclusive.[8, 9] Nevertheless, we do not routinely use phenformin in patients who have diseases which may hinder metabolism or excretion of the drug (hepatic or renal diseases), or who have complicating processes (extensive vascular disease) that may be associated with hypotension and tissue underperfusion.

COMMON TREATABLE AND PREVENTABLE
COMPLICATIONS OF DIABETES MELLITUS

As is the case in nearly all areas of diabetes mellitus, controversy exists over whether the more serious complications of diabetes mellitus, such as the various forms of renal disease and the destruction of vision can be prevented or forestalled by proper management. It is beyond the scope of this review to deal with the efficacy of the various modes of treatment believed by some to be of benefit in these serious instances. There is no doubt, of course, that some patients receiving even the best, most careful, and meticulous care, develop the full complement of tragic sequelae in relentless and irreversible fashion. There are by contrast, however, certain common problems which are indeed preventable and treatable in the vast majority of patients.

In general, physicians caring for patients with diabetes should encourage special precautions to prevent infections, to which, as a group, these patients appear extraordinarily susceptible. For example, death attributed to pyelonephritis occurs four times more frequently in diabetic patients than in nondiabetic patients.[21] Renal papillary necrosis, a serious and frequently lethal complication, is more frequently encountered in patients with diabetes mellitus and can usually be traced to instrumentation of the genitourinary tract. Urethral catheterization should be used only in very special circumstances and with exceptional caution in patients with diabetes mellitus. Other kinds of infections likely to be encountered include skin infection, vulvovaginitis, pneumonia, periodontal disease, and, particularly, tuberculosis. In our clinic, we routinely obtain a chest x-ray at least annually on each patient with diabetes mellitus.

Virtually all of these disparate infections are capable of drastically altering the status of carbohydrate metabolism, opening the way for severe hyperglycemia and frequently ketosis. During treatment for such infections, individuals ordinarily treated with oral therapy may require insulin until the infection is brought under control. Every effort should be made by the physician to educate the patient to these problems.

At the University of Miami and in other centers, there has been considerable interest in regular foot care for diabetic patients. Our experience has shown that the routine foot care delivered to a large number of patients on a regular basis in the clinic pays enormous dividends. A general philosophy that all feet, prior to the point of actual gangrene, are salvagable, is probably not far from the truth. That amputation has been performed too often and too extensively on too many patients in the past is now quite clear. There is every reason to believe that a concerned physician, examining all patients' feet on a regular basis, can significantly reduce the amputation rate in his patients.

A foot clinic is in operation at the University of Miami, and the actual administration of care is done by a trained nurse. Patients with diabetic ulcers are dealt with in this clinic in the context of the overall diabetes outpatient unit. The nurse simply debrides the callus around the ulcer and the surrounding tissue with a single-edge razor blade. Such a patient requires weekly visits to the foot clinic during his months of treatment, and in the interim is instructed to soak the affected foot in a high pail of lukewarm water containing a small amount of pHisoHex or other surgical soap. This should be done three or four times daily for 30 minutes at a time. It is usually all that is needed to control infection and keep the foot completely clean. A regimen of such soaks, combined with scrupulous drying of the feet and toes between soaks, and weekly visits to the nurse in the foot clinic, has yielded extremely gratifying results. Figure 2 shows a series of photographs of stages in the healing of a deep diabetic ulcer in a patient's foot over the ensuing weeks after its presentation.

The essential points to be borne in mind are: (1) the dividends in terms of salvaged feet are very striking indeed and, (2) care of this nature can be routinely made available in the office of any physician, administered safely and highly effectively by an office nurse.

Another complication of diabetes mellitus, far less frequently seen than those mentioned above, and generally far less serious, is the hyperlipemia of diabetes. These hypertriglyceridemias occur infrequently and are generally associated with persistent hyperglycemia or acute ketoacidosis. In general, lowering the blood glucose level and reversing the ketosis, usually with insulin, drastically reduces the hyperlipidemia. The mechanism whereby this hyperglycemia produces hyperlipidemia is

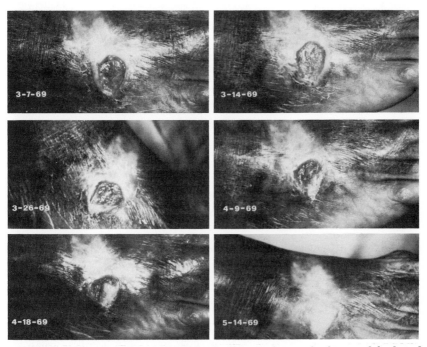

Figure 2. Sequential stages of healing of a diabetic ulcer on the dorsum of the foot of an elderly woman with diabetes. The lesion occurred following injury of the lower aspect of a previously healed elongated scar. The healed area is depigmented. The photo dated 5–14–69 shows new skin covering the entire ulcerated area. (Photos made by Parkland Memorial Hospital Diabetic Foot Clinic and Medical Illustrations Department, University of Texas Southwestern Medical School, Dallas, and reproduced with permission.)

complex, but the clinical expression of the problem is generally easily reversed. These entities are discussed more fully in a subsequent report.[5]

REFERENCES

1. Ahrens, E. H., Hirsch, J., Insull, W., Tsaltas, T. T., Blomstrand, R., and Peterson, M. L.: The influence of dietary fats on serum lipid levels in man. Lancet, 1:943, 1957.
2. Albrink, M. J., Lavietes, P. H., and Man, E. B.: Vascular disease and serum lipids in diabetes mellitus. Ann. Intern. Med., 58:305, 1963.
3. Bell, E. T.: A postmortem study of vascular disease in diabetics. Arch. Path., 53:444, 1952.
4. Berson, S. A., and Yalow, R. S.: Some current controversies in diabetes research. Diabetes, 14:549, 1965.
5. Bloom, M., Mintz, D. H., and Field, J. B.: Insulin-induced post-hypoglycemic hyperglycemia as a cause of "brittle" diabetes: Clinical clues and therapeutic implications. Amer. J. Med., 47:891, 1969.
6. Bricker, L. A.: A clinical approach to the hyperlipidemias. MED. CLIN. N. AMER., 55:403, 1971.
7. Clawson, B. J., and Bell, E. T.: Incidence of fatal coronary disease in non-diabetic and in diabetic persons. Arch. Path., 48:105, 1949.
8. Craig, J. W., Millner, M., Woodward, H., Jr., and Merik, E.: Influence of phenethylbiguanide on lactic, pyruvic, and citric acids in diabetic patients. Diabetes, 9:186, 1960.
9. Ewy, G. A., Maher, J. F., Pabico, R. C., and Mintz, D. H.: Lactate acidosis associated with phenformin therapy and localized tissue hypoxia: Report of a case treated by hemodialysis. Ann. Intern. Med., 59:878, 1963.
10. Fajans, S. S., Levine, R., and Moss, J. M.: The diagnosis of diabetes: The fasting blood glucose test and the oral glucose tolerance test. Gen. Pract., 39:133, 1969.
11. Grodsky, G. M., Bennett, L. L., Smith, D., and Nemechek, K.: The effect of tolbutamide and glucose on the timed release of insulin from the isolated perfused pancreas. In Butterfield, W. J. H., and Van Westering, W., eds.: Tolbutamide after Ten Years. New York, Excerpta Medica Foundation, 1967, p. 11.
12. Keys, A., Anderson, J. T., and Grande, F.: Serum cholesterol response to changes in the diet. IV. Particular saturated fatty acids in the diet. Metabolism, 14:776, 1965.
13. Knowles, H. C., Jr., Guest, G. M., Lampe, J., Kessler, M., and Skillman, T. G.: The course of juvenile diabetes treated with unmeasured diet. Diabetes, 14:239, 1965.
14. Kreishberg, R. A., Boshell, B. R., DiPlacido, J., and Roddam, R. F.: Insulin secretion in obesity. New Eng. J. Med., 276:314, 1967.
15. LeCompte, P. M.: Vascular lesions in diabetes mellitus. J. Chron. Dis., 2:178, 1955.
16. Lipman, R. L., Schnure, J. J., Bradley, E. M., and Lecocq, F. R.: Impairment of peripheral glucose utilization in normal subjects by prolonged bed rest. J. Lab. Clin. Med., 76:221, 1970.
17. McDonald, G. W., Fisher, G. F., and Burnham, C.: Reproducibility of the oral glucose tolerance test. Diabetes, 14:473, 1965.
18. Menert, H.: Experimental investigation of the mode of action of biguanides. In Ostman, J., ed.: Diabetes. Proceedings of the Sixth Congress of the International Diabetes Federation. Amsterdam, Excerpta Medica Foundation, 1969.
19. Patel, D. P., and Stowes, J. M.: Phenformin in weight reduction of obese diabetics. Lancet, 2:282, 1964.
20. Recommended Dietary Allowances. A report of the Food and Nutrition Board, National Academy of Science, National Research Council. Publication No. 1146, 6th ed., 1964.
21. Robbins, S. L., and Tucker, A. W.: The causes of death in diabetes. New Eng. J. Med., 231:865, 1944.
22. Samols, E., and Marks, V.: Interpretation of the intravenous glucose test. Lancet, 1:462, 1965.
23. Siperstein, M. D., Unger, R. H., and Madison, L. L.: Studies of muscle capillary basement membranes in normal subjects, diabetic and prediabetic patients. J. Clin. Invest., 47:1973, 1968.
24. Taylor, C. B., Yogi, M., Wood, J., and Cox, G.: Cholesterol vs. neutral fat in cholesterolosis in monkeys. Fed. Proc., 18:510, 1959.
25. Tyberquein, J. M., and Williams, R. H.: Metabolic effects of phenethylbiguanide, a new hypoglycemic compound. Proc. Soc. Exper. Biol., 96:29, 1957.
26. Unger, R. H., Madison, L. L., and Carter, N. W.: Tolbutamide-phenformin in ketoacidosis-resistant patients. J.A.M.A., 174:2132, 1960.

Department of Medicine
University of Miami School of Medicine
P. O. Box 875, Biscayne Annex
Miami, Florida 33152

Treatment of Uncomplicated Peptic Ulcer Disease

*Eugene R. Schiff, M.D.**

The therapeutic approach to the patient with a peptic ulcer is hampered by a poor understanding of the pathogenesis of this disease. Along with the lack of knowledge as to the cause of peptic ulcer, one is further frustrated by the failure to convincingly demonstrate that what is currently considered "adequate medical therapy" either enhances healing, decreases the incidence of complications, or prevents recurrence. Nevertheless, the physician is faced with the responsibility of optimally treating this relatively common disease with its attendant morbidity. The sparse controlled double-blind prospective studies assessing the various modes of current therapy are of little solace to the symptomatic patient or to his physician, who must make the best of what is available.

Although the cause of peptic ulcer is not known, it is apparent that the presence of gastric acid and pepsin is a prerequisite for ulcer formation. The development of ulceration seems to be dependent on the degree of acid secretion relative to the resistance of the mucosal barrier. The conversion of pepsinogen to the proteolytic enzyme pepsin is pH-dependent. At a pH range of 1.5 to 3.5, pepsin activity is maximal, and at pH levels greater than 7, pepsin activity is nil. For these reasons, current medical and surgical therapy is oriented primarily around measures directed toward the reduction of gastric acidity, hopefully to a level at which pepsin activity is insignificant. An understanding of the normal control of gastric acid secretion gives the physician some rationale for currently advocated therapy.

GASTRIC SECRETION OF ACID

Hydrochloric acid is secreted by the parietal cells located in the body of the stomach, and its secretion is controlled primarily by the interaction of stimulators and inhibitors. The major stimulators of acid secretion are acetylcholine and gastrin. Acetycholine directly stimulates the

---

*Assistant Professor of Medicine, University of Miami School of Medicine; Staff Physician, Gastroenterology, Miami Veterans Administration Hospital and Jackson Memorial Hospital

parietal cells to release hydrochloric acid, and is the sole mediator of gastrin release from the antrum. Gastrin, a hormone carried in the bloodstream to the parietal cells, acts synergistically with acetylcholine in stimulating acid secretion. Gastrin release is inhibited by acidification of the antrum via an unknown mechanism. The major inhibitors of acid secretion are the hormones secretin and cholecystokinin, which are released from the duodenum into the bloodstream and act on receptor sites in the parietal cells.

Afferent impulses that initiate reflex arcs, centrally or locally, ultimately result in the postganglionic release of acetylcholine. These impulses are triggered by psychic stimuli, such as the sight, smell, taste, or thought of food, by gastric distention, and by chemical substances such as alcohol and amino acids. The afferent and efferent impulses travel via the vagus nerve or the local cholinergic pathways in the walls of the stomach. Release of the inhibitory hormones secretin and cholecystokinin is initiated by acid, fat, or hyperosmolar solutions entering the duodenal lumen.

Thus, there are many potential physiologic pathways that may be modified in an attempt to reduce gastric acidity. Measures may be directed toward eliminating chemical or mechanical stimuli of acid secretion; impeding cholinergic pathways medically or surgically; eliminating gastrin-secreting cells; removing or destroying parietal cells; and finally, neutralizing acid in the gastric lumen. The use of synthetic inhibitory hormones has not been studied in a clinical setting but may offer a therapeutic avenue in the future. Newer therapeutic agents which have been introduced are not directed at reducing acid secretion, but have pharmacologic properties that may inactivate pepsin or perhaps enhance the integrity of the mucosal barrier.

Peptic ulcerations may develop in the esophagus, stomach, duodenum, jejunum, or a Meckel's diverticulum. The following discussion will focus on the therapy of uncomplicated duodenal and gastric ulcer disease, and is drawn from what little is known of the pathophysiology of the disorder, as well as the accumulated clinical experience of several investigators in the field.

DIAGNOSIS

Of paramount importance to the institution of proper treatment of peptic ulcer is the establishment of a correct diagnosis. Care must be taken to rule out malignant gastric ulcer and the Zollinger-Ellison syndrome masquerading as a garden variety of duodenal ulcer. Furthermore, predisposing factors such as stressful environmental situations or suspected ulcerogenic drugs (phenylbutazone, reserpine, indomethacin, and corticosteroids) should be eliminated if possible.

The diagnosis of peptic ulcer frequently can be made by history alone. It is usually not difficult to elicit from the patient a history of recurrent episodes of abdominal pain over a period of several years or more with seasonal variation. The pain may be nonspecific, but characteristically is burning or gnawing in nature; it is sharply localized, usually in the epigastrium, maximal in intensity prior to mealtime, and readily relieved by the ingestion of food or alkali. The patient may be awakened at night by the pain, but it is unusual for him to experience it on awakening in the morning. If the pain tends to persist throughout the day, ulcer penetration may have developed.

Associated with the characteristic distress, there may be a history of vomiting, melena or hematemesis, or both, or sudden onset of a more severe and persistent abdominal pain. These complications should alert the physician to the possibility of pyloric obstruction, gastroduodenal hemorrhage, or a perforation, respectively. Signs and symptoms of diarrhea or steatorrhea associated with a history of ulcer-like pain may represent the Zollinger-Ellison syndrome. Physical findings are generally negative or nonspecific in the patient with uncomplicated benign peptic ulcer.

X-Ray Examination

The most helpful diagnostic tool is the upper gastrointestinal tract series. A competent radiologist will detect approximately 95 per cent of gastric or duodenal ulcers. Although the incidence of gastric carcinoma is decreasing in this country, approximately 5 per cent of gastric ulcers are malignant. It is obviously of great importance to ferret out the malignant ulcers for definitive surgical resection as soon as possible.

The radiologist can usually make the differentiation between a benign and a malignant ulcer. A gastric ulceration that does not project outside the gastric lumen is suggestive of an ulcer within a mass. This finding may be the result of inflammation only, but should raise the possibility of neoplasm. A nodular collar surrounding the ulcer or the failure of radiating folds to extend close to the crater margin also favor the diagnosis of a malignant lesion.

Large gastric ulcers are more likely to be malignant, in contrast with prepyloric or gastric ulcers associated with duodenal ulcer disease. The presence of jejunal or post-bulbar ulcerations on x-ray examination should immediately raise the possibility of an underlying Zollinger-Ellison syndrome. The majority of patients with the Zollinger-Ellison syndrome initially show x-ray findings of a typical duodenal ulcer. Associated large gastric folds, as well as evidence of increased gastric secretion, are common.

Gastric Analysis

Gastric analysis for determination of the basal and maximal acid output has two practical applications in the management of patients with peptic ulcer disease: (1) to determine the presence or absence of achlorhydria in the patient with gastric ulcer, and (2) to demonstrate basal hypersecretion of gastric acid in the range highly suspect for the Zollinger-Ellison syndrome.

The demonstration of histamine-fast achlorhydria in a patient with gastric ulcer would most certainly indicate that the ulcer is malignant. Spot checks of random gastric aspirations should be performed on all gastric ulcer patients. If pH values are greater than 6, histamine stimulation should be resorted to in order to confirm or refute the presence of achlorhydria. Gastric ulcers developing in the absence of gastric acid secretion are malignant. However, most malignant gastric ulcers develop in the presence of gastric acidity, so that the presence of acid does not by any means rule out an underlying malignant ulcer.

The second practical application of gastric secretory studies is in the patient with apparent uncomplicated duodenal ulcer disease, in whom the possibility of an underlying Zollinger-Ellison syndrome exists. Gastric secretory studies are rarely performed on the vast majority of patients with duodenal ulcer disease. If the Zollinger-Ellison syndrome is present, eventually the patient's poor response to conventional therapy will (hopefully) alert the physician to suspect this relatively rare disorder.

Unfortunately, the patient with the Zollinger-Ellison syndrome usually presents having previously undergone a surgical procedure which normally would have substantially improved the ulcer disease but instead has resulted in recurrence. In the patient with previous gastric surgery, gastric secretory studies are frequently more difficult to interpret. The technical problems of inadequate gastric aspiration and alkaline reflux of intestinal juices into the gastric lumen will tend to falsely lower the results. One must also take into consideration an anticipated drop in gastric secretion as a result of gastric resection or vagotomy.

To avoid this diagnostic dilemma, a plea is made to perform gastric secretory studies in all duodenal ulcer patients in whom surgery is anticipated. If the basal acid output is greater than 15 mEq. per hr. or the basal acid output is greater than 60 per cent of the maximal acid output, the Zollinger-Ellison syndrome should be suspected. Since some duodenal ulcer patients without the Zollinger-Ellison syndrome may have similar degrees of acid hypersecretion, measurement of serum gastrin levels may be required to establish the correct diagnosis.[19]

Radioimmunoassay of serum gastrin levels is currently performed in only a few laboratories, but it is anticipated that this determination will become more readily available at large medical centers.

Gastroscopy

With the advent of fiberoptic equipment, renewed enthusiasm for endoscopy has evolved. Gastroscopy is not fruitful in the patient with an uncomplicated duodenal ulcer. The most practical application of gastroscopy has been in the evaluation of the acute upper gastrointestinal bleeder. If peptic ulcer disease is present in the patient with hematemesis or melena, endoscopy is helpful in determining whether or not the ulcer is the actual site of bleeding. In the patient with a history suggestive of peptic ulcer disease, but in whom radiological studies are negative, gastroscopy may detect a gastric ulcer missed on x-ray examination.

Gastroscopy is indicated for further evaluation of a gastric ulcer which shows equivocal radiologic evidence of malignancy. Endoscopic findings of an ulcer with poorly defined irregular margins is suggestive of a malignant lesion. At the time of gastroscopy, a biopsy specimen or washings for cytology, or both, may be taken of suspicious areas. Photographs provide a permanent record of the lesion and may be particularly helpful in follow-up evaluation of a healing gastric ulcer.

Cytology

Cytologic examination of gastric washings has been shown to be greater than 90 per cent accurate in differentiating benign from malignant gastric ulcers. Early detection of the malignant gastric ulcer by this means may lead to earlier justification of appropriate therapy.[3] The specimens are obtained by means of simple saline lavage, followed by immediate processing. Unfortunately, gastric cytology is not done as frequently as indicated in many centers primarily because of a shortage of experienced cytopathologists.

MEDICAL TREATMENT

The overall medical regimen should be tailored to make the individual patient as comfortable and relaxed as possible. In some individuals sedation may be required, whereas in others it is unnecessary. Ideally, all patients with gastric ulcer should be hospitalized to insure maximal medical therapy in an attempt to achieve rapid healing and confirm the benignancy of the lesion. The patient should be given some insight into the nature of his disease, in particular its tendency to recur. Although smoking may impede the healing of gastric ulcers, any pharmacologic benefit achieved by cessation of smoking during treatment of an acute ulcer usually does not offset the associated anxiety and tension generated by such a change. Ulcerogenic drugs should be eliminated if possible. Salicylates should be avoided since acetylsalicylic acid has been shown to produce gastrointestinal bleeding, even in the absence of a previous gastric lesion. The bleeding probably results from local gastric erosions combined with a systemic platelet dysfunction.[27, 30]

Diet

The role of diet in the therapy of peptic ulcer remains controversial.[17] The ideal diet should be nutritious and nondestructive to the mucosa. It should not stimulate gastric secretion of acid, and should neutralize gastric acidity. Food constituents, proteins in particular, tend to neutralize gastric acidity, but at the same time stimulate acid secretion.

Milk, the time-honored food antacid, lowers gastric acidity but produces postprandial gastric hypersecretion. If milk feedings are taken frequently, hypersecretion of acid is counter-balanced by neutralization of the gastric contents. In contrast, milk taken just prior to bedtime will stimulate acid secretion during the night while the patient is sleeping. Milk should be utilized as a source of nutrition and not primarily as an antacid.

Antacid preparations are available that are more effective than milk in decreasing gastric acidity, and have the added advantage of not significantly stimulating gastric acid secretion. In situations where oral feedings are initiated on a trial basis, following complications of ulcer disease such as hematemesis, small frequent feedings of milk would seem reasonable. If milk feedings are utilized, skimmed milk is preferable in view of the higher incidence of coronary artery disease seen in patients treated with frequent milk feedings.

Buchman and co-workers evaluated the effect of a bland versus a regular diet on the clinical course of patients hospitalized with active duodenal ulcer disease.[2] Both groups received frequent milk feedings and antacid therapy. These investigators could not demonstrate any difference in the response obtained that could be related to either a bland or a regular diet.

Based on the failure of any investigator to demonstrate convincingly the clinical advantage of particular dietary modifications, the more recent trend has been toward the institution of three regular meals daily. The patient may take interval feedings to prevent hunger. Food that the patient associates with dyspepsia should be avoided. Since alcohol and caffeine-containing beverages are potent stimulators of acid secretion, they should be eliminated from the diet if possible.

Antacids

The mainstay of ulcer therapy is the proper use of antacids. Although antacids unquestionably relieve peptic ulcer pain, there is no incontrovertible evidence that they either enhance the healing rate or decrease the frequency of ulcer disease.[21] Ideally, one attempts to raise the gastric pH above 6 to inactivate pepsin; but this is rarely achieved.

There are in general two types of antacids that are commonly used: calcium carbonate and aluminum hydroxide preparations (with or without magnesium). Therapeutic doses of calcium carbonate will suppress gastric acidity and peptic activity to a greater extent than aluminum hydroxide.

Recently Fordtran demonstrated that 3 to 5½ hours after administration of calcium carbonate, rebound gastric hypersecretion of acid occurs, the mechanism of which is unclear.[13] It is not a result of alkalinization of the antrum. Both aluminum-magnesium hydroxide and sodium bicarbonate failed to induce rebound gastric hypersecretion in spite of achieving early neutralization of gastric contents, comparable to that of the calcium carbonate, within the first 30 minutes following administration of either drug. The stimulus for the rebound acid secretion is most likely mediated by calcium absorption. Rebound gastric hypersecretion, alkalosis, as well as the potential development of renal failure secondary to hypercalcemia and nephrocalcinosis, make calcium carbonate a less attractive antacid. In contrast, aluminum hydroxide preparations are relatively free of adverse effects, although large doses rarely cause a phosphorus depletion syndrome as a result of an intraluminal limitation of phosphorus absorption.[18] This adverse effect is easily averted by insuring an adequate phosphorus content in the diet. Magnesium-containing antacid preparations should not be used if renal failure is present, in order to avoid hypermagnesemia.

Antacids should be given following meals. Fordtran and Collyns demonstrated that when antacids are given 1 hour after eating, they will lower gastric acidity for 3 hours.[14] In contrast, studies done on fasting individuals show that antacids exert their neutralizing effect usually for less than 40 minutes, primarily as a result of rapid gastric emptying.

Liquid antacids are preferable and should be given in adequate doses, generally 15 to 30 ml. The frequency of antacid administration is governed primarily by the severity of the pain. The patient should be given antacids at least 1 hour after meals and at bedtime, but in treatment of an acute ulcer it may be necessary to give antacids hourly while the patient is awake to make him pain-free. The choice of aluminum hydroxide preparation is largely arbitrary and usually governed by the relative cathartic or constipating side effects.

If ulcer pain does not remit with hourly aluminum hydroxide administration, Spiro recommends a trial of calcium carbonate, 4 gm. hourly.[24] In addition, aspiration of gastric juice at bedtime may facilitate therapy, particularly in the patient with night pain who does not respond to an antacid regimen. Although no evidence supports the role of antacids in enhancing the healing of an ulcer, in an attempt to hasten the healing of a gastric ulcer and substantiate the benignancy of the lesion, antacids are given hourly while the patient is awake. Ideally, a minimal antacid regimen should be continued indefinitely since the aluminum hydroxides are relatively harmless and conceivably may exert a prophylactic effect.

Anticholinergics

Anticholinergics are used in the treatment of peptic ulcer in an attempt to inhibit acetylcholine stimulation of parietal cell secretion as well as antral release of gastrin. These agents are effective in reducing gastric acid secretion nocturnally, in the basal state, and during the postprandial period. Nevertheless, it has not been convincingly demonstrated that anticholinergics alter the clinical course of patients with ulcer disease.

Long-term administration of anticholinergics has been reported to decrease the incidence of recurrence as well as bleeding in duodenal ulcer patients.[23, 25] If in fact there is a beneficial effect of long-term anticholinergic therapy, it is not a result of a decrease in the functional parietal cell mass. Norgaard et al. assessed the effect of 6–18 months of poldine (Nacton) and glycopyrrolate (Robinul) on gastric acid secretion.[20] They found no significant effect of either anticholinergic drug, as compared to a placebo, on maximal acid output, quantitated 48 hours after cessation of the test substance.

To achieve decreased acid secretion, anticholinergics must be given in doses that produce the well-known side-effects of dry mouth and blurred vision. It is not clear whether in combination with antacids they reduce gastric acidity beyond that achieved by antacids alone. One must weigh the necessary side effects of anticholinergics against any potential benefit of these drugs when given in conjunction with antacid therapy, particularly when taken during the daytime when the patient is awake and active.

Fordtran studied the effect of anticholinergics on gastric acidity when given in conjunction with calcium carbonate.[14] There was no significant difference in the effect on acid secretion of the anticholinergic given 30 minutes prior to a meal followed by calcium carbonate one hour after the meal, as compared to a placebo given in a similar sequence with calcium carbonate. It does seem reasonable to give anticholinergics at bedtime, in particular in the patient with nocturnal pain, in order to decrease acid secretion at a time when the patient is not taking antacid and will not be bothered by unpleasant side-effects.

Responsiveness to a given dose of an anticholinergic is highly variable among patients and, therefore, the effective pharmacologic dose must be determined individually. This is easily accomplished by using tincture of belladonna, starting with 8 to 10 drops, and then gradually increasing the dose until side-effects develop. During the daytime, the anticholinergic should be given 30 minutes prior to mealtime in order to achieve decreased acid secretion in the postprandial period.

Anticholinergics are contraindicated in the presence of glaucoma or urinary retention. Relative contraindications include gastroesophageal reflux, severe coronary artery disease, pyloric obstruction and recent hemorrhage. Although the use of anticholinergics in the treatment of gastric ulcer has not been investigated, they probably have no place in the therapeutic approach to this disease unless there is demonstrable hypersecretion of acid.

Other Forms of Therapy

Carbenoxolone is a licorice derivative, extensively studied in Great Britain, and reported to be effective in the treatment of peptic ulcer disease. The pharmacologic mechanism of the drug is not clearly understood, but may primarily be an antipeptic action.[16] The results of most studies seem to indicate that carbenoxolone is effective in enhancing the healing rate of gastric ulcers in ambulant outpatients.[6, 9, 10] It offers no therapeutic advantage in the treatment of gastric ulcer over hospitalization alone.

It has been assessed in the treatment of duodenal ulcer disease, utilizing position release capsules in an attempt to achieve release of the drug in the duodenum. The results thus far have been contradictory and would indicate a need for further investigation before advocating its use in the treatment of duodenal ulcer disease.[1, 5]

The major adverse side effects constitute a mineralocorticoid-like action consisting of edema, hypertension, and hypokalemia, and can be mitigated by restricting the dose to 50 mg. three times daily.[7] Glycyrrhizinic acid is the component of carbenoxolone responsible for the adverse side-effects. A deglycyrrhizinized preparation of the drug has been shown to retain the therapeutic effectiveness without the adverse side-effects.[29] Carbenoxolone is not yet marketed in this country and its advantage over conventional therapy is yet to be proved.

Amylopectin sulfate is a drug with demonstrable antipeptic activity independent of acid neutralization. There is also evidence that the drug confers a protective action on the gastric mucosal barrier. Amylopectin sulfate has been evaluated in the treatment of peptic ulcer disease, and recent reports have been favorable. Zimmon et al. reported, in a double blind controlled study, accelerated healing of chronic gastric ulcers in hospitalized patients treated with this drug.[31] Sun and Ryan compared the effects of amylopectin sulfate alone and in combination with anti-cholinergics, anticholinergics alone, and placebo alone on the recurrence rate of duodenal ulcers.[26] Patients selected for this study had recently been treated for an acute duodenal ulcer and had evidence of complete healing of the ulcer prior to institution of maintenance therapy. They were subsequently followed for 1 year on one of the drug regimens and observed for recurrent ulcer disease.

These investigators showed a striking difference in recurrence rates among the study groups. The recurrence rate was lowest in those patients treated with amylopectin alone (16 per cent) or in combination with anticholinergic (12 per cent), as compared to those receiving therapy with anticholinergics alone (39 per cent) or placebo alone (75 per cent). These early favorable claims await confirmation by other investigators.

Estrogens have been shown to have a beneficial effect on the clinical course of duodenal ulcer disease. The results of studies by Truelove[28] imply that estrogens may enhance the healing of duodenal ulcers, as well as reduce the recurrence rate. A similar beneficial effect of estrogens is not demonstrable in patients with gastric ulcer disease.[8] Unfortunately, the associated side-effects of feminization in men and endocrinological dysfunction in women makes the use of estrogens for peptic ulcer disease impractical. The mode of action of estrogens in enhancing the healing of peptic ulcers is unknown.

Gastric freezing, once in vogue as a mode of ulcer therapy, has no place in the treatment of peptic ulcer disease. Ruffin et al. carried out a double-blind evaluation of gastric freezing in duodenal ulcer patients.[22] They found no significant difference in relief of pain, suppression of acid secretion, or recurrence rate in the patients treated with gastric freezing as compared to patients undergoing a sham procedure.

SURGERY

In general, the high recurrence rate and frequency of complications, as well as the possibility of an underlying malignancy, warrant early surgical intervention in the patient with chronic gastric ulcer disease. If, in the face of adequate medical therapy, a gastric ulcer fails to heal at an acceptable rate as assessed radiologically, i.e. 50 per cent at 3 weeks or 90 per cent at 6 weeks, to eventual complete healing, gastric surgery should be strongly considered. The complications of perforation, unrelenting pyloric obstruction, and recurrent or persistent hemorrhage are usually clear indications for surgery.

The majority of patients undergoing gastric surgery for peptic ulcer fall into the category of "intractable" disease. A proportion of the so-called intractable patients indeed have persistent symptomatology, resulting frequently from penetration of the ulcer, and will require surgical repair. However, most of the "intractable" patients have a long history of exacerbation and remission of ulcer disease, and a point is reached in the clinical course when the patient, the physician, or both become intractable. At this time the physician has to weigh the short-term and long-term risks of continuing medical therapy, against a surgical approach. The surgical risks must be considered in terms of operative mortality and postgastrectomy morbidity in the light of a given procedure performed by a particular surgeon in a particular institution.

The various modes of surgical therapy are directed primarily at reducing acetylcholine stimulation by vagotomy, eliminating gastrin by antrectomy, or removing parietal cell mass by subtotal gastrectomy. Currently, vagotomy and a drainage procedure, pyloroplasty or gastroenterostomy, is the surgical therapy of choice for duodenal ulcer in most institutions, and is being popularized by some for gastric ulcer.[11] Gastric resection with removal primarily of the antrum, as well as the ulcer, is still the therapy of choice for gastric ulcer. In general, the mortality and morbidity is less, but the recurrence rate is more, in vagotomy with a drainage procedure as compared to the various types of gastric resections. Mortality approximates 1 per cent in vagotomy and drainage procedures as compared with 5 per cent in a resective procedure.

These figures vary widely, depending primarily on the experience of the surgeon with a given procedure. In the surgical series reported by Goligher et al., amazingly there was no operative mortality among 507 men with duodenal ulcer, 239 of which underwent vagotomy and gastroenterostomy, 116 vagotomy and antrectomy, and 107 subtotal gastrectomy.[15] Eisenberg et al. reported similarly encouraging results from vagotomy and drainage procedures in 455 patients with duodenal ulcer disease.[12] In this series the elective mortality rate was less than 1 per cent, the emergency mortality rate 1.85 per cent, and the recurrence rate was 3.6 per cent.

In addition to operative mortality, vagotomy and all of these surgical procedures permanently alter gastric function and may result in significant morbidity characterized by dumping, malabsorption, malnutrition, or diarrhea.

GASTRIC IRRADIATION

In the patient with recurrent peptic ulcer who is a poor operative risk because of coexistent pulmonary, cardiac, or hepatic disease, gastric irradiation should be considered. Clayman et al. have demonstrated, in a large series of duodenal and gastric ulcer patients, that irradiation of the fundus utilizing total doses of approximately 1600 to 2000 R. will significantly reduce acid secretion as well as recurrence rate.[4] Gastric irradiation should be reserved primarily for the patient over 45 years of age who has responded unfavorably to medical therapy and is a poor candidate for surgery.

REFERENCES

1. Amure, B. O.: Clinical study of Duogastrone in the treatment of duodenal ulcers. Gut, 11:171, 1970.
2. Buchman, E., Kaung, D. T., Dolan, K., and Knapp, R. N.: Unrestricted diet in the treatment of duodenal ulcer. Gastroenterology, 56:1016, 1969.

3. Cantrell, E. G.: Why use gastric cytology? Gut, 10:763, 1969.
4. Clayman, C. B., Palmer, W. L., and Kirsner, J. B.: Gastric irradiation in the treatment of peptic ulcer. Gastroenterology, 55:403, 1968.
5. Cliff, J. M., and Milton-Thompson, G. J.: A double-blind trial of carbenoxone sodium capsules in the treatment of duodenal ulcer. Gut, 11:167, 1970.
6. Cocking, J. B., and MacCaig, J. N.: Effect of low dosage of carbenoxolone sodium on gastric ulcer healing and acid secretion. Gut, 10:219, 1969.
7. Doll, R., Langman, M. J. S., and Shawdon, H. H.: Treatment of gastric ulcer with carbenoxolone: Antagonist effect of spironolactone. Gut, 9:42, 1968.
8. Doll, R., Langman, M. J. S., and Shawdon, H. H.: Treatment of gastric ulcer with oestrogens. Gut, 9:46, 1968.
9. Doll, R., Hill, I. D., and Hutton, C. F.: Treatment of gastric ulcer with carbenoxolone sodium and oestrogens. Gut, 6:19, 1965.
10. Doll, R., Hill, I. D., Hutton, C., and Underwood, D. J.: Clinical trial of a triterpenoid liquorice compound in gastric and duodenal ulcer. Lancet, 2:793, 1962.
11. Duthie, H. L.: Vagotomy for gastric ulcer. Gut, 11:540, 1970.
12. Eisenberg, M. M., Woodward, E. R., Carson, T. J., and Dragstedt, L. R.: Vagotomy and drainage procedure for duodenal ulcer: The results of 10 years experience. Ann. Surg., 170:317, 1969.
13. Fordtran, J. S.: Acid rebound. New Eng. J. Med., 279:900, 1968.
14. Fordtran, J. S., and Collyns, J. A. H.: Antacid pharmacology in duodenal ulcer, effect of antacids on postcibal gastric acidity and peptic activity. New Eng. J. Med., 274:922, 1966.
15. Goligher, J. C., Pulvertaft, C. N., de Dombal, F. T., Conyers, J. H., Duthie, H. L., Feather, D. B., Latchmore, A. J. C., Shoesmith, J. H., Smiddy, F. G., and Wilson-Peper, J.: Five-to-eight-year results of Leeds/York controlled trial of elective surgery for duodenal ulcer. Brit. Med. J., 2:781, 1968.
16. Henman, F. D.: Inhibition of peptic activity by carbenoxolone and glycyrrhetinic acid. Gut, 11:344, 1970.
17. Ingelfinger, F. J.: Let the ulcer patient enjoy his food. In Controversy in Internal Medicine. Philadelphia, W. B. Saunders, 1966.
18. Lotz, M., Zissman, E., and Bartter, F. C.: Evidence for a phosphorus depletion syndrome in man. New Eng. J. Med., 278:409, 1968.
19. McGuigan, J. E., and Trudeau, W. C.: Immunochemical measurement of elevated levels of gastrin in the serum of patients with pancreatic tumors of the Zollinger-Ellison variety. New Eng. J. Med., 278:1308, 1968.
20. Norgaard, R. P., Polter, D. E., Wheeler, J. W., and Fordtran, J. S.: Effect of long-term anticholinergic therapy on gastric acid secretion with observations on the serial measurement of peak histalog response. Gastroenterology, 58:750, 1970.
21. Piper, D. W.: Antacid and anticholinergic drug therapy of peptic ulcer. Gastroenterology, 52:1009, 1967.
22. Ruffin, J. M., Grizzle, J. E., Hightower, N. C., McHardy, G., Shull, H. and Kirsner, J. B.: A co-operative double-blind evaluation of gastric "freezing" in the treatment of duodenal ulcer. New Eng. J. Med., 281:16, 1969.
23. Ruffin, J. M., and Cayer, D.: The role of anticholinergic drugs in the treatment of peptic ulcer disease. Ann. N.Y. Acad. Sci., 99:179, 1962.
24. Spiro, H. M.: Clinical Gastroenterology. New York, MacMillan Company, 1970.
25. Sun, D. C. H.: Long-term anticholinergic therapy for prevention of recurrences in duodenal ulcer. Amer. J. Digest. Dis., 9:706, 1964.
26. Sun, D. C. H., and Ryan, M. L.: A controlled study on the use of propantheline and amylopectin sulfate (SN-263) for recurrences in duodenal ulcer. Gastroenterology, 58:756, 1970.
27. Thorsen, W. B., Western, D., Tanaka, Y., and Morrissey, J. F.: Aspirin injury to the gastric mucosa. Arch. Intern. Med., 121:499, 1968.
28. Truelove, S. C.: Stilbesterol, phoenobarbitone, and diet in chronic duodenal ulcer. A factorial therapeutic trial. Brit. Med. J., 2:559, 1960.
29. Turpie, A. G. G., Runcie, J., and Thomson, T. J.: Clinical trial of deglycyrrhizinized liquorice in gastric ulcer. Gut, 10:299, 1969.
30. Weiss, H. J., Aledort, L. M., and Kochwa, S.: The effect of salicylates on the hemostatic properties of platelets in man. J. Clin. Invest., 47:2169, 1968.
31. Zimmon, D. S., Miller, G., Cox, G., and Tesler, M. A.: Specific inhibition of gastric pepsin in the treatment of gastric ulcer. Gastroenterology, 56:19, 1969.

Veterans Administration Hospital
1201 N.W. 16th Street
Miami, Florida 33125

The Treatment of Chronic Hypertension

Hugh R. Gilmore, III, M.D.*

Hypertension may be defined as a disease or condition identified by an elevation of blood pressure, associated with increased morbidity and mortality, and best treated by a reduction of the blood pressure. The truth of that statement remains inviolate in spite of the many qualifications, exceptions, and outright objections to such a definition. The jeopardy to health of high blood pressure is undeniable, and it matters little whether there is actually a discrete disease named "essential hypertension" or whether the individual is merely in the upper range of a population "standard distribution curve" and hence is not suffering fron an actual disease but merely from the effects of a "normally" elevated blood pressure. Furthermore, causing a reduction in an already elevated blood pressure—whatever the cause—apparently results in lower mortality and morbidity. This point deserves special emphasis when one considers the possible harmful effects of treatment, including the greatly feared possibility of precipitating a stroke or acute myocardial infarction by an abrupt lowering of the blood pressure, or the less feared but more real possibility of serious reactions to antihypertensive drugs.

Although cases of acute myocardial infarction or stroke following reduction in blood pressure are often mentioned, the cause and effect relationship cannot be established, and when any group of treated patients at any level of blood pressure are compared to a similar control or untreated group, the treated group invariably is found to have done better. This difference is actually more difficult to show in groups of mildly or moderately hypertensive patients than in severely hypertensive patients.[1-3] An easily remembered figure from the Framingham Study is that a systolic blood pressure greater than 160 for individuals from 39 to 59 years of age causes approximately a 3 to 4-fold increase in the risk of coronary heart disease.

Another danger in the reduction of blood pressure is the precipitation or aggravation of uremia. One should be particularly watchful of

---

*Clinical Associate Professor of Medicine, Division of Cardiology, Department of Medicine, University of Miami School of Medicine, Miami, Florida

renal function during the early stages of the treatment of severe hypertension. If renal function deteriorates as the blood pressure is lowered, obviously a re-evaluation of the treatment program must be made and corrective changes instituted. Drugs which reduce renal function the least should be selected. In fact, short-term dialysis may be indicated as an adjunct to therapeutic blood pressure reduction.[6, 11] We have found that patients with hypertension and poor renal function respond best to small doses of diuretics plus a combination of hydralazine (Apresoline) and methyldopa (Aldomet), titrated upward until effective. More vigorous therapy usually is not tolerated.

It is frequently stated that the measurement of blood pressure in the doctor's office has little meaning; i.e., casual blood pressures are not useful and only the basal blood pressure has sufficient validity. Actually, the two measurements are clearly related, and the basal blood pressure usually just reflects a somewhat lower figure than the casual blood pressure. It is unrealistic to expect either patients or physicians to repeatedly obtain basal blood pressures, except for certain specific purposes. In fact, most of our information regarding incidence, prevalence, natural history, and response to treatment is based on casual blood pressure measurements.

Of course, the blood pressure must be measured accurately, it should be taken in several positions, and done repeatedly under the same conditions before valid conclusions can be made. The initial measurements should be made in both arms and one leg with the patient at rest, in comfortable surroundings. At subsequent visits, measurements should be made in the same arm, and at least with the patient supine and standing so that orthostatic changes can be observed. Measurements should be made at least three times, or until two measurements are approximately the same. The pulse rate should be recorded with every change in body position.

The significance of elevated blood pressure lies in its ability to produce or accelerate cardiovascular disease. The natural history of hypertension, therefore, is a function of its complications, which unfortunately are not predictable early in the course of the disease.[7, 8, 10] However, it is possible to make some useful conclusions about chronic hypertension. The prognosis is worsened by the following factors: (1) height of the systolic pressure; (2) height of the diastolic pressure; (3) worse in males than in females; (4) funduscopic abnormalities, including arteriole narrowing, hemorrhages, exudates, or papilledema; (5) manifestations of any form of cardiovascular disease, including angina pectoris, abnormal electrocardiogram, cardiac enlargement by x-ray or physical examination, or the presence of a stroke due to either occlusion or hemorrhage; (6) the presence of any renal disease or, in fact, any abnormal renal function test; (7) Negro race.

These important observations have led to various classifications or gradings of hypertension according to its severity. Hence mild, moderate and severe hypertension have been described, depending on the elevation of systolic or diastolic or, in fact, mean blood pressure compared to an arbitrary scale of severity. In such classifications, greater weight is generally given to diastolic pressure or to calculation of the mean blood pressure; systolic pressure appears to have less prognostic significance. Of perhaps greater usefulness is the early description by Keith, Wagner, and Barker[5] of the correlations between funduscopic changes and prognosis. The most comprehensive classification to find wide usage is that of Smithwick,[9] which incorporates into a numerical score all of the above factors and evidence of other peripheral organ damage. Although classification of hypertension according to severity must remain somewhat arbritrary and therefore subject to error, its usefulness in studying the natural history and the results of therapy makes it a valuable tool, and it should be carried out to some extent in office practice.

Before considering the use of drugs in the treatment of hypertension, one should accomplish the following:

1. Diagnosis should be established by a minimum of three separate, careful measurements of blood pressure under resting conditions with the patient in several positions, particularly lying supine and standing. In "chronic" hypertension these measurements should be made at approximately weekly intervals.

2. Other causes of hypertension should be excluded.

3. The patient should be adequately examined with particular attention to the optic fundus, cardiac size and function, including electrocardiogram and chest x-ray, and evaluation of kidney function, including at least a urinalysis and BUN or creatinine determination.

4. The findings and proposed program should be discussed with the patient to his full satisfaction.

This last point is worth emphasizing since it will frequently prevent future problems. The patient may be unduly alarmed by the knowledge that he has high blood pressure. He needs reassurance and encouragement to undergo what probably will be a life-long therapeutic program. It is useful to point out that the role of hypertension as a risk factor in cardiovascular disease is of approximately the same magnitude as that of smoking cigarettes.

It should be emphasized to patients that a single measurement of his blood pressure is not the criterion by which control and treatment will be regulated. If such an attitude is allowed to become established, the patient will anxiously await the measurement of blood pressure at each visit to the doctor's office and attach excessive importance to minor fluctuations. It is not usually wise for the patient to share in the knowledge of his daily readings, but rather for the doctor to state simply that the patient's progress is satisfactory, or that the patient's progress is unsatisfactory and additional adjustments will have to be made in the therapeutic program.

So-called "home blood pressures" are extremely helpful in certain individual cases. These may be carried out either by a member of the patient's family or a visiting nurse. Such a program is not satisfactory for all patients, however, and the physician should use care in selecting patients for this approach.

The treatment of hypertension should then progress along the following lines.

1. Proper living habits, including dietary control to achieve or maintain optimum weight, should be encouraged. Other risk factors for cardiovascular disease should be assessed and corrected. A measurement of serum cholesterol and triglycerides in order to aid dietary management should not be neglected. Discussion of smoking and exercise habits should be accomplished.

2. Drug therapy. Great experience has now been accumulated in the use of drugs for the control of blood pressure. Perhaps the most important single concept to keep in mind is that the response of the individual patient is not predictable. Although, in general, the more severe the hypertension, the more likely the need for multiple drugs or the use of highly potent drugs will be, in some patients dramatic response may occur to a relatively minor drug.

Each of the following drugs may by itself lower the blood pressure of an individual patient to normal, but more often a combination of drugs will be needed. Therefore a systematic "building block" approach should be used. For each drug, titration of dosage may be necessary and should be carried out with careful clinical observation, usually not increasing the dose at more than weekly intervals.

Such an approach makes the diuretics a logical starting point, since they have of themselves an effective hypotensive effect; even more important, they cause considerable potentiation of the other antihypertensive drugs. The selection of a diuretic agent lies between any of the thiazides and furosemide (Lasix). Ethacrynic acid is equally effective but has greater gastrointestinal side-effects.

Hypokalemia is the most common unfavorable side-effect of a diuretic, but rarely occurs to a significant degree in patients who are maintaining a normal diet and who are not on digitalis. Dosage is usually one tablet daily, given preferably in the morning in order that any diuretic action take place during the patient's waking hours. If the dosage is increased to twice daily, some additional hypotensive action will often be achieved. The second tablet should then be given in the early afternoon to avoid causing nocturia. Hypokalemia may be avoided by the use of supplements of potassium or by the addition of a potassium-retaining diuretic such as triamterene or spironolactone. Maximum hypotensive effect is obtained by the use of approximately 1 to 1.5 gram of chlorothiazide or its equivalent daily, with perhaps slight potentiation by the addition of triameterene or spironolactone. Doses above this level will not result in a greater lowering of blood pressure. If satisfactory reduction of the patient's blood pressure is not achieved, additional drugs must be added in approximately the following order.

If sedation is indicated for anxiety or tenseness, phenobarbital or a minor tranquilizer should be added. Of the tranquilizers available, reserpine is sometimes more effective than the others in blood pressure reduction. It has more side-effects, such as nasal stuffiness, nightmares, or even severe emotional depression, and its use is no longer as common as in the past. However because it is so effective in certain patients it will be described at length below.

More potent antihypertensive drugs are added in approximately the following order:

1. Hydralazine (Apresoline), 40 to 400 mg. per day in 3 or 4 divided doses.
2. Alpha methyldopa (Aldomet), 250 to 3000 mg. per day in 3 or 4 divided doses.
3. Guanethidine (Ismelin), 10 to 200 mg. per day given in a single dose.
4. Propranolol (Inderal), 40 to 160 mg. per day in 4 divided doses.

The following are used much less frequently:

5. Pargyline (Eutonyl)
6. Ganglionic blocking drugs, Veratrum compounds, sympathectomy.

Short summaries of individual drugs follow.

Diuretics

The development of potent oral diuretics has caused a remarkable change in the treatment and prognosis of hypertension. As mentioned above, they are the keystone of most therapeutic programs. Mechanism of action is initially but transiently related to salt and water excretion with a decrease in circulating blood volume. However, chronic studies have shown that the long term reduction in blood pressure is probably secondary to alterations in sodium ion concentration in arteriolar muscle cells. Furosemide or thiazides may be used in appropriate doses for long periods of time. A rise in BUN in patients with abnormal renal function may occur and is often related to hypokalemic alkalosis. Hyperuricemia with clinical gout and diabetes mellitus may occur while on these drugs. Skin rash, hematological disorders and pancreatitis have also been reported.

Rauwolfia Alkaloids

The most widely used is reserpine. The exact mechanism of action is unknown. Peripheral resistance is lowered, probably by central as well as peripheral action. At both sites the action may be due to the liberation of catecholamines from storage sites, resulting in tissue depletion. Bradycardia, sedation, and increased gastric acidity occur. Its central nervous system side-effects have already been mentioned.

ADMINISTRATION. For hypertensive crises, reserpine is given intramuscularly in doses of 1 to 2 mg. The onset of action is usually in about 2 hours, with a duration of 4 to 12 hours. Intravenous administration does not produce effects faster but may be used. Doses above 2 mg. are probably not more effective in lowering blood pressure. Certainly doses above 5 mg. are not needed since they cause only an increase in sedation. Marked orthostatic hypotension and sedation almost invariably occur when reserpine is used parenterally; hence, its prolonged parenteral use is not feasible.

Reserpine is given orally in doses of 0.1 and 0.25 mg., one to four times daily. Usually 0.25 mg. once daily is satisfactory. Onset of action is very slow, often requiring several weeks to become effective. Following discontinuation of the drug, its effects may last for 1 to 6 weeks. Hence, its use as a fixed dose in combination with diuretics and other drugs is undesirable.

Patients on reserpine who undergo anesthesia or surgery have low tissue levels of norepinephrine and therefore may be more subject to vascular collapse, or at least less responsive to those drugs which depend for their effect upon the release of tissue norepinephrine. The response to intravenously administered norepinephrine will however be normal or even increased. Reserpine should not be used during pregnancy because it increases respiratory complications in the fetus.

Hydralazine

This drug is unique in that it causes a reduction in blood pressure while causing an increase or at least no decrease in cardiac output. It has central and peripheral actions resulting in tachycardia and direct vasodilation on the arterial side of the circulation. In fact, its major action is probably directly on the smooth muscle of the arterioles. There is at least a temporary increase in renal blood flow with no change in glomerular filtration rate; hence this drug is frequently recommended for patients with poor or borderline renal function. Because the drug by itself is of only mild to moderate potency, it should always be combined with other drugs. In addition to the diuretic, the use of reserpine, propranolol or guanethidine will usually result in a reduction in side-effects such as tachycardia, as well as potentiate the hypotensive effects of hydralazine.

ADMINISTRATION. When given intravenously, its maximum effect occurs in 20 to 40 minutes and lasts for several hours. An initial oral dose of 10 mg. four times a day is gradually increased until a desirable effect has occurred. Doses above 400 mg. are rarely used because of the danger of a lupus-like syndrome. Side-effects are not common but angina pectoris may occur with the tachycardia.

Alpha Methyldopa

This drug interferes with the metabolic decarboxylation of DOPA and thus interferes with the formation of dopamine, a precursor of norepinephrine. Thus a weak compound of alpha methylnorepinephrine is formed and competes with norepinephrine for adrenergic terminals, thus creating a weaker response. However, its mechanism of action in reducing blood pressure remains uncertain, since it reduces cardiac output, peripheral resistance, and pulse rate.

ADMINISTRATION. The drug may be used intravenously in doses of 250 to 1000 mg., with onset of action in 4 to 6 hours and duration of action of 10 to 16 hours. Orally, a total daily dose of 0.5 to 3 gm. should be given in four divided doses. Upon discontinuance of the drug, effects may continue for approximately 48 hours. Side-effects include mild sedation, orthostatic hypotension, and rarely weakness, headache, dizziness, nasal stuffiness, dry mouth, weight gain, or edema. Because of its sedative-like action, its combination with reserpine is usually not desirable.

Guanethidine

This is the most potent and most commonly used antihypertensive drug. Its mode of action is to depress postganglionic nerve responses, apparently by causing the slow release of norepinephrine at the neuro-effector junction, resulting in a depletion of norepinephrine stores. It therefore blocks both alpha and beta receptors. Thus a chemical sympa-thectomy is carried out, with reduction in cardiac output, reduction of pulse rate, and decrease in peripheral resistance. Guanethidine is blocked at the blood-brain barrier and there is no central nervous system depression.

ADMINISTRATION. Guanethidine is rarely used intravenously since it may cause an initial rise in blood pressure unless the tissue stores of norepinephrine have been previously depleted by the use of reserpine. Oral dosages should be started at 10 mg. daily. Because the onset of action usually takes 2 to 3 days and the duration is up to 7 to 10 days, the dosage may be given once daily, preferably at bedtime, and increased no more frequently than every 3 to 4 days until satisfactory levels of blood pressure are obtained.

The head end of the patient's bed should be elevated as much as he will tolerate it in order to reduce the major complication of orthostatic hypotension. The other major complaint is inhibition of ejaculation or the development of impotence in the male. This is a common and severe complaint, and coupled with the complaint of orthostatic hypotension usually limits the dose of this drug that can be used. Hence, it is usually well to have previously placed the patient on a diuretic and other less potent hypotensive agents. Guanethidine may aggravate congestive heart failure and should never be used with monoamine oxidase inhibitors.

Pargyline

This is a non-hydrazine inhibitor of monoamine oxidase. The exact mechanism of action for its reduction of blood pressure in man is un-known. Its effect on the central nervous system is that of an antidepres-sant. It takes up to a week to reach a peak effect. Following discontinuation, its effects may last for 6 weeks.

ADMINISTRATION. The initial dose of 25 mg. once daily by mouth should be titrated upward at weekly intervals until a satisfactory effect is obtained. Dosage rarely exceeds 100 mg. per day. Side-effects and undesirable reactions are common. Important among them are ortho-static hypotension, constipation, weight gain, and insomnia. The risk of severe adverse reactions when other drugs such as sympathomimetics, barbiturates, antidepressants, or the consumption of beer, wine, and certain cheeses has precluded its widespread use. Furthermore, if side-effects occur, they may persist for days after discontinuing the drug.

Propranolol

This drug is currently the only beta-adrenergic compound available for clinical use. When blood pressure is reduced by propranolol, the mechanism of action appears to be predominantly due to beta-adrenergic blockade. However, its direct quinidine-like depressant effect on the myocardium may play a role. Decrease in heart rate, prolonged mechanical systole, and a modest reduction in peripheral resistance are common with this drug. Its use in hypertension has generally been reported to be disappointing; however, in selected patients dramatic improvement has occurred. It is known to be helpful in the medical management of pheochromocytoma. It may also be the drug of choice in the so called "hyperkinetic heart syndrome." Its use in combination with other hypertensive agents has been insufficiently explored, but it appears that the combination of propranolol and hydralazine may be extremely useful since the side-effects of each drug are partially neutralized by the other, and the hypotensive effects are augmented.

ADMINISTRATION. The oral dose is initiated with 10 mg. 4 times daily and progressively increased at approximately weekly intervals to 40 mg. 4 times daily. Dosages above this level have not been used to any extent.

REFERENCES

1. Effects of treatment on morbidity in hypertension. Report of Veterans Administration Cooperative Study Group. J.A.M.A., 213:1143, 1970.
2. Effects of treatment on morbidity in hypertension. Report of Veterans Administration Cooperative Study Group. J.A.M.A., 202:1028, 1967.
3. Farmer, R. G., et al.: Effect of medical treatment in severe hypertension. Arch. Int. Med., 112:118, 1963.
4. Goodman, L. S., and Gilman, A., eds.: The Pharmacological Basis of Therapeutics. New York, The MacMillan Co., 3rd ed., 1965.
5. Keith, N. M., Wagener, H. P., and Barker, N. W.: Some different types of essential hypertension: their course and prognosis. Amer. J. Med. Sci., 197:332, 1939.
6. Mroczek, et al.: The value of aggressive therapy in the hypertensive patient with azotemia. Circulation, 40:247, 1969.
7. Perera, G. A.: Natural history of hypertension. Amer. Heart J., 42:421, 1952.
8. Perry, H. M., Jr., et al.: Studies on control of hypertension. VIII. Mortality, morbidity and remissions during 12 years of intensive therapy. Circulation, 33:958, 1966.
9. Smithwick, R. H.: The effect of sympathectomy upon the mortality and survival rates of patients with hypertensive cardiovascular disease. In Bell, E. T., ed.: Hypertension. Minneapolis, University of Minnesota Press, 1951.
10. Sokolow, M., and Perloff, D.: The prognosis of essential hypertension treated conservatively. Circulation, 23:697, 1961.
11. Woods, J. M., and Blythe, W. B.: Management of malignant hypertension complicated by renal insufficiency. New Eng. J. Med., 277:57, 1967.

Department of Medicine
University of Miami School of Medicine
P.O. Box 875, Biscayne Annex
Miami, Florida 33152

Hypertensive Emergencies

Carlos A. Vaamonde, M.D.,* Noble J. David, M.D.,** and
Roger F. Palmer, M.D.***

The physician responsible for the care of the patient with hypertension is frequently confronted with "hypertensive crises" or emergencies. One of these is hypertensive encephalopathy, characterized by severe elevation of the diastolic blood pressure in association with headache, nausea, and vomiting and changing neurological signs (mental confusion, weakness, hemiparesis, convulsions, coma). The other is the accelerated phase of hypertension, or *malignant hypertension,* characterized by the association of severe diastolic hypertension with advanced retinopathy and renal failure. Hypertension of this severity if uncontrolled for any length of time will frequently lead to uremia, cerebral hemorrhage, acute left ventricular failure, dissecting aneurysm, and death.

Perhaps the most important thing we have learned from the study and treatment of these hypertensive emergencies is that lowering the blood pressure results in a definite increase in life-span of the hypertensive patient.

A nephrologist, a neurologist, and a clinical pharmacologist have joined in a discussion of the hypertensive "crisis." Although differentiation of malignant hypertension from hypertensive encephalopathy may at times be difficult, we have elected to discuss them separately.

MALIGNANT HYPERTENSION

There is confusion concerning the definition of malignant hypertension. Some workers have considered papilledema in a patient with high blood pressure as the sole criterion for the diagnosis, while others have defined the term on the basis of the level of the diastolic blood pressure

---
*Associate Professor of Medicine, University of Miami School of Medicine; Chief, Nephrology Section, Miami Veterans Administration Hospital
**Professor of Neurology, University of Miami School of Medicine; Chief, Neurology Service, Miami Veterans Administration Hospital
***Professor and Chairman, Department of Pharmacology, and Professor of Medicine, University of Miami School of Medicine

alone. We would like to consider malignant hypertension in much broader terms, as describing a clinical situation characterized by an acute and, if untreated, almost always fatal form of hypertensive disease. In general, this rapid deterioration is associated with papilledema, progressive renal failure, and cardiac and central nervous system manifestations.[9]

This syndrome is usually accompanied by a histological lesion — malignant nephrosclerosis — characterized by proliferative endarteritis of the afferent arteriole and small interlobular arteries of the kidney, with commonly associated necrosis of the arteriole and glomeruli.

It is important to bear in mind some exceptions to this definition. Some patients will have a rapidly progressive course characterized by severe diastolic hypertension, papilledema, or cerebral vascular deterioration without azotemia and without the histologic features of malignant nephrosclerosis. We have also seen patients with a fulminating clinical course with uremia and malignant nephrosclerosis but without papilledema.

Since early and adequate treatment of this severe form of hypertensive disease reverses vascular changes and is associated with a definite prolongation of life span, it appears reasonable to rely on such less restrictive criteria in approaching the diagnosis of malignant hypertension.

The incidence of malignant hypertension is not clearly established; problems of definition and case selection are mostly responsible for this. It has been suggested that as low as 1 per cent[1, 4] and as high as 6 or 8 per cent[2, 10] of patients with benign essential hypertension will develop malignant hypertension. Thus, while the arteriolar nephrosclerosis accompanying essential hypertension is the most common background for the development of malignant hypertension (42 per cent of the patients studied by Kincaid-Smith et al.),[4] accelerated hypertension may be superimposed upon a variety of diseases associated with hypertension: 21 per cent of the patients of Kincaid-Smith had chronic pyelonephritis; 6 per cent had polyarteritis nodosa or scleroderma; and 16 per cent had a variety of other renal and endocrine disorders (unilateral renal artery stenosis, postpartum hypertension, radiation nephritis, congenital renal disease, hydronephrosis, Cushing's syndrome, nephrocalcinosis, aldosterone tumor). Rarely, malignant hypertension may start de novo in patients recently known to be normotensive.

While malignant hypertension does not present a uniform clinical picture, there are certain characteristics that allow fairly accurate diagnosis.[9] Abrupt onset of severe headache, or a sudden increase in its intensity, may be the first or most distressing symptom. Blurring of vision is very common, and sometimes visual symptoms precede any others. Often they are associated with papilledema and may be attributed to it, but it is important to recognize that sometimes no such correlation exists. Similarly, anorexia, nausea, vomiting, and abdominal pain may be associated with uremia but may also be present in its absence. Unexplained weight loss is a relatively common finding; it may precede any other clinical manifestation of malignant hypertension. Physical examination reveals high blood pressure and perhaps an enlarged heart. The results of neurologic examination vary from normal findings to a host of neurologic abnormalities associated with cerebral vascular disease. In most instances, *severe hypertensive retinopathy* (cotton-wool exudates and linear and flame-shaped hemorrhages) and bilateral papilledema are observed.

The urinary findings are characteristic: a rather abrupt onset or a striking increase in previously present proteinuria; microscopic or gross hematuria; hyaline, granular, and red blood cell casts. Renal failure may not be present at the onset, depending on the background in which malignant hypertension develops, but generally ensues and often progresses with great rapidity.

As stated before the most important thing that we have learned from the study of malignant hypertension is that lowering the blood pressure, by whatever means, reverses the vascular changes in the eyegrounds or elsewhere and slows or arrests the progressive deterioration in renal function.[5] The result is demonstrable healing of the damaged blood vessels and a definite increase in life span. This has been amply demonstrated in recent years.[3, 6, 11, 13] In 1959, Harington, Kincaid-Smith, and McMichael[3] reported their 7 year experience in 82 patients with malignant hypertension treated with ganglionic blocking drugs, as compared to 105 untreated patients. The treated patients had an over-all survival rate of 50 per cent at 1 year, 33 per cent at 2 years, and 25 per cent at 4 years, as compared with a 90 per cent mortality rate in the first year and almost zero survival at 4 years in the untreated group.

The high mortality rate during the first year was largely in the group with grossly impaired renal function: 13 per cent had survived at 1 year in this group, as compared with 73 per cent survival over the same period in those with an initial BUN under 60 mg. per 100 ml. At 5 years, 30 per cent of the treated patients without initial azotemia were alive, while only 10 per cent of those with severe azotemia were living. More recently, the study of Perry and associates[11] reports 65 per cent survival at 5 years in nonazotemic patients with malignant hypertension (NPN less than 30 mg. per 100 ml), while only 25 per cent of the patients with azotemia survived. From these and similar studies it is clear that there is considerable prognostic significance in the level of renal function at the time of diagnosis of accelerated hypertension.

The specific management of hypertensive emergencies with pharmacologic agents will be discussed below; some important generalities of treatment will be discussed first.

One of the chief problems in the management of malignant hypertension is to recognize that it is a real medical emergency. Too many physicians do not treat malignant hypertension with resolution. Each day that passes without adequate reduction in arterial pressure enhances the possibility of severe or irreversible damage to vital organs. Concern for an etiologic diagnosis in an unknown patient (perhaps with the exception of pheochromocytoma) or concern for the final outcome in a complicated case should come after, not before, control of the elevated blood pressure.

Treatment of malignant hypertension should be performed in the hospital, preferably within the confines of an intensive care unit. The selection of the antihypertensive agent is, in general, not critical, provided that a therapeutic effect is obtained. There is no particular "best" drug for the treatment of high arterial pressure. One of the great mysteries of hypertension is the way in which some patients respond well to one drug, and some to another, without any other obvious difference between the patients. Thus, it is best to use a small variety of drugs, those that the physician knows best—their mode of action, side-effects, and interaction with other agents.

Argument still exists in relation to how rapidly the arterial pressure should be reduced in patients with malignant hypertension. There are those physicians who prefer immediate but gradual reduction, and those who favor immediate acute reduction. These different approaches will obviously be reflected in the choice of drugs. If the clinical situation permits, a gradual lowering of the blood pressure can be obtained in few hours by the use of parenteral reserpine or methyldopa. In many instances this will be sufficient. In others, because of lack of response to initial treatment or a complicated clinical situation (encephalopathy, heart failure, pulmonary edema), more rapidly effective drugs are needed (ganglion-blockers, diazoxide, etc.). Many of these drugs require constant monitoring of the blood pressure and the rate of administration. If this cannot be done satisfactorily, it is preferable not to use these powerful agents.

Fluid overload frequently tends to make these patients resistant to antihypertensive therapy. Thus, in the overexpanded hypervolemic patient, restriction of fluids is mandatory. This is a point to remember, since many patients receive intravenous antihypertensive medications in the form of drip infusion of isotonic or hypotonic glucose or sodium chloride solutions. In addition, some of these potent antihypertensive agents have renal sodium-retaining properties of their own.[6] A potent diuretic, such as furosemide or ethacrynic acid, will be helpful in relieving the excess fluid and in preventing the salt retention induced by most antihypertensive agents. Rarely, dialysis may be required for the removal of excess fluid in an unresponsive patient.

Occasionally, marked extracellular fluid volume depletion may make patients with severe hypertension relatively more sensitive to antihypertensive agents. This possibility should be kept in mind when combining potent antihypertensive drugs with diuretics or dialysis in nonedematous patients that are initially resistant to treatment.

The preservation of renal function in patients with accelerated hypertension during hypotensive therapy poses a basic dilemma. This is particularly relevant when renal failure is already present. It is a common experience that reduction of blood pressure beyond certain critical levels, which often cannot be defined other than empirically in the individual patient, may in itself cause progression of renal failure.

Renal function may be expected to deteriorate following successful lowering of the blood pressure, although this does not always occur. For example, cardiac output and renal blood flow may be lowered by a reduction in blood pressure, leading to further deterioration in renal function. Fortunately, this is usually a transient phenomena.

There is much in the literature expressing doubt that treatment of the accelerated renal phase of hypertension favorably alters the course of the disease in patients whose renal function has already deteriorated to the point where a BUN higher than 60 mg. per 100 ml. is sustained in the absence of dehydration, heart failure, or other reversible causes of uremia. This view has recently been challenged by several authors.[6, 11, 13] Woods and Blythe,[13] for example, treated 20 patients with malignant hypertension with a combination of antihypertensive medications and chronic dialysis, and concluded that reduction of blood pressure in patients with malignant hypertension and renal insufficiency (BUN between 50 and 148 mg. per 100 ml.) does not necessarily result in deterioration of renal function, and improves survival rates. More recently, it has been suggested that aggressive antihypertensive treatment of malignant hypertension (diazoxide and furosemide) may even result in some degree of improvement of the renal function impairment.[6]

In view of these recent experiences, it seems clear that previous views must be modified. Patients with malignant hypertension and elevated BUN levels should be treated vigorously with antihypertensive medications, along with meticulous attention to the management of renal failure. The latter may include dialysis if this is necessary for the adequate treatment of renal failure. Thus dialysis may be indicated because the presence of resistant fluid retention or azotemia, or to allow more aggressive treatment of the hypertension per se. Fortunately, this appears necessary only in a small group of patients. The role of bilateral nephrectomy in the treatment of accelerated hypertension is presently limited to patients with end-stage renal disease maintained in chronic dialysis programs or awaiting renal transplantation.[12]

In conclusion, malignant hypertension should always be considered as a medical emergency. Its clinical course may be ameliorated and the survival rate improved by treatment designed to cause a sustained reduction in arterial pressure. While patients with moderate to marked renal insufficiency have a less favorable prognosis, even in this group treatment is beneficial.

HYPERTENSIVE ENCEPHALOPATHY

The inclusion of a neurologist in a discussion of hypertensive encephalopathy promptly raises several questions. In this particular case, it provokes an apology, because my experience, whether representative or not, has included rather few patients with what I call hypertensive encephalopathy over the past few years. There may, of course, be several reasons for this, the first of which is that the internist may be recognizing and treating this disorder without bestirring his neurologic colleagues to share the experience. Perhaps a more optimistic reason for the decreasing incidence for neurology consultations for this condition is the fact that better control of the so-called benign essential hypertension and more powerful available medications to interrupt the course of malignant hypertension have materially reduced the incidence of this disorder.

In the milieu of an academic hospital where the house staff is in training, the neurologist is called upon most frequently to see patients in whom the question of hypertensive encephalopathy is raised, but in whom the most likely neurologic diagnosis is another form of cerebrovascular disease associated with hypertension. Thus, we are most often able to offer help in a diagnostic way in clarifying the semantic and conceptual vagueness which at times besets the student concerning the diagnostic criteria for hypertensive encephalopathy.

At the outset it might be well to outline some of the conditions that are commonly misdiagnosed as hypertensive encephalopathy. Among these are hypertensive patients who have seizure disorders either due to cortical scars of vascular origin or of some other etiology. In some patients, large, edematous cerebral infarctions or lesions causing obtundity because of their location high in the brain stem, suggest the diagnosis, since the diastolic pressure is also elevated. Of course, until it is recognized that gross bleeding has occurred, massive intracerebral hemorrhage is common in hypertensive patients and may be confused with hypertensive encephalopathy. Other disorders, such as pseudotumor cerebri, cerebral torulosis with hydrocephalus and papilledema, and even rapidly growing intracranial tumors, particularly of the glial and infiltrative variety, will require further examination and testing to be distinguished from hypertensive encephalopathy.

I recognize hypertensive encephalopathy as an acute condition, not one that lingers on into a subacute form of prolonged confusion, nor any chronic picture of permanent dementia. Its course is settled in short order by either recovery or death of the patient. Hypertensive encephalopathy has as its common denominator the arteriolar disease associated with high diastolic hypertension and culminating in necrotizing arteriolitis not only in the brain but in the eye, the kidney, spleen, and other organs as well. We generally think of it as part of the syndrome of malignant hypertension, and are reluctant to accept it without hemorrhages, exudates, and usually papilledema in the eye grounds. The other diagnostic possibilities mentioned above, if these qualifications obtain, would have to be ruled out by other tests.

Whether the basic process is toxemia of pregnancy, acute glomerulonephritis, one of the collagen vascular disease, or the idiopathic hypertensive disease of adult life in its malignant phase, the histopathology of the resulting hypertensive encephalopathy is very similar. Necrotizing arteriolitis with diapedesis, petechial hemorrhages, and edema into brain tissues leads to swelling and, in over half the cases, increased intracranial pressure as judged by lumbar manometrics. The spinal fluid may be at the upper limits of normal or slightly increased in protein content. Gross blood is rarely present although mild degrees of xanthochromia may be observed.

Given the vagaries of regional involvement to a greater or lesser extent, one can understand the appearance of variable focal signs and symptoms such as monoparesis, upgoing toes, reflex asymmetries, and visual disturbances, and focal onset of seizures in patients with hypertensive encephalopathy; but, in the main, these are not the dramatic features of the illness. Rather, the clinical picture is dominated by severe and intractable headaches, nausea, vomiting, confused mental status, and usually rather intense apprehension even in the obtunded sufferer. One would be reluctant to diagnose this condition were it not acute and were the sensorium perfectly normal. Of course, convulsions, fever, and coma may ensue with death of the patient due to uncontrolled cerebral changes.

It is a happy fact that the physician now has at his disposal a vastly more effective array of medicines to reverse this state than he has had at any previous time in medical history. With any kind of luck, if the diagnosis is clear and the patient is still conscious and has not suffered cerebral hemorrhage, this syndrome should be reversible. The vascular disease itself, of course, remains, and eventually may go on to kill the patient with some other insufficiency such as uremia.

The two most important points a neurologist can contribute are (1) strict adherence to the proper diagnostic criteria so that one can be certain that one is in fact treating hypertensive encephalopathy, and (2) early initiation of treatment with vigorous and constant monitoring until the patient's acute brain syndrome due to arteriolar damage reverses itself.

TREATMENT OF HYPERTENSIVE EMERGENCIES

There has been considerable debate about the optimum method of treating acute hypertensive emergencies. However, all agree that appropriate and immediate therapy is indicated. It has been pointed out in the previous sections that the complications attendant upon hypertensive crisis are reversible, and the degree of reversibility is a function of how soon treatment is begun.

We would like to outline a mode of therapy employed at the University of Miami based on our previous experience with dissecting aneurysms of the aorta. In over 65 cases of dissecting aneurysm of the aorta treated by medical means here and elsewhere a treatment program has evolved.[7] This program has proved effective in reducing blood pressure immediately and effectively in almost all cases, and has produced few side effects when properly monitored.[8]

When the diagnosis is established, an intravenous drip of trimethaphan (arfonad) is begun. The head of the bed is elevated to an angle of 30 to 40 degrees. The bed is not broken, so that the patient is on a flat surface; yet the head of the bed is at a 30 degree angle to the floor. This is to achieve the maximum effect of the drugs. Indeed, it is almost mandatory for the management of some patients.

A 500 mg. ampoule of trimethaphan is added to a liter of dextrose solution, and the drip is begun at a rate of 1 or 2 ml. per minute. The onset and offset of action is rapid. Unfortunately trimethaphan's effectiveness is lost in about 48 hours. So at the same time 1 mg. of reserpine is given intramuscularly and 50 mg. of guanethidine orally. These three drugs form the regimen of the triple therapy. Reserpine is not effective immediately but trimethaphan is. Guanethidine requires 3 or 4 days for its onset of action.

Reserpine's onset of action is in about 4 hours. After this time trimethaphan is stopped to evaluate what effect the 1 mg. of reserpine has had. If the blood pressure is down on the basis of the reserpine, then the trimethaphan is discontinued. If on the other hand, the blood pressure has risen, then another milligram of reserpine is given and the trimethaphan is restarted.

In another 4 hours the trimethaphan is stopped to see the effect of the 2 mg. total dose of reserpine, and the procedure is repeated, depending upon the state of the blood pressure. These procedure is summarized in Table 1. The necessary dose of reserpine (usually the total dose of reserpine on the first day) is repeated every day until the guanethidine takes effect, which is in about 4 days. At this time, the reserpine can be discontinued and the patient maintained on guanethidine on an outpatient basis. Usually, at some point a thiazide diuretic, preferably hydrochlorthiazide, 50 mg. twice a day, is begun. If there are no complications, the patient is almost ready to be discharged.

We feel that when this regimen is properly applied, hospital stay is shortened for the treatment of acute hypertensive "crisis." Occasional patients will present who are refractory to trimethaphan. These are usually those with severe renovascular hypertension.

If trimethaphan is ineffective, then sodium nitroprusside is begun. Sixty mg. are dissolved in a liter of dextrose in water. The transfer is made aseptically, but the nitroprusside is not sterilized. A drip is started at 1 to 2 ml. per minute. One advantage of nitroprusside is that the patient rarely becomes refractory to it; although thiocyanate levels can increase significantly, they rarely pose a problem. Nitroprusside in solution becomes inactivated with time, and this inactivation is accelerated

Table 1. *Procedure for Initiating Therapy in Acute Hypertensive Emergencies*

1. Place patient in an intensive care unit.
2. Elevate head of bed 30° (footboards are necessary).

3. Begin I.V. trimethaphan (Arfonad) 0.5 to 2 mg. per min. (500 mg. in 1 liter of D-5-W at a rate of 1 to 4 ml. per min.). Reduce blood pressure over 1 hour to 110 to 120 mm. Hg diastolic.
   Give I.M. reserpine, 1 mg.
   Give 25 mg. guanethidine orally b.i.d., and continue each day.
4. After 3 to 4 hours stop trimethaphan.
   If blood pressure is still elevated give another 1 mg. of reserpine I.M. and restart trimethaphan.
   Repeat above procedure every 3 or 4 hours until blood pressure is at satisfactory level without trimethaphan.
5. Continue total first day's dose of reserpine on the second day, then taper over the next 3 days as guanethidine takes effect.
6. Regulate guanethidine dosage on an outpatient basis.

by exposure to light. Therefore, a paper bag or some other device is used to prevent photo-oxidation.

It must be recalled that ganglionic blocking agents will produce ileus and pupillary dilation. Bladder atony is common, and the patient must be catheterized. Catheterization is useful in these situations since the urinary flow is an index of renal perfusion, and urinary flow is kept at a level between 20 and 40 ml. per hour. A central venous pressure catheter is introduced to guide fluid therapy and to detect early signs of congestive heart failure, a rare complication.

Frequent neurological examinations are given during the course of therapy. However, an obtunded patient results most often as a result of the reserpine therapy, rather than an intrinsic part of the encephalopathy, and one must not be alarmed by seeing an obtunded patient with normal neurological signs. This is most likely a result of reserpine and will clear in a few days.

With trimethaphan and nitroprusside, close monitoring is essential. Lapses in attention to monitoring can result in rapid infusions of the drug to the point of shock, usually resulting in stroke or acute tubular necrosis.

With the potent pharmacologic agents available, there is no reason why the acute hypertensive "crisis" cannot be managed effectively. We have not mentioned the use of other drugs, as hydralazine, pentolinium, or bethanidine. Our position is that although these drugs may be effective in a majority of patients, they are not effective in all patients. We think that the regimen described here will be effective in virtually all patients, and it has the advantage of being reliably and uniformly effective in lowering the blood pressure immediately to a level predetermined by the physician.

REFERENCES

1. Bechgaard, P.: The natural history of benign hypertension. In Bock, K. D., and Cottier, P. T.: Essential Hypertension. Berlin, Springer Verlag, 1960, p. 198.
2. Goldring, W., and Chasis, H.: Hypertension and Hypertensive disease. New York, The Commonwealth Fund, 1944.
3. Harington, M., Kincaid-Smith, P., and McMichael, J.: Results of treatment in malignant hypertension. Brit. Med. J., 2:969, 1959.
4. Kincaid-Smith, P., McMichael, J., and Murphy, E. A.: The clinical course and pathology of hypertension with papilloedema (malignant hypertension). Quart. J. Med., 27:117, 1958.
5. McCormack, L. J., Béland, J. E., Schneckloth, R. E., and Corcoran, A. C.: Effects of antihypertensive treatment on evolution of renal lesions in malignant hypertension. Amer. J. Path., 34:1011, 1958.
6. Mroczek, W. J., Davidov, M., Gabrilovich, L., and Finnerty, F. A. R.: The value of aggressive therapy in the hypertensive patient with azotemia. Circulation, 40:893, 1969.
7. Palmer, R. F., and Wheat, M. J.: Treatment of dissecting aneurysms of the aorta. Ann. of Thorac. Surg., 4:38, 1967.
8. Palmer, R. F., and Wheat, M. J.: Treatment of impending rupture of the aorta with dissection. Advances Int. Med. (in press).
9. Papper, S., and Vaamonde, C. A.: Nephrosclerosis. In Strauss, M. B., and Welt, L. G.: Diseases of the Kidney. Boston, Little, Brown & Co., 1971, 2nd ed.
10. Perera, G. A.: Hypertensive vascular disease; description and natural history. J. Chron. Dis., 1:33, 1955.

11. Perry, H. M., Schroeder, H. A., Catanzaro, F. J., Moore-Jones, D., and Camel, G. H.: Studies on the control of hypertension. VIII. Mortality, morbidity, and remissions during 12 years of intensive therapy. Circulation, 33:958, 1966.
12. Vertes, V., Cangiano, J. L., Berman, L. B., and Gould, A.: Hypertension in end-stage renal disease. New Eng. J. Med., 280:978, 1969.
13. Woods, J. M., and Blythe, W. B.: Management of malignant hypertension complicated by renal insufficiency. New Eng. J. Med., 277:57, 1967.

University of Miami School of Medicine
P.O. Box 875, Biscayne Annex
Miami, Florida 33152

Renal Failure

*Solomon Papper, M.D.**

When a patient's renal function is inadequate to maintain the volume and composition of his internal environment, he is said to be in "renal failure." These circumstances may result from a large variety of diseases of the kidney; thus, the term "renal failure" is similar to "heart failure" in that a level of organ function is described, rather than a specific disease. Traditionally, the subject is divided in accordance with the rapidity with which the renal function deteriorates, i.e., "acute" versus "chronic."

ACUTE FAILURE OF RENAL FUNCTION

Acute renal failure is generally, but not invariably, accompanied by oliguria. The syndrome of acute renal failure may be due to any one of three general conditions (1) Hypoperfusion of the kidney causes impaired renal function without parenchymal damage. This is sometimes referred to as "pre-renal azotemia" and is usually due to shock or severe dehydration. If renal hypoperfusion is severe enough, acute tubular necrosis may result. (2) Obstruction to the flow of urine may cause oliguria and acutely impaired renal function. This is sometimes referred to as "post-renal azotemia." (3) A variety of renal parenchymal diseases may cause acute renal failure. These include acute glomerulopathies (e.g., post-streptococcal, systemic lupus erythematosus), acute vascular disorders (e.g., malignant nephrosclerosis, polyarteritis nodosa, hypersensitivity angiitis), severe fulminant pyelonephritis (perhaps with papillary necrosis), acute tubular necrosis, and an acute activation of chronic renal disease.

ACUTE TUBULAR INSUFFICIENCY

Acute tubular necrosis is the most common cause of acute renal failure. We prefer the term acute tubular insufficiency (ATI), since the

---

*Professor and Co-Chairman, Department of Medicine, University of Miami School of Medicine; and Chief, Medical Service, Veterans Administration Hospital, Miami, Florida.

condition need not be accompanied by frank necrosis of tubular cells. ATI may be caused by (1) nephrotoxic agents or (2) severe ischemia.

Many chemicals have the potentiality of causing ATI. Organic solvents (e.g., carbon tetrachloride) have traditionally been common offenders. In recent years, we have been especially impressed with antibiotics (amphotericin, cephaloridine, colistin, gentamicin, kanamycin, methicillin, neomycin, polymixin, and sulfonamides) as causes of ATI. Heavy metals may produce ATI. Hemoglobinuria and myoglobinuria may be accompanied by ATI, although the mechanism is probably not simple direct tubular toxicity of hemoglobin or myoglobin. It may well be that other chemical agents now in use or to be used as drugs, in industry and for environmental control, will be shown to be nephrotoxic.

Ischemic ATI generally occurs in a clinical setting that has resulted in shock. In infants and in the aged, severe dehydration without gross shock may produce ATI.

Large, edematous kidneys have one of two types of lesions. The "nephrotoxic" lesion tends to be faily uniform in type with necrosis especially of proximal cells sparing the basement membrane. The "ischemic" lesion is irregular in distribution and tends to involve the basement membrane.

The mechanism of oliguria in ATI has not been established, but it is most likely that there is severe reduction in glomerular filtration rate (GFR) despite the absence of morphologic abnormality in the glomerulus.

The diagnosis of ATI is generally not difficult. In many instances, there is a setting that predisposes to ATI, i.e., the patient has been in shock or been exposed to a nephrotoxic agent. In some instances, the history of chemical exposure requires quite detailed inquiry and search. In other instances, no cause of ATI is evident. Most patients are oliguric, but total anuria is uncommon in ATI. The true *absence* of urine is more suggestive of obstruction or even acute glomerulonephritis, vascular disorder, or papillary necrosis than of ATI.

In some instances, the oliguric phase is very transient; in others, it may be completely absent (so-called "high output failure"). Thus a rising blood urea nitrogen concentration (BUN) in the presence of a liter or more of urine daily does not exclude ATI. The urine often appears dark and "dirty." The urine is not concentrated, and because of the tubular lesions, sodium cannot be conserved. Thus the urine tends to be close to isosmotic (specific gravity less than 1.020 and osmolality of 280 to 320 mOsm. per Kg.) and urinary sodium concentration in a random urine sample generally in excess of 40 mEq. per liter. Modest proteinuria, red blood cells, and white blood cells are common observations.

A very common clinical situation requiring diagnostic separation is that of distinguishing between hypoperfusion without ATI and hypoperfusion where ATI has already occurred. Obviously, shock or severe dehydration, or both, serve as the clinical background for either situation. Examination of random urine specimens is very helpful, especially the urinary sodium concentration (Table 1).

When the data are not discriminating, or while waiting for the determination, one may try to distinguish the two conditions on the basis of

Table 1. *The Urine in Renal Hypoperfusion Versus Acute Tubular Insufficiency**

	HYPOPERFUSION	ACUTE TUBULAR INSUFFICIENCY
Urine solute concentration	concentrated	isosmotic
Urine Na^+ concentration	< 40 mEq/L	> 40 mEq/L
Creatinine $\frac{U}{P}$ ratio	> 15	< 15

*From Papper, S.: Clinical Nephrology. Boston, Little, Brown & Co. (in press). Reproduced with permission.

the patient's ability to respond to a diuretic stimulus. With already existent ATI, no diuresis can be expected. One may use a single intravenous injection of 25 to 50 gm. of 20 per cent mannitol, ethacrynic acid (40 to 80 mg.), or furosemide (50 to 100 mg.) to induce diuresis. Failure to respond should not be followed by repeated use of these drugs.

As indicated previously, ATI must also be distinguished from obstruction. This may be difficult since both conditions may or may not be accompanied by oliguria, and both may not be able to conserve sodium normally. In the absence of a known cause of the acute renal failure, cystoscopy with unilateral retrograde study should be done without delay. ATI also must be distinguished from acute glomerulopathy, acute vascular disorders, acute papillary necrosis, and an acute exacerbation of chronic renal disease.

It is platitudinous but correct to state that the best *treatment* of ATI is to prevent exposure to nephrotoxic agents and avoid renal ischemia. If exposure has taken place, the likelihood of ATI can probably be reduced by the very early initiation of diuresis with mannitol, ethacrynic acid, or furosemide, as described.

The Oliguric Phase

Once the *oliguric* phase of ATI has developed, there are two guiding therapeutic principles that form the basis of an effective program. First, ATI cannot be cured by treatment, but spontaneous cure can occur. Second, the patient must be kept alive long enough to undergo spontaneous cure. The physician must take the leadership in orienting nursing personnel, relatives, and even the patient to himself as a human being and not simply as a vehicle to the production of urine volume. This can be achieved only if the physician places the urine volume in reasonable perspective.

Within the framework of therapeutic principles, individualization is essential, as it is in all clinical medicine. If the patient has had severe and extensive trauma, with or without infection, it is reasonable from the outset to assume that the destruction of tissue and the catabolic state will result in rapid rise in blood urea and that hyperkalemia may be a problem fairly early. Under such conditions, we would be ready to perform hemodialysis early and, on the occasion of the first dialysis, put in place a plastic arteriovenous fistula on the basis that multiple, frequent dialyses are likely. On the other hand, a previously healthy man whose tubular necrosis is due to carbon tetrachloride and who has no extrarenal adverse effects of the toxin might be treated less vigorously, although with as much care.

During the oliguric phase, meticulous attention to the details of day-to-day care are mandatory.

Fluids and Electrolytes

Initially, fluid and electrolyte therapy should be estimated to provide whatever is necessary to replace previous losses. Thereafter, daily replacement is geared to estimated and projected losses. On the average, one may assume that the net water loss from the body under these conditions is about 500 ml. daily. Obviously, this is larger with fever, vomiting, etc. All losses (gastrointestinal, renal) should be measured daily and replaced along with appropriate solutes. One of the best ways to have these losses under thorough surveillance is by daily, accurate determination of body weight, anticipating a loss of 200 to 500 gm. (½ to 1 lb.) daily in the fasting individual. In addition, we determine serum and urine electrolytes daily to be certain that the composition of body fluid is maintained.

Caloric Intake

Ideally, one would like to provide adequate total calories without protein. At present, this is not feasible except with intravenous fat preparations, which present sufficient problems that general use has not occurred. But 100 gm. of carbohydrate daily will reduce protein breakdown by 50 per cent, and should be provided for its "protein-sparing" effect. This is best achieved by distribution of the carbohydrate over the 24 hour period. Whether it is worth giving more than 100 gm. of carbohydrate short of meeting total caloric needs is doubtful.

If the patient's fluid losses are 1000 ml. per day or more, it is a simple matter to replace this and provide 100 gm. of carbohydrate daily as a 10 per cent solution of glucose. However, if the fluid losses are less, so that the glucose would have to be provided as a 15 per cent or even more concentrated solution, sclerosis of veins may occur, and more important, there are hazards of infection and thrombosis. Rather than assume this risk, we prefer to provide less total glucose, given as a 10 per cent solution within the limits of not exceeding fluid losses, recognizing that this approach may, in certain instances, mean earlier or more frequent dialysis.

In our experience, very few patients can tolerate oral feedings for any period of time; rather than deal with nausea and vomiting, we have tended to elect the intravenous route from the outset.

While some have used anabolic steroids to minimize the catabolic phase, we have not been impressed that this is of practical value.

Hyperkalemia

Hyperkalemia in the oliguric patient may be an important problem, especially if there is tissue damage or infection. One essential form of treatment is to ensure that *no* potassium is received as food or medication. The hazard of hyperkalemia is cardiac arrhythmia and death. Potassium is best monitored by both electrocardiogram (ECG) and the measurement of potassium concentration in serum. Except at the extremes of hypokalemia and hyperkalemia, the electrocardiogram does not correlate completely with serum values.

The earliest ECG change seen in patients with hyperkalemia is the tall, peaked T wave with a narrow base. Next one notes depressed S-T segments and decreased amplitude of the R wave with a deeper S wave. A still later, more readily defined stage consists of prolongation of the P-R interval, followed by diminution or disappearance of P waves. There may be widening of the QRS segment. In more severe situations, the S-T is fused into the ascending limb of the T wave, and, just before cardiac arrest, a sine wave appearance occurs.

We use daily measurement of serum potassium and electrocardiograms so long as the patient is oliguric. If the ECG or serum potassium level show any change, these determinations may be made several times daily. With severe hyperkalemia (7 mEq. per liter) or definite ECG changes, immediate lowering of the serum potassium level is essential. This may be accomplished rapidly with the intravenous administration of 1 liter of 10 per cent glucose, with or without 40 units of regular insulin, or with 200 ml. of molar bicarbonate or 1000 ml. of isotonic bicarbonate. These measures will increase the intracellular movement of potassium. However, the effects are transient, and repeated use results in expansion of extracellular fluid volume.

Sodium polystyrene sulfonate resin (Kayexalate) is more effective, although less rapid, and should be started once the infusion of glucose or bicarbonate has been instituted (or simultaneously). We give 30 gm. of the resin in 200 ml. of water as a retention enema (30 to 45 minutes). This procedure can be repeated every 2 to 4 hours until the serum potassium is normal. While each gram of resin takes up approximately 1 mEq. of potassium as well as some hydrogen and calcium, it may release in exchange as much as 3 or 4 mEq. of sodium. Therefore, the hazard of the continued use of resin is sodium overload. Whenever serum potassium reaches 5.5 mEq. per liter, we use resins continuously to prevent further rise. When potassium is exceedingly difficult to control with these measures and sodium overload is a problem, it is better to use dialysis than to procrastinate.

Acidosis

Acidosis is treated when the patient is symptomatic (Kussmaul breathing) or when the serum bicarbonate level is below 15 mEq. per liter. This can generally be accomplished in a 70 kg. man by giving 120 to 150 mEq. of sodium bicarbonate intravenously over 6 or 8 hours, either hypertonically in 3 ampules of 50 per cent sodium bicarbonate, or isotonically in 1000 ml. of 1/6 M sodium bicarbonate. Either method may be expected to result in an increase of serum bicarbonate of 5 to 6 mEq. per liter. The choice of hypertonic versus isotonic correction of the acidosis should be based on other aspects of fluid and electrolyte balance, especially total fluid requirements and serum sodium concentration. When intravenous sodium bicarbonate is given under such circumstances, it is wise to administer 30 gm. of calcium gluconate intravenously at the same time in order to avoid the development of hypocalcemic tetany. If treatment with sodium bicarbonate is necessary to the point of fluid overload in the oliguric patient, dialysis is indicated.

Anemia

Anemia is treated with packed red blood cells when the patient has symptoms referable to anemia. Seldom does one have to maintain the hematocrit above 25 per cent.

Hypertension

Hypertension is seldom a problem. However, in the case of hypertension and cardiomegaly, heart failure, or encephalopathy, we lower the blood pressure. Even without these complications, we generally use antihypertensive drugs when the diastolic blood pressure is 110 mm. Hg or greater.

Dialysis

The indications for dialysis generally agreed upon are: (1) the development of uremic symptoms, (2) uncontrolled hyperkalemia, and (3) uncontrolled, symptomatic acidosis. We use earlier and more frequent dialyses in patients with trauma or infection, or both, and in elderly patients who have undergone surgery. In these instances, we use dialyses often enough to prevent the BUN from rising above 100 mg. per 100 ml. When this is done, these particularly sick patients can be nourished properly (including protein), can be ambulated, their convalescence hastened, and infections diminished. Peritoneal dialysis may be used except when *very* rapid dialysis is required or when one may expect frequent dialyses.

While peritoneal dialysis can be accomplished in almost any hospital, the procedure may be associated with important technical problems. Aside from the physician's skill, trained nursing care is critical for proper dialysis.

The physician adheres strictly to aseptic technique. We do not "routinely" use antibiotics or heparin in the dialysate. Under ordinary circumstances, our dialysate is an electrolyte solution containing 1.5 gm. of glucose per 100 ml. If there is hyperkalemia, potassium is not added to the dialysate. If serum potassium is normal, 3 to 4 mEq. of potassium chloride is added to each liter of dialysate. Two liters of dialysate at 38° C. is allowed to remain in the peritoneal cavity for 30 to 45 minutes. If we wish to remove fluid, every other consideration is the same, except that we use dialysate containing 4.25 gm. of glucose per 100 ml. Under these circumstances, blood sugar should be monitored.

If all goes well, about 20 exchanges of 2 liters each can be done in 24 hours, lowering the BUN by 50 per cent. We generally dialyze for 48 hours.

After the catheter is removed, its tip is stained and cultured.

Complications range from minimal to fatal; many are preventable. There may be mechanical problems such as pain, leakage, inadequate drainage, breakage and intraperitoneal loss of the catheter, dissection of the abdominal wall, wound evisceration, and perforation of a viscus. There may be infection, including generalized peritonitis. If the fluid and electrolyte balance is not properly managed, there may be a variety of distortions: hyponatremia, hypernatremia, hypokalemia, hyperkalemia, hyperglycemia, fluid overload, dehydration, etc.

The fact that peritoneal dialysis is readily available does not negate its potential hazards.

Antibiotics

Antibiotics are probably best reserved for evidence of infection with an identified organism, rather than used prophylactically. When infection has developed, the choice of antibiotic and its dose will depend not only on the sensitivity of the organism but on the route of excretion of the drug as well.

Drug Dosage

In renal failure, the dose requirement of many drugs may be significantly reduced; this depends on renal clearance, other routes of elimination, volume of distribution, and the relation of toxicity to blood level. The maintenance dose of digitalis preparations should be reduced. For digoxin in a patient with a GFR of less than 10 ml. per min., maintenance doses are about 40 to 50 per cent of the usual doses. With a reduced GFR, but one greater than 10 ml. per min., treatment with intermediate doses of digoxin must be individualized. After the customary initial doses, certain antibiotics must be given in reduced doses: tetracycline, kanamycin, streptomycin, colistin, polymyxin, penicillin G, lincomycin, and cephalothin. Other antibiotics require no reduction in dosage: chloramphenicol, erythromycin, methicillin, oxacillin, and novobiocin. The many details of this important subject obviously cannot be covered in a paper of this type: the reader is referred elsewhere.[2, 3, 7]

THE DIURETIC PHASE

The oliguric phase may last a variable period of time—from a few days to as long as a month, but generally less than 2 weeks. The onset of the diuretic phase does not abruptly terminate all the problems of renal failure. For several days after diuresis begins, renal function remains very poor; the BUN may continue to rise, infection may develop, and the uremic syndrome may develop or become worse. Dialysis may be indicated even though diuresis is already underway. As the diuretic phase develops, however, the major hazard is excessive loss of fluid, sodium, and potassium. The losses may reach major proportions, and we have seen urine volumes of 10 liters a day during this period.

Several factors may be relevant in the production and maintenance of the diuretic phase. One is that the patient may have had a positive fluid balance during the oliguric phase, and this accumulated fluid is delivered as renal function is restored. The high urea content in the blood also acts as an osmotic diuretic. A defect in concentrating ability may account for some of the diuresis.

Ultimately, efforts to "keep up" with the diuresis may actually perpetuate it, making it difficult to know whether the administered fluids are "replacement" for obligatory losses, or the large urine volumes are due to the large amount administered. In this instance, fluid administration may be curtailed for 6 to 8 hours to determine what happens to the role of urine flow on an hourly basis. If it remains high, one may assume that the losses are due to renal factors; if the volume decreases significantly under these circumstances, it is reasonable to suspect iatrogenic diuresis.

In the diuretic phase, if one "replaces" the urinary losses of sodium and potassium in volume and content, the problems of hypokalemia and hyponatremia do not occur. We prefer, then, to continue daily measurement of weight, urine volume, and serum and urine electrolytes until stability has been attained.

PROGNOSIS

Recovery from acute tubular insufficiency is determined in part by the presence and nature of any underlying disease. The patient with extensive trauma, infection, and shock has a worse prognosis than the healthy man who had exposure to carbon tetrachloride. It is believed that the "nephrotoxic" renal lesion which does not destroy the basement membrane provides a better outlook than the "ischemic" one which is patchy but tends to destroy the tubular cell basement membrane. And finally, meticulous attention to the details of management make a difference. Statistics are difficult to interpret because of all the variables. Overall mortality rates, for whatever they may or may not mean, are generally given as approximately 40 per cent. In patients who undergo clinical recovery, renal function studied years later is either normal or very near normal.

CHRONIC FAILURE OF RENAL FUNCTION

PATHOPHYSIOLOGY

There are two major theoretical approaches to overall pathophysiology in chronic renal failure.

1. The "traditional" view has been to regard the net renal function

as the composite function of *all* of the nephron units, each of which is diseased. The degree and precise anatomic locus of disease vary among the nephrons.

2. In more recent years, Bricker has presented experimental evidence to support what is often referred to as the Bricker hypothesis, or the "intact nephron" hypothesis. In this perspective, the diseased kidney consists of two populations of nephrons: (a) one group of nephrons that is nonfunctioning because of significant destruction of any portion of the nephron, and (b) normally functioning units. In this context, net renal function is the result of a reduction in the number of appropriately functioning nephrons, rather than the result of a variously diseased total nephron population.

Also consistent with this view is the evidence of orderly functional adaptation in the diseased kidney. For example, sodium balance is generally maintained despite marked deterioration in renal function. Excretory adjustments, serving the interests of homeostasis, also occur in the instances of hydrogen ion, phosphate, potassium, and other solutes.

OVERALL COURSE OF DETERIORATED RENAL FUNCTION

To gain an overview of the course of deterioration in renal function in chronic renal disease, it may be helpful to look at the relationship of blood urea nitrogen (BUN) or serum creatinine level to the GFR. The curve described is a square hyperbola (Fig. 1). Several points are apparent in such a relationship: (1) There may be a considerable decrease in GFR (lowered to as little as 25 per cent of normal) before the BUN or serum creatinine level becomes elevated above the normal range. A BUN of 18 mg. per 100 ml. (normal up to 20) or a creatinine level of 1.8 mg. per 100 ml. (normal up to 2.0) may, in a particular individual, represent a normal GFR; in others whose "base-line normal" values were lower,

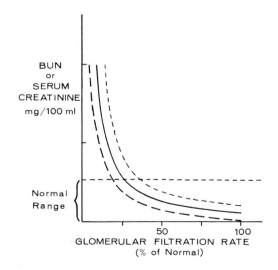

Figure 1.   The relationship of BUN or serum creatinine to glomerular filtration rate. (From Papper, S.:   Clinical   Nephrology. Boston, Little, Brown & Co., (in press), reproduced with permission.

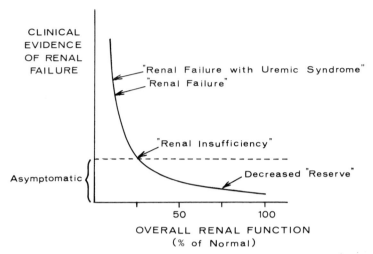

Figure 2. The relationship of clinical evidence of renal failure and renal function. Some authors use the terms listed to describe various progressive stages of renal functional impairment. *From* Papper, S.: Clinical Nephrology. Boston, Little, Brown & Co. (in press), reproduced with permission.

these values may be associated with a substantial reduction of the GFR. (2) At the portion of the curve approaching a normal GFR, relatively large reductions in GFR are not accompanied by major increments in BUN or serum creatinine level. (3) At the steep end of the curve, on the other hand, relatively small decrements in the GFR are accompanied by large increases in BUN or serum creatinine level.

Since the total functions of the kidney are decreased in diffuse end-stage parenchymal renal disease, we may view this same curve in more general clinical terms (Fig. 2). (1) Renal function may deteriorate without producing clinical symptoms over variable periods of time. Depending on the course of illness in a particular patient, this may be a matter of months or many years. (2) When there is considerable renal function still present, events which temporarily reduce renal function (dehydration, heart failure, infection) have relatively little impact on the clinical picture. (3) In the steep portion of the curve, even small decrements in renal function result in further rapid and significant deterioration of the clinical state of the patient.

Therefore, in the patient with renal failure, therapy must be directed toward maximum function of the entire nephron population in its diseased state (traditional view) or toward maximum function of the residual normal nephron population (intact-nephron hypothesis).

METABOLIC CONSEQUENCES OF RENAL FAILURE

Glucose intolerance is common in renal failure. It is seldom sufficiently severe to have clinical relevance. Its major clinical importance is in its possible confusion with diabetes mellitus. Uremic glucose intolerance is corrected by frequent hemodialyses, suggesting that some dialyzable material(s), presently not identified, is responsible for the observed disturbance. Glucose intolerance in uremia is associated with peripheral insulin antagonism, increased basal plasma insulin levels, and delayed insulin secretion in response to glucose loading.

Protein metabolism has attracted considerable interest in uremia for many years. The uremic individual may be able to maintain positive nitrogen balance (or at least avoid negative balance) while taking diets sufficiently low in protein to produce negative balance in the normal individual. There is evidence that this difference is explained by the re-utilization of urea nitrogen for the production of non-essential amino acids in the uremic state.

Hyperuricemia is common and, in the individual patient, does not correlate well with the degree of renal failure.

Categories of Clinical Manifestations

Patients with renal failure may be asymptomatic or may have symptoms of three general varieties.

1. They may have symptoms quite specifically referable to disorders of fluid and electrolyte excretion, such as coma due to hyponatremia. The clinical manifestations are reversed with correction of the underlying cause (e.g., hyponatremia), and are not improved with dialysis per se unless the underlying fluid and electrolyte disturbance is corrected during dialysis.

2. There are some manifestations of chronic renal failure that are not direct consequences of altered excretion. Nor are they entirely attributable to retained "waste" products, since dialysis may result in only partial improvement or no improvement at all. They may perhaps be regarded as resulting primarily from disordered regulatory functions. We refer to anemia, hypertension, renal osteodystrophy, and metastatic calcification.

3. Finally, patients with renal failure may have a symptom complex involving the gastrointestinal, cardiovascular, and central nervous systems, as well as other generally less prevalent manifestations. These symptoms are referred to as "uremic symptoms" and are believed to be due to some dialyzable substance(s) which accumulates in the blood.

We will now consider these three groups of clinical manifestations in order.

Fluid and Electrolyte Abnormalities and Treatment

Sodium Excretion. Even in patients with marked renal functional impairment, sodium balance may be maintained. In the context of the intact nephron hypothesis, maintenance of sodium balance is accounted for on the basis of increased sodium excretion per individual nephron. As renal function deteriorates and the number of functioning nephron units decreases, excessive sodium excretion commonly occurs. Generally, this is modest in amount (20 to 40 mEq. daily), but sometimes major proportions are achieved, i.e., "salt-wasting" (100 to 200 mEq. daily).

The explanation for this phenomenon is not fully established. The loss of body sodium is frequently aggravated by gastrointestinal losses secondary to the vomiting which commonly occurs in uremic patients. Sodium is lost with water, resulting in decreased extracellular fluid volume (ECFV). The latter causes further reduction in the GFR. If sodium losses occur in association with a limited capacity for water excretion, hyponatremia may result. Dietary sodium restriction in itself represents some significant hazard to the patient with chronic renal failure.

In many instances, as the number of functioning nephrons decreases, and despite adaptive mechanisms, the capacity of the kidney to excrete sodium may be reduced; one then faces the hazards of salt overload. Commonly, the kidney has reduced "flexibility;" i.e., its capacity to eliminate sodium is restricted to a relatively narrow range. *The dietary prescription of sodium must be determined for each individual patient. Sodium should be given in the maximum tolerable amounts in order to maintain the ECFV.* The maintenance of adequate, but not excessive, sodium intake thereafter depends on careful following of the patient, his body weight, serum sodium concentration, urinary sodium excretion, and GFR.

WATER. The observed abnormalities in water excretion may be explained largely in the context of the intact nephron hypothesis. There is evidence indicating that the defect in concentrating ability is related not necessarily to disease of the collecting duct or loop of Henle, but rather to a large solute (urea) load per remaining normal nephron. The large distal delivery of fluid may interfere with the opportunity to form or maintain an hyperosmotic interstitium. As the number of nephrons diminish, the "flexibility" in water excretion may be reduced to a narrow range. In this instance, the extremes of water overload and dehydration may readily occur.

Water excess and salt-wasting (renal and extrarenal) are the major causes of hyponatremia in patients with renal failure. Water deficiency (dehydration), with salt deficiency (ECFV diminished) are *major* and *common* reversible causes of reduced renal function in patients with chronic renal failure, and establish a potentially hazardous perpetuation of adverse circumstances.

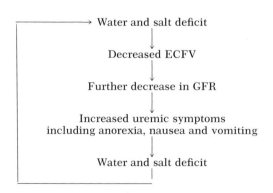

How much water should be prescribed? The traditional figures given approximate 3.5 liters daily, to assure a urine volume of 2.5 to 3 liters daily. This is derived from two types of data: (1) In the "average" diet, a volume that large would be required to deliver an isosmotic urine, and (2) maximum urea clearance occurs at a urine flow of 2 ml. per min., or an output of 2880 ml. of urine daily.

In some patients, however, the amount of water that can be excreted is less than two liters per day. The calculation of the amount of fluid given must be individualized on the basis of weight change, serum sodium concentration, urine volume, and maintenance of maximum GFR. It is very important in *any* water prescription to emphasize nocturnal water drinking. *Whatever the optimal volume of total water ingestion, it should be distributed over 24 hours.* Obviously, patients with an inability to concentrate the urine have nocturia; and if this loss is not replaced, nocturnal dehydration may occur. The physician is well advised to *prescribe* water (i.e., time and amount) as "medicine" and not simply give the general advice to "force fluids." Thirst has so many determinants in man that it cannot always be relied upon to reflect physiologic need.

SODIUM AND WATER.   The maintenance of a good state of salt and water intake is essential to patients with chronic renal failure. A reduced state of hydration and extracellular fluid volume results in a further lowering of the GFR in a patient at the steep end of the curve (Figs. 1 and 2) and can cause marked clinical deterioration.

POTASSIUM.   While hyperkalemia is a common problem in acute renal failure, it is not ordinarily a feature of chronic renal failure because the remaining nephrons undergo an adaptive phenomenon characterized by augmented potassium secretion per nephron. One view is that this compensatory system is due to functional hyperaldosteronism. Under the following circumstances, the secretory mechanism for potassium may be exceeded in chronic renal failure, with resultant hyperkalemia: (1) exacerbation of the underlying renal disease, leading to severe oliguria; (2) excessive potassium intake, including potassium-containing medication; (3) acute intercurrent illness and catabolic state liberating more potassium into the blood than the limited kidney function can handle. Steroid administration and its catabolic influence may have the same result. The treatment of hyperkalemia has been discussed.

ACIDOSIS.   Acidosis obviously develops in renal failure because hydrogen ion excretion does not keep pace with the acid load requiring excretion. The major mechanism in this occurrence is a reduction in ammonia (NH_3) production. Another mechanism is the reduction of titratable acid (largely phosphate) secondary to a reduction in the GFR, resulting in less buffer available for hydrogen ion secretion. In most patients, acidosis stabilizes at some given level. This indicates that at some point acid production and acid elimination are equal. The mechanism for this stabilization is not completely understood. In addition to some adaptive increase in acid excretion, buffering with the alkaline bone salts (calcium carbonate) may also play a role in stabilizing the acidosis.

Patients with modest acidosis (> 15 mEq. of HCO_3^- per liter) generally do not require treatment. Patients with symptomatic acidosis (Kussmaul respiration) should be treated. We also generally treat patients with less than 15 mEq. of bicarbonate in the serum even if they are not symptomatic, While we cannot be certain of the merits of this approach, it is done with the hope of preventing symptoms.

In the latter instance, oral alkali treatment may be employed. For example, Shohl's solution continues to be a valuable alkalizing agent. The solution is made up of 140 gm. of citric acid and 98 gm. of sodium citrate dissolved in water up to a volume of 1 liter. Each ml. contains 1 mEq. of sodium. A total daily dose of 25 to 75 ml. of the solution in three divided doses, dissolved in water or ginger ale, generally suffices. The patient with severe acidosis with Kussmaul respiration should be treated with intravenous administration of sodium bicarbonate, as described for patients with acute renal failure.

PHOSPHATE. Serum phosphate levels remain within the normal range, despite reduced filtration, until GFR falls below 25 per cent of normal. This is accomplished by decreased tubular reabsorption of phosphate per nephron. The observed phosphaturia per nephron is primarily attributable to increased secretion of parathyroid hormone ("secondary" hyperparathyroidism). The latter presumably occurs in response to hypocalcemia.

CALCIUM. Hypocalcemia is the rule in patients with chronic renal failure and is due to two factors, vitamin D resistance and hyperphosphatemia.

Vitamin D serves to enhance the absorption of calcium from the gastrointestinal tract, and there is evidence that it makes the bone more responsive to the action of parathyroid hormone. Chronic renal failure is often accompanied by vitamin D resistance. There is evidence that this is due to an increased turnover rate of the vitamin, increased accumulation of a biologically inactive metabolite of the vitamin, and increased urinary excretion of an active metabolite.

Hyperphosphatemia is a factor in lowering serum calcium. There is good evidence supporting the older concept that the solubility product of calcium phosphate is exceeded in the presence of hyperphosphatemia, with resultant precipitation of calcium phosphate in the body and lowering of serum calcium.

Selected Consequences of Chronic Renal Failure

ANEMIA. The anemia of chronic renal failure may be divided into two components. (1) The smaller component can be corrected by dialysis and is, therefore, presumably attributable to material(s) retained in the plasma as a result of failure of renal excretory function. In this category, we include the reduced life span of the red blood cells, as well as blood loss due to uremic ulceration of the bowel. (2) The major cause of the normocytic, normochromic anemia is the marrow's inability to respond to the generally small amount of bleeding and mild hemolysis. The failure of the bone marrow is due to a deficiency in erythropoietin. Dialysis does not alter this situation.

Purpura is common in chronic renal failure. The major problem is altered platelet function due to retention of nitrogenous material, probably guanidinosuccinic acid. This can be corrected by dialysis.

There is no known merit in treating asymptomatic anemia. Currently there is *no* known reason to treat the anemia for the purpose of improving renal function. On the other hand, the hazards of transfusion reaction, hepatitis, and congestive heart failure are real. The best treatment, when required, is transfusion of red blood cells *only*, in an amount and with a frequency that relieves the symptoms of anemia. It is seldom necessary to maintain the hematocrit above 25 per cent.

Cobalt and testosterone have been used with some success in the treatment of anemia and presumably work by stimulating erythropoietin. However, the side-effects outweigh the doubtful advantages of an unpredictable response.

HYPERTENSION. Hypertension in chronic renal disease is inadequately understood. Whatever the mechanism, it is known that in certain patients the hypertension of renal failure may be lowered by reducing the volume of extracellular fluid. It is possible that when dialysis results in a lowering of the blood pressure, or in making the blood pressure more responsive to antihypertensive medications, it does so by reduction in fluid volume rather than by the removal of a pressor agent. On the other hand, in some patients only bilateral nephrectomy results in reduction of the blood pressure.

Hypertensive encephalopathy, superimposed malignant hypertension, and frank heart failure are reasons to lower blood pressure in patients with chronic renal failure. In the absence of these manifestations, the role of treatment is controversial. Some do not treat this asymptomatic state because of uncertain benefit and because lowering the blood pressure may induce impaired renal perfusion and further decrease the GFR. The opposite opinion considers the possibility that a high blood pressure leads to nephrosclerosis and, thereby, lowers renal function.

We are inclined to treat patients whose diastolic pressure is above 110 mm. Hg even in the absence of complications. We are reluctant to discuss the specific details of drug therapy because so much is opinion, the drugs available change rather quickly, and there are many routes to the same end-point. It should be emphasized that *any* drug that lowers blood pressure with or without reducing the ECFV may be followed by further decrease in renal blood flow and GFR. In some instances, hypertension is helped by dialysis when other measures fail; and sometimes only bilateral nephrectomy is effective.

BONE LESIONS (RENAL OSTEODYSTROPHY). While former clinical impression has been that bone complications are infrequent in the adult, more recent experience, at least in chronic dialysis programs, has suggested that they are common.

Two clinically important types of bone lesions occur in chronic renal failure.

Osteomalacia (or Rickets, in the Child). This condition is one of inadequate mineralization of normal osteoid tissue. Renal osteomalacia is probably due largely to vitamin D resistance. Some patients have bone pain; and on X-ray one sees, in the pelvis and in the scapula, the linear radiolucent lesions of inadequately mineralized bone.

The treatment of renal osteomalacia is reserved for patients with related symptoms, because treatment carries a risk of serious complications of its own. We suggest the administration of vitamin D (50,000 to 150,000 units daily) and calcium gluconate (4 to 12 gm.).

Two precautions are essential in treatment with vitamin D. (a) Serum phosphate should be lowered before treatment, because elevation of the serum calcium level in the presence of an elevated phosphate level may result in metastatic calcification. This lowering of the phosphate level may be accomplished by a low-protein diet (such diets are also low in phosphate) or the administration of aluminum hydroxide gel (30 ml., four times daily), or both, until the serum phosphate is within the normal range. Phosphate is bound in the gut by aluminum hydroxide and is not absorbed. (b) Serum calcium must be monitored regularly and frequently to be certain that hypercalcemia does not result.

Osteitis Fibrosa. This lesion consists of osteoclastic reabsorption of bone and its replacement with fibrous tissue. The lesion may be localized and result in cyst-like radiographic lesions (osteitis fibrosa cystica), or it may take the form of generalized demineralization. Subperiosteal bone resorption in the phalanges is very helpful and reasonably early evidence of this lesion. It is virtually certain that it is due largely to the associated secondary hyperparathyroidism. The lesion may coexist with osteomalacia, and fractures may occur.

Treatment logically should be aimed at decreasing parathyroid activity by raising the serum calcium levels with vitamin D and calcium gluconate, as described in the case of osteomalacia. Unfortunately, this often is unsuccessful in patients with osteitis fibrosa. Parathyroidectomy is preferred for severe osteitis fibrosa.

The Uremic Syndrome

The term "uremia," although in use for a long time, remains differently defined by various authors. We use the term to describe a clinical syndrome unique to renal failure.

A uremic patient might have symptoms and signs referable to altered fluid and electrolyte excretion as well as to disordered regulatory systems. However, in order for us to designate the clinical complex as "uremia," we require that the patient have manifestations directly related to the accumulation of dialyzable substances and generally successfully treated with dialysis. "Uremic symptoms" most particularly involve the gastrointestinal, nervous, and cardiopulmonary systems.

PATHOGENESIS OF UREMIC SYMPTOMS. Since the "uremic symptoms" are relieved by dialysis, it is reasonable to assume that the symptom complex is due to some dialyzable substance(s) which accumulates in the blood. While urea itself has been incriminated, there is much evidence to the contrary. It is entirely possible that there is no single uremic "toxin," but rather several materials that act to disturb one or another biological system. At present, the particular offending material(s) remains unidentified.

UREMIC SYMPTOMS. *Gastrointestinal Symptoms.* Anorexia, nausea, vomiting, and hiccoughs are the common gastrointestinal manifestations. Frequently, nausea and vomiting occur in a characteristic fashion strongly resembling "morning sickness" of pregnancy. Nocturnal hydration often results in marked improvement because it prevents the sequence of a nocturnal decline in renal function, increase in renal failure, and further accumulation of the material leading to nausea and vomiting. If nocturnal hydration is of no avail, chlorpromazine may be of help in alleviating symptoms, including the hiccoughs. If this fails, a low-protein diet may result in improvement; and finally, dialysis will almost always produce remarkable improvement, if not complete disappearance, of the symptoms. Aside from personal discomfort, the great hazard of anorexia, nausea, and vomiting is the resultant dehydration and salt deficit which reduce extracellular volume and further lower GFR, thus aggravating renal failure.

Another feature of involvement of the gastrointestinal tract in uremia is ulceration anywhere from the mouth to the anus. Ulcerations may cause pain, blood loss, and perforation.

Nervous System. The uremic patient has a wide spectrum of nervous system manifestations. He may be fully alert almost to the time of death. On the other hand, he may be anxious, irritable, agitated, have delusions, hallucinations, and report frightening dreams. Some patients become paranoid, and some depressed; others present a cheerful demeanor that seems inappropriate to the circumstances. The patient may be lethargic, sleep a great deal, be somewhat confused, and lose his ability to concentrate. And there are patients who are drowsy during the daytime, but whose nights are spent in confused agitation. Many patients ultimately become comatose. Without dialysis, they die.

Muscle twitching is very common, even in comatose patients. Grand mal seizures, including some with neurological localization, may occur. Here the differential diagnosis is important because of the several etiologies of convulsions in uremia and their therapeutic implications. Convulsions may be due to hyponatremia, hypertensive encephalopathy, hypocalcemic tetany, or the uremic state. Hypocalcemic tetany is quite uncommon in uremia, except where excessive bicarbonate has been administered. Apparently the low serum protein and acidosis combine to result in generally adequate defense against tetanic seizures. While one may treat a single uremic convulsion with amobarbital (Amytal) or diphenylhydantoin (Dilantin), there is a high likelihood of recurrence unless dialysis is undertaken.

Cardiopulmonary System. We have already discussed hypertension and shall not refer to it now. One of the most common cardiac "uremic manifestations" is fibrinous pericarditis. Frequently, there are no symptoms and the only indication is the presence of a pericardial friction rub. On occasion, however, the pericarditis is associated with severe substernal pain. Rarely there may be sufficient pericardial fluid to produce tamponade.

Similarly, patients may have a uremic "pleuritis" with only a pleural friction rub or associated pain. Distinguishing this lesion from pulmonary embolism has obvious clinical importance. Both pericarditis and pleuritis respond to dialysis.

The "uremic lung" refers to a radiographic observation characterized by bilateral opacification extending as "bat wings" from the hilum to the periphery of the lung fields, not involving the apices or bases. In some patients, this finding is attributable to left heart failure; but in others, it is likely that, for some unexplained reason, uremia produces increased pulmonary capillary permeability and transudation of fluid.

Other Uremic Symptoms. Very often the appearance of the patient is so characteristic that he can be identified on sight as having chronic renal failure. These patients have increased pigmentation which, in association with the anemia, gives a characteristic color that appears to be a combination of beige, tan, and, in some light, a bit of green. In addition, the patient's face is often puffy (even in the absence of edema); this and the special discoloration convey an almost characteristic appearance.

Pruritis may be mild or very distressing. In some patients, the pruritus disappears with dialysis; in others this is not the case. In some of these patients, there appears to be a relation between calcium deposition in the skin and pruritus. Parathyroidectomy can result in relief in such instances.

TREATMENT OF "UREMIC SYMPTOMS." We have already considered treatment of (a) the fluid and electrolyte disturbances secondary to renal failure, and (b) the disorders of the non-excretory regulatory mechanism—anemia and hypertension. (c) While we have mentioned some specific treatments that might help certain aspects of the unique "uremic symptoms," we have not yet considered the general treatments available for this group of symptoms.

Low-Protein Diet. A diet low in protein has been proposed intermittently for many years in the treatment of patients with renal disease. The major rationale is that we might reduce the accumulation of protein-metabolic end-products responsible for the uremic symptoms.

In the past, low-protein diets tended to be low in calories and deficient in essential amino acids. Under these circumstances, already malnourished patients suffer further deterioration. In recent years, two Italian investigators, Giovannetti and Giordano, recognized that by adding essential amino acids and adequate total calories to a diet containing 20 gm. of protein, the BUN declined even further and negative nitrogen balance became less negative, or even positive. These authors interpreted their results to mean that in uremia, under appropriate dietary circumstances, urea is available for metabolic utilization.

This low-protein diet with adequate calories and essential amino acids has resulted in good clinical response in many patients. Along with a lowering of the BUN (and presumably the symptom-producing material(s)), there is improved general well-being, especially marked relief of gastrointestinal symptoms and sometimes of all specific "uremic symptoms."

There are limitations to this dietary program. Acceptability of the diet may be a problem. While the BUN may remain in the 50 to 60 mg. per 100 ml. range and the patient may be without gastrointestinal symptoms, serum creatinine may rise to 20 with progressive acidosis, bleeding tendency, uremic coma, and death. Thus in patients taking this diet, the BUN may be quite misleading, and there is an even stronger argument to measure serum creatinine concentration. In addition in this setting, gastrointestinal symptoms may not be a forewarning of increasing uremia.

In some patients and under certain conditions, 20 gm. of protein daily may be too low, with resultant malnutrition. Good clinical response then may be achieved with 30 to 40 gm. of protein each day.

We tend to use this dietary approach in patients with uremic symptoms when other measures have failed, and prior to chronic dialysis.

Chronic Intermittent Dialysis. The patient with end-stage renal disease, renal failure, and severe uremic symptoms may have a pleasurable and useful life with chronic intermittent dialysis.

Dialysis can be expected to eliminate or markedly ameliorate the central nervous system, gastrointestinal, cardiopulmonary, and bleeding manifestations we have described as "uremic symptoms." By altering the dialyzing bath fluids, one can more readily deal with the fluid and electrolyte disturbances of renal failure, such as acidosis and hyponatremia. Hypertension may be improved and more readily managed by better control of the volume of the extracellular fluid. In addition, pruritus may disappear. Libido and sexual potency, frequently diminished or absent in uremia, often return completely or at least improve significantly during chronic dialysis. All in all, the patient feels much better.

Despite marked improvement, certain problems persist. The anemia is not eliminated because erythropoietin deficiency remains. Peripheral neuropathy may get worse or make its initial appearance after dialysis has been instituted. There is reason to believe that this is not the case if dialysis is carried out more frequently. With chronic dialysis, severe renal osteodystrophy may manifest itself despite correction of so many other abnormalities. There are several reasons for this. Dialysis apparently does not improve Vitamin-D resistance. Dietary restrictions including protein (and phosphate) may be liberalized because the patient feels well, resulting in some elevation in serum phosphate, consequent lowering of serum calcium, and secondary hyperparathyroidism. Increased metastatic calcification has also been observed. This is presumably due, at least in part, to increased phosphate, for the reasons already given.

Several steps may be taken to deal with the calcium and phosphorus problems that develop in patients undergoing chronic, intermittent dialysis. An initial approach is to decrease the level of phosphate by dietary change (low protein and phosphate diet) and by the administration of phosphate-binding gels as previously described. *After* this has been accomplished, serum calcium can be increased to 10 mg. per 100 ml. by increasing the calcium in the bath solution. In some instances, vitamin D and calcium gluconate may also be given. This treatment can avoid metastatic calcification and suppress the parathyroid glands, resulting in bone healing.

There are now instances in which the parathyroid gland seemingly becomes autonomous and is not suppressed by increased calcium levels. This is sometimes referred to as "tertiary" hyperparathyroidism, and parathyroidectomy is advised. On the other hand, at least some of these apparently autonomously functioning, overactive glands subside spontaneously, albeit slowly, over a matter of many months after transplantation.

One of the main problems of chronic dialysis relates to the indwelling arterial-venous cannulas used to form a shunt. The shunt has a tendency to clot, and the sites in the skin may become infected.

Other important problems relate to the emotional impact of devoting so much time to a program in which a human being becomes entirely dependent upon a machine. Some patients are in fine spirits because they feel better, can work, and feel productive; and they accept all the problems inherent in this kind of treatment. Others do become depressed; and indeed, suicide has occurred.

In general, patients are dialyzed two or three times weekly for 6 to 12 hours. Patients may now be trained and equipped to carry out dialysis at home. This involves a room, a sturdy family, money, and training.

There are social problems related to chronic dialysis. One problem is cost. Chronic dialysis in a center currently costs approximately $10,000 per year per patient. Home dialysis costs the same the first year and then about $3,000 to $5,000 per year. Another problem relates to the limitations of center dialysis. In a center with accommodations for 15 patients in the program, for the sixteenth patient, it is as if there were no program at all.

Another central problem in chronic dialysis is the selection of patients for the program. Patients should have end-stage disease, require dialysis to survive, and have sufficient stability to live with the program. One of the difficult aspects is to choose from among the eligible candidates. Many centers have an anonymous committee to evaluate the social aspects of the several applicants. This raises the philosophic question of how does one (anyone) evaluate the "worth" of any man compared with another.

Finally, for the future, improved technical development should reduce the complexity and cost of operation. Even at the present level, 87 per cent of patients on dialysis programs survive one year; 77 per cent survive 2 years and 67 per cent survive 3 years!

Transplantation. In the transplantation program, a patient with end-stage renal disease is given a kidney from a living donor or from a cadaver. In most recipients, bilateral nephrectomy is carried out because of reasons that incriminate the kidney itself as a source of antirenal antigen in certain glomerular diseases. It is pointless, in a very rapidly moving scene, to go into detail concerning the present state of the art. It suffices to say that the results clearly justify this as a therapeutic procedure.

Recent overall international data gave 60 to 70 per cent effective 2-year results with living sibling or parent donors and close to 30 to 40 per cent with cadaver donors. In certain centers, as in Denver, there is a 90 per cent survival in 1 year with living donors; in Australia, 65 per cent in 1 year with cadaver kidneys. The major problem now relates to the rejection phenomenon, and the side effects of its treatment with immunosuppressive agents and corticosteroids. The prospects are good and will be better as tissue typing and histocompatibility become better and as immunosuppressive agents improve. In addition, kidney banks will presumably be formed someday to solve the problem of availability of organs.

SUMMARY OF TREATMENT CONSIDERATIONS IN CHRONIC RENAL FAILURE

1. Search for reversible, treatable chronic diseases of the kidney, and wherever possible, institute appropriate therapy. Examples include (a) infectious disease (pyelonephritis, tuberculosis, infective endocarditis), (b) hypercalcemic nephropathy, (c) hypokalemic nephropathy, (d) renal disease due to drugs and chemicals, and (e) obstructive nephropathy.

2. Search for *reversible factors* adversely influencing the course of irreversible renal disease. At times, these reversible factors are more important determinants of life and comfort than the underlying renal disease itself. (a) Urinary tract infection is commonly superimposed on renal disease of any cause and may serve further to impair renal function. Other reversible factors include (b) water deficit, (c) sodium deficit, (d) hypokalemia, and (e) heart failure.

Sometimes patients with chronic renal failure, who have been getting along reasonably well, suddenly become much worse, especially exhibiting central nervous system symptoms. It may be impossible to know if this represents the terminal phases of the chronic disease or an acute exacerbation, or the intervention of some of the reversible factors mentioned above. In these instances, peritoneal or extracorporeal dialysis may be undertaken to gain time for more accurate assessment of the situation.

3. Maintain the internal environment as nearly normal as possible, consistent with clinical considerations rather than the aesthetic value of the chart. (a) Prevent dehydration and salt deficit as well as fluid overload. Determine sodium and water needs and capability in each patient individually. (b) Treat acidosis only if the patient is symptomatic, or if serum bicarbonate levels are below 15 mEq. per liter. When treating, avoid excessive replacement because of the hazards of volume overload and tetany. (c) Prevent hypokalemia and hyperkalemia. (d) Anemia is treated when there are clinical indications and then by transfusion of red blood cells. Seldom does one have to keep the hematocrit above 25 per cent. (e) Hypertension should be treated when there is cardiomegaly, heart failure, encephalopathy, or accelerated (malignant) hypertension.

(We tend also to treat patients whose diastolic blood pressure exceeds 110 mm. Hg, even if they are asymptomatic.) (f) Renal osteodystrophy should be treated if the patient is symptomatic. Severe osteomalacia is treated carefully with vitamin D and calcium. Severe osteitis fibrosa may best be treated with parathyroidectomy. (g) Uremic symptoms may be treated with measures to maximize renal function, protein restriction, dialysis, and transplantation.

4. The presence of renal failure alters treatment with a variety of drugs that depend on the kidney for excretion.

5. The hospital environment does not necessarily serve the best interests of the patient. We have often been dismayed by the difficulties some patients encounter in obtaining water, especially at night. In addition, because of gastrointestinal symptoms, patients may have a gastrointestinal radiographic series with overnight dehydration. This is a major hazard. Patients with chronic renal failure can fast overnight but should receive parenteral hydration before and during a gastrointestinal series. In many hospitals, "routine" laboratory tests require fasting. For some reason, this is often translated into the interdiction of fluids and the patient becomes dehydrated.

Sometimes the concept of "routine" is extended to include a "routine renal workup." This is conceptually unsound and potentially dangerous. For example, to do a concentration test with dehydration is useless, because for reasons already considered, the patient with chronic renal failure cannot elaborate a concentrated urine, and furthermore, overnight dehydration is hazardous. To do a "routine intravenous pyelogram" will not be revealing because of poor function, and the dehydration and purgation is extremely hazardous. If pyelograms are needed, they can be done safely *with* hydration. It is our custom to keep patients with chronic renal failure at home in a good, trained environs, and admit them to the hospital only for good reason.

6. Patients with chronic renal failure need considerable attention from their physicians, as do all patients with chronic illness. Periodically, they become despondent and weary of being sick and being different. Frequently, the patients are young adults whose despair is augmented by an inability to care for children optimally, by the indignities of being deprived of a good job, and by sexual inadequacy. Patients with chronic renal failure will stop drinking water regularly, forego their diet, etc., and develop irreversible renal failure and death. One thing the physician can do is to see the patient often, demonstrate his interest in small details – food, appetite, fluids, sleep, etc. – while listening to the patient's feelings and his fears. One can frequently prevent harmful rebellion by this type of interest and awareness of the earliest evidence of depression.

ACKNOWLEDGMENT

This article is modified from the section on Failure of Renal Function in the author's book Clinical Nephrology, shortly to be published by Little, Brown & Co., and is used with the permission of the publisher.

REFERENCES

Acute Renal Failure
1. Epstein, F. H.: The treatment of reversible uremia. Yale J. Biol. Med., 27:53, 1954.
2. Hollenberg, N. K., and Epstein, M.: The use of drugs in the patient with uremia. Mod. Treat., 6:1011, 1969.
3. Maher, J. F.: Drug therapy in patients with renal failure. The Kidney, 3:1970.
4. Merrill, J. P.: Acute renal failure. *In* Strauss, M. B., and Welt, L. G., eds.: Diseases of the Kidney. Boston, Little, Brown (in press).
5. Muehrcke, R. C.: Acute Renal Failure: Diagnosis and Management. St. Louis, C. V. Mosby, 1969.
6. Oken, D. E.: Diagnosis and treatment of acute renal failure. Mod. Treat., 6:927, 1969.
7. Papper, S.: Clinical Nephrology. Boston, Little, Brown (in press).
8. Schreiner, G. E.: Acute renal failure. *In* Black, D. A. K., ed.: Renal Disease. Philadelphia, F. A. Davis, 2nd ed., 1967.

Chronic Renal Failure
9. Hampers, C. L.: Treatment of chronic uremia. Mod. Treat., 6:1036, 1969.
10. Merrill, J. P., and Hampers, C. L.: Uremia. New Eng. J. Med., 282:953, 1014, 1970.
11. Papper, S.: Clinical Nephrology. Boston, Little, Brown (in press).
12. Schwartz, W. G., and Kassirer, J. P.: Medical management of chronic renal failure. Amer. J. Med., 44:786, 1968.
13. Seldin, D. W., et al.: Metabolic consequences of renal failure and their management. *In* Strauss, M. B., and Welt, L. G., eds.: Diseases of the Kidney. Boston, Little, Brown (in press).

Department of Medicine
University of Miami School of Medicine
P. O. Box 875, Biscayne Annex
Miami, Florida   33152

Diuretic Drug Therapy of Edema

Eliseo C. Perez-Stable, M.D., *
and Barry J. Materson, M.D. **

Diuretic drug therapy is an empirical approach to the management of patients with a variety of diseases characterized by renal salt and water retention and formation of edema. These drugs increase renal sodium and water excretion but do not attack directly the primary etiology of the extracellular fluid (ECF) overload, and should be considered as symptomatic therapy. This is, nevertheless, of great importance, because in many instances there is no other treatment and diuretic therapy of the edema may not only make the patient feel better but also improve his functional capacity.

The clinician now has at his disposition potent and effective natriuretic drugs which are capable of drying practically every patient with edema if the renal function is preserved. However, in this process he may induce serious disturbances in the volume and composition of the body fluids and create a more complicated situation.[15] These complications of diuretic therapy have been justifiably emphasized in recent articles. However, we believe that many of these complications can be prevented if the clinician has a clear understanding of the mechanism of action and effects of the natriuretic drugs, and consequently plans his therapy according to the expected changes in body fluids that he will induce.

The purpose of this article is to present a practical approach to the clinical use of diuretic drugs for the treatment of edema which may allow the patient to obtain the maximum benefit of diuresis with minimal or no complications.

MECHANISM OF ACTION

The common denominator of the mechanism of action of all diuretic drugs is their ability to impair tubular reabsorption of sodium. The

*Professor, Department of Medicine, University of Miami; and Assistant Chief, Medical Service, Veterans Administration Hospital, Miami, Florida
**Instructor, Department of Medicine, University of Miami; and Research Associate, Veterans Administration Hospital, Miami, Florida

known facts and theories of the cellular and biochemical mechanisms of this effect have been reviewed in other publications and will not be considered here. We will review briefly the renal excretion of sodium in normal and abnormal conditions and illustrate how this excretion can be influenced by diuretic drugs.

Urinary excretion of sodium is the result of the interaction of two main factors: glomerular filtration and tubular reabsorption. Sodium is filtered through the glomerulus at the same concentration as that in plasma. Assuming a glomerular filtration rate of 100 ml. per min. and a plasma concentration of sodium of 140 mEq. per liter, the amount of sodium filtered in 24 hours is about 24,000 mEq. From this enormous load the tubules have to reabsorb enough sodium to maintain homeostasis. Sodium excretion varies from less than 1 to more than 300 mEq. per day.

It has been postulated that a mechanism of glomerular tubular balance allows the kidney to accomplish this regulation of sodium balance.[17] In general, tubular reabsorption and glomerular filtration will change in similar directions. A decrease in filtration will provoke a decrease in reabsorption and vice versa. Tubular reabsorption may vary independently from glomerular filtration.[2] The exact mechanism responsible for this fine adjustment has not yet been completely clarified, but recent investigations suggest a paramount role of proximal tubular reabsorption.[1, 12]

For the purpose of this article, we may schematically consider tubular reabsorption of sodium to take place in four sites as shown in Figure 1. Site 1 is located in the proximal tubule and is responsible for 60 or 70 per cent of tubular sodium reabsorption. Site 2 is in the ascending loop of Henle, where 15 or 20 per cent of sodium reabsorption occurs. Sites 3 and 4 are located in the distal tubule, where 6 to 8 per cent of the filtered sodium is reabsorbed.

Recent investigations suggest that an increase of sodium reabsorption in site 1 is the most important factor in salt and water retention in patients with edema.[5, 18] Acetazolamide has some action at this level by inhibiting carbonic anhydrase, but this is a self-limited, weak diuretic. Furosemide[11] may have some action in this site. Mercurials probably act here also, although there is no conclusive evidence for this.

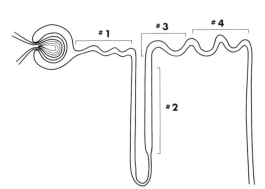

Figure 1. Theoretical sites of action of diuretic drugs.

The most potent diuretics, furosemide and ethacrynic acid, have their main action at site 2 and can block up to 20 or 25 per cent of the filtered sodium. Thiazide derivatives act at site 3 and are able to block the sodium remaining after more proximal reabsorption.

From an inspection of Figure 1 one can appreciate that more proximally acting diuretics have the potential for blocking reabsorption of a greater fraction of the filtered sodium than those which act more distally. Under conditions of maximal sodium reabsorption, so little sodium may reach the distal sites that even effective blockade of those sites can cause little increase in sodium excretion. This may account, in part, for the efficacy of ethacrynic acid or furosemide in patients whose edema is refractory to thiazides.

In site 4, reabsorption of sodium takes place as if sodium were exchanged directly for potassium or hydrogen. In reality, potassium is secreted following an electrochemical gradient, and the tubular reabsorption of sodium is important because it creates the necessary electronegativity to allow the potassium or hydrogen to be secreted from the interior of the tubular cell to the tubular lumen. Here is where aldosterone regulates potassium and where spironolactone acts, probably by competing for receptor sites with aldosterone. Triamterene also acts at this site but by a mechanism independent of the action of aldosterone. Spironolactone and triamterene are additive in their natriuretic and potassium-sparing effects.

This schematic conception of the site of action of diuretic drugs is very helpful to the clinician. First, it explains the differences in potency of diuretics on the basis of how proximally they act. Second, an inspection of Figure 1 will show that all drugs blocking sodium reabsorption in sites 1, 2, and 3 will leave more sodium to be reabsorbed at site 4; this will favor more potassium and hydrogen secretion. Therefore, by using diuretics which block sodium reabsorption at site 4, one can not only enhance the natriuretic effect of drugs which act more proximally, but also decrease potassium and hydrogen losses.

Third, a patient may be refractory to the use of one diuretic but still sensitive to another diuretic which acts by a different mechanism or at another site. The most potent possible diuretic, which does not now exist, would be one which exerted its main action in the proximal tubule and could be combined with other drugs acting at the more distal sites.

EFFECTS OF DIURESIS

The goal of the use of diuretic drugs is to establish a negative balance of water and sodium in order to correct an extracellular fluid volume overload, but without inducing serious disturbances in the volume and composition of body fluids. To accomplish this the clinician should have a clear idea of the effects of diuretics on the volume and composition of both ECF and the resultant urine.

Any given diuretic has two major effects on the kidney: it increases urine volume output and increases excretion of urine electrolytes.

Changes in Volume

Plasma Volume

The increased urine volume must, of necessity, originate from plasma ultrafiltered at the glomerulus. That is, the immediate source of urine is intravascular. This inevitably means that plasma volume must be reduced at least transiently. The hematocrit and serum protein concentration rise and, as a sequel to the latter, the plasma oncotic pressure rises. The volume reduction also causes a decrease in intravascular hydrostatic pressure.

Flow of extracellular fluid between capillaries and the interstitial spaces is governed by Starling's law which, in essence, states that the direction of flow is a resultant of the gradients of hydrostatic and oncotic pressure across the capillary wall.

Increased intravascular volume causes increased hydrostatic pressure and, because of dilution of serum proteins, reduced oncotic pressure. This favors transudation of fluid into the tissue spaces, i.e., edema formation. When diuretic-induced plasma volume contraction occurs with reduction of hydrostatic pressure and increase in oncotic pressure, the Starling forces favor transfer of edema fluid back into the intravascular compartment, where it becomes accessible to the glomerulus for urinary elimination.

Unfortunately, the physiological kinetics of this fluid transfer is less than ideal.[14] Plasma ultrafiltration occurs at a faster rate than interstitial fluid transfer, which is more rapid than the movement of trapped fluid out of serosal spaces. Uninterrupted use of potent modern diuretics may not allow time for re-equilibration of body fluids and thereby induce an undesired plasma volume contraction even in the face of edema and continuing diuresis.

Plasma volume contraction is easy to detect at the bedside. Blood pressure will be reduced and there may be an orthostatic pressure drop. Pulse pressure will be narrowed and the pulse rate increased. BUN and creatinine levels will rise because of decreased GFR. Central venous pressure by neck vein observation or direct measurement will be very low. At this point the clinician must cease efforts at diuresis even in the face of continued presence of edema or fluid trapped in serosal spaces, and permit equilibration between the volume compartments to take place. If one is aware of this possible induced plasma volume contraction, it usually can be obviated by judicious modification of diuretic therapy.

Total Body Water

One follows a patient's water balance by the fundamental parameter of body weight. Because rapid changes in body weight are due to fluid balance rather than body tissue mass fluctuations, one can assume that daily gain or loss of each kilogram or pound of body weight reflects a net change of 1 liter or 1 pint, respectively, of body water. If accurate measurements of urinary output are made then one can determine the real

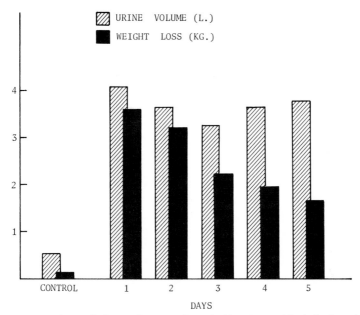

Figure 2.   Daily weight loss and urine volume in 10 patients with cirrhosis and ascites after infusion of 100 mg. of intravenous ethacrynic acid twice a day. Difference between urine volume and weight loss represents actual water intake.

intake of fluid (usually sodium free) above that prescribed by subtracting kilograms of body weight lost from liters of urine excreted.

$$\text{Fluid intake (L.)} = \text{urine volume (L.)} - \text{weight loss (Kg.)}$$

Figure 2 shows combined daily weights and 24-hour urine volumes of 10 patients with cirrhosis and ascites in our series. These patients had water intake restricted to 700 ml. per day. Note the close correlation between weight and output during the control days and the first 2 days after the initiation of massive diuresis. By the third day the patients were drinking some excess water, and by the fifth day flagrant violation of fluid restriction is obvious.

Changes in Composition

The ideal diuretic agent, which does not now exist, would be capable of increasing the volume of urine with a composition identical to that of extracellular fluid. Deviation from the ideal urine electrolyte composition is the rule with diuretics and presents a more difficult problem than volume.

The urine composition during diuresis in different disease states has been established.[10, 19] The urine electrolyte composition at the peak of diuresis after the intravenous administration of a potent diuretic to a group of 11 patients with cirrhosis and ascites studied by us is

Table 1. *Urinary Concentration of Electrolytes After
Administration of a Potent Diuretic to 11 Patients
With Cirrhosis and Ascites*

	CONTROL	PEAK DIURESIS
Urine flow (ml. per min.)	0.51	15.0
Sodium (mEq. per liter)	35.2	112.0
Chloride (mEq. per liter)	33.9	132.0
Potassium (mEq. per liter)	81.1	20.6

presented in Table 1. However, the 24 hour urinary electrolyte output
is more important for management of the patient.

Our study of 10 additional patients with cirrhosis and ascites over
five days of intermittent diuretic administration elicited the mean 24
hour urine electrolyte composition shown in Table 2. The daily potassium
losses are especially large because of the inevitable rebound hyperaldosteronism which results from reduction of plasma volume by
diuretics. Note that chloride excretion is approximately equal to the
sum of sodium and potassium excretion. Therefore, chloride excretion
exceeds sodium excretion by the amount of potassium excretion – about
50 mEq. per liter.

Hyponatremia

A frequent complication of diuretic therapy is hyponatremia. This
occurs despite the fact that urine sodium concentration is less than
that of plasma. Assuming that the patient's sodium is restricted, this is
an indication that the net sodium loss is proportionally greater than net
water loss owing to continued intake of salt-free water. The clinician
can determine the true volume as explained previously.

The following formula is useful for conceptualizing problems of
salt and water balance:[3, 9]

$$Na_x \propto \frac{Na_E + K_E}{TBW}$$

where Na_S = serum sodium concentration (mEq. per liter)
Na_E = total exchangeable sodium
K_E = total exchangeable potassium
TBW = total body water

Table 2. *Mean 24 Hour Urine Electrolyte Composition After
Intravenous Ethacrynic Acid During 5 Days in 10 Patients
with Cirrhosis and Ascites*

	DAY 1	DAY 2	DAY 3	DAY 4	DAY 5
Sodium (mEq. per liter)	81	92	78	71	67
Potassium (mEq. per liter)	49	51	48	53	47
Chloride (mEq. per liter)	128	141	125	126	131

Since daily water balance is equal to daily changes in body weight, we can interpret the formula as follows: changes of serum sodium are proportional to changes in the ratio of the sum of sodium and potassium balance to water balance.

Inspection of the formula reveals that if total body water increases markedly (as in extracellular fluid overload), total exchangeable sodium must increase proportionally if the concentration of serum sodium is to be maintained in the normal range. This indeed happens in most untreated ECF overloaded patients because they continue to eat salt and because of the stimuli to the kidneys to retain sodium. If such a patient is subjected to diuresis but water is not restricted, he may tend to maintain his total body water by replacing his sodium-rich urine output volume for volume with sodium-free water.

It can be seen in the formula that if TBW is reduced proportionally less than Na_E, then hyponatremia must ensue. In this situation note that increase in TBW is due to an increase in ECF which contains most of the Na_E. Therefore, if ECF is markedly increased, total body Na will be increased even in the face of Na_S so low as to produce symptoms.

Another mechanism for hyponatremia is the induction of a negative balance of potassium. This may be seen from inspection of the formula.

The implications of these observations are clear. If a patient has too much sodium and too much water, then the goal must be to reduce them both in a proportion such that the serum sodium concentration is not significantly altered. Hyponatremia can be corrected by causing excretion of urine with a sodium concentration less than plasma and avoiding redilution by excess water intake. Therefore, in patients with massive edema or ascites, both salt and water intake must be restricted.

Potassium Depletion

All diuretics which act proximal to the distal exchange site cause an increase in potassium and hydrogen ion excretion and will eventually cause hypokalemic metabolic alkalosis.

The critical role of chloride in correction of metabolic alkalosis and potassium deficiency has been demonstrated by Schwartz[6] and others.[8] Any attempt to prevent the alkalosis induced by diuretic agents has to take into account the fact that chloride losses in these circumstances are grossly equal to the losses of sodium and potassium. In the extracellular phase the ratio of chloride to sodium is 0.75:1; therefore, renal excretion at a ratio of 1:1 or greater entails a loss of chloride in relation to sodium, and if only the chloride lost with potassium is replaced, hypochloremia may result. This is the rationale for our postulation that for an electrolyte replacement solution to be effective it should contain chloride in excess of potassium.

CLINICAL USE OF DIURETIC DRUGS

Diuretic drugs are part of the overall therapeutic plan for the edematous patient, and are not necessary in all instances. Many patients are quite comfortable with mild edema and require no natriuretic agents. They should not be treated for purely cosmetic reasons.

Diet modification plays an important role in the treatment of edema. In general the kidneys tend to retain sodium, and it is imperative to restrict salt intake, preferably below the limit of renal sodium retention for each patient; this enables the patient to achieve a negative sodium balance. For example, if a given patient excretes 30 mEq. of sodium daily and is placed on a diet containing 10 mEq. of sodium, a negative sodium balance of 20 mEq. daily will be established. After 1 week the patient will have achieved a net loss of 140 mEq., which represents the loss of 1 liter of extracellular fluid or 1 kilogram of body weight, assuming that the serum sodium is unchanged.

Many edematous patients will respond to this approach alone. However, strict sodium restriction is unpleasant and many patients are unwilling or unable to adhere to their diet. Also, especially with patients in severe cardiac or liver decompensation, the magnitude of sodium retention may be well below 10 mEq. per day. It is important to keep in mind that a low-sodium diet is also a low chloride diet, and if diuretic drugs are used it will be necessary to supplement chloride to avoid hypochloremic alkalosis. The advantage of dietary treatment is that it is less complicated and is not associated with the side-effects induced by diuretic drugs.

We favor the intermittent use of diuretics to permit time between doses for re-equilibration of body fluids between compartments and to allow normal homeostatic mechanisms to operate as explained in the previous section.

We have previously discussed the disturbances in body fluid composition induced by diuretic drugs, but they also may have direct toxic effects, which are less predictable but can be anticipated. The ototoxicity of both ethacrynic acid and furosemide has been well established. Most such cases occur in patients with renal failure or in those who receive high dosages. Nearly all cases of tinnitus and deafness have been reversible but a few have not.

Both ethacrynic acid and furosemide are membrane-active drugs and may induce transient cardiac arrhythmias when given rapidly intravenously. An association between gastrointestinal bleeding and use of intravenous ethacrynic acid has been noted by a computer survey of drug use and toxicity;[16] this has not been documented further. Hyperglycemia and hyperuricemia are well-known side-effects which have been discussed elsewhere. Both are simple to manage and generally do not necessitate cessation of drug therapy. Mercurials may cause renal tubular damage and should not be used in patients with impaired renal function.

Discussion of the clinical use of diuretics may be conveniently divided into treatment of hospitalized patients and treatment of clinic or office patients.

Hospitalized Patients

Patients with ECF overload syndromes are hospitalized for one or more of the following reasons: hospital-dependent diagnostic investigations of the primary disease, treatment of the primary disease, or because the ECF overload has produced symptoms incompatible with continued outpatient function. The rest and dietary restriction associated with hospitalization may effect favorable changes in the hemodynamic status of the patient and induce a diuresis. With the exception of emergencies, the physician can observe his patient for 2 or 3 days before starting him on natriuretic agents.

In general it is better to begin treatment with a moderately potent diuretic such as hydrochlorothiazide in doses of 50 or 100 mg. daily and increase to a maximum of 200 mg. in two divided doses. If this regimen is ineffective, one can change to the more potent diuretics such as ethacrynic acid or furosemide in low initial doses of 50 and 40 mg. respectively, and gradually increase the dosage until a response is ob-obtained. Spironolactone (Aldactone) or triamterene (Dyrenium), combined with other diuretics, may be useful in some patients to increase diuresis and to reduce or obviate the need for potassium supplementation. During the diuresis the physician must watch carefully for changes in body weight, serum electrolyte concentration, and urine volume.

Refractory Edema

There are patients who do not respond to a regimen as outlined above. In general they are recognized as having refractory edema. Advanced heart failure and severely decompensated cirrhosis of the liver are more common examples of the clinical situation. In an attempt to solve this problem we have devised the protocol listed in Table 3. The rationale of this regimen has been explained in the sections on mechanism of action and effects of diuretic drugs. This aggressive approach to the management of edematous states should be reserved only for patients who do not respond to conventional treatment.

We have been particularly successful in the treatment of resistant ascites in cirrhotic patients and have practically abolished the need for abdominal paracentesis which has well known complications such as bleeding, peritonitis, shock, and protein depletion. We prefer instead a pharmacological paracentesis achieved by using potent diuretics in single, well-spaced doses. Both ethacrynic acid and furosemide achieve a rapid peak effect which declines rapidly and is gone by 5 or 6 hours. If no more than two doses are given daily at least 6 hours apart there is adequate time for re-equilibration of plasma volume as fluid is "pulled" from edema and ascites pools. We generally limit massive diuresis by this protocol to 2 or 3 days, followed by a few days of rest, and then proceed until the desired amount of fluid has been removed. When patients have no peripheral edema, or when the edema is removed by diuresis and the ascites remains, this protocol for rapid diuresis is more likely to induce plasma volume contraction and must be used with even greater caution.[14]

The question of whether or not oral forms of these diuretics can be substituted for the intravenous drugs and achieve equal effect remains unanswered. This problem is being explored currently by our group.

As discussed earlier, it is essential that potassium replacement be given with chloride as the reabsorbable anion. For this reason potassium

Table 3. *Protocol for Rapid Diuresis*

1. Restrict sodium to 10 mEq. a day and water intake to 600 ml.
2. Weigh daily at the same time each morning before breakfast after evacuation of bladder and bowel.
3. Accurately measure urine output and calculate real fluid intake by subtracting weight loss in kg. from urine volume in liters.
4. Administer furosemide (160 mg. I.V.) or ethacrynic acid (100 mg. I.V.) twice a day, at least 6 hours apart.
5. Administer 30 ml. (48 mEq. of K and 66 mEq. of Cl) of electrolyte replacement solution immediately after each liter of urine is voided.
6. Monitor daily serum electrolytes, BUN, creatinine, and signs of volume depletion; adjust electrolyte replacement and duration of diuretic administration according to results.

preparations such as Kaon, K Triplex, and K-lyte, which contain non-reabsorbable anions and no chloride, are unsatisfactory for potassium replacement. We use potassium chloride (KCl) as a flavored 10 or 20 per cent solution, given orally, either in or with a small (60 to 70 ml.) water "chaser." Commercial potassium chloride preparations include Kaochlor liquid (Warren-Teed, 20 mEq. per 15 ml.), Kay Ciel Elixir (Cooper, 20 mEq. per 15 ml.) and Kato Powder (Ingram, 20 mEq. per powder measure). K-20 (Hart) is a flavored powder but must be dissolved in 6 oz. of water.

We have prepared an electrolyte replacement solution, the contents of which is shown in Table 4. Although we add flavoring (as do the proprietary preparations), it is most difficult to disguise the unpleasant taste of potassium. However, our patients seem to tolerate it well. We generally administer 30 ml. (48 mEq. of K) just prior to diuresis and then give an additional dose immediately after the excretion of each liter of urine. This is adequate for most patients. However, it is essential that the serum electrolytes be monitored daily during rapid diuresis, since this dose will be either too high or too low for a few patients.

Many clinicians prefer to reduce or eliminate the need for potassium replacement by using spironolactone (Aldactone) or triamterene (Dyrenium). Spironolactone has the disadvantage of delayed onset of action and may cause painful gynecomastia.

Triamterene has a different mechanism of action from spironolactone and has an additive effect. This can cause lethal hyperkalemia if triamterene and spironolactone are used together. Some proprietary drugs combine spironolactone or triamterene with a diuretic. The physician must be aware of this if he adds a potassium-retaining drug separately.

Table 4. *Composition of Electrolyte Replacement Solution*

	1 ML.	30 ML.
Potassium (mEq.)	1.6	48
Chloride (mEq.)	2.2	66
Calcium (mEq.)	0.6	18

A rare patient with cirrhosis may have a peculiar renal tubular acidosis as described by Shear and Gabuzda.[13] These patients have elevated serum chloride levels and, since they have impaired acid secretion, they may secrete even more potassium than usual. They are extremely susceptible to hypokalemia and hepatic encephalopathy, even in the face of normal or high chloride and normal or reduced bicarbonate levels. At least some of the potassium replacement in these patients is best done with one of the non-chloride containing preparations.

An occasional cirrhotic patient will prove refractory to all efforts at diuresis and yet have so much ascites and peripheral and penile edema that he suffers from skin infections, decubitus ulcers, immobility, and even urinary outlet obstruction. We treat these patients electively in the manner described by Eknoyan et al.,[4] by withdrawing ascitic fluid, running it through a filter and reinfusing it into a peripheral vein while simultaneously administering diuretics. We place a plastic catheter in the peritoneal space, connect it to standard intravenous tubing which runs through a peristaltic infusion withdrawal pump, thence through a standard blood transfusion filter and tubing, and into the vein. Figure 3 shows the results in one patient. Note the marked increase in sodium excretion and GFR. Considerable volume and weight can be removed rapidly by this method (18 to 25 lb. per day in our series) with good patient tolerance and safety.

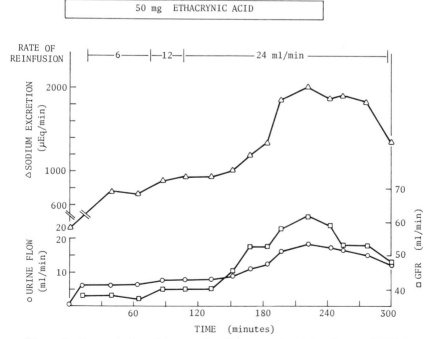

Figure 3. Demonstration of increased sodium excretion, urine flow, and GFR in a cirrhotic patient who was treated with simultaneous reinfusion of autologous ascitic fluid and a diuretic.

After the patient has achieved maximum benefit from his hospital treatment, it is well for the physician to observe him on the appropriate dose of oral diuretics (if still required) and a more liberal salt intake. Most patients can be taught to maintain their weight and keep track of their urine output. They require careful outpatient followup.

Acute Pulmonary Edema

Frequently the volume of plasma which needs to be removed in order to achieve cardiac compensation in acute pulmonary edema is on the order of only a few hundred milliliters. If an effective diuresis can be achieved, it can be highly therapeutic, since the urine excreted is derived directly, often within minutes, from the plasma volume. We prefer furosemide intravenously in a dose of 20 to 40 mg. (one or two 2-ml. ampoules). Furosemide requires no time for preparation and mixing, is given in a volume so small that of itself it does not contribute to volume overload, and may be less likely to cause cardiac arrhythmias than ethacrynic acid.

If there is sufficient renal blood flow, there is good evidence that both furosemide and ethacrynic acid effect a redistribution of renal blood flow to the cortical nephrons, which are better suited for salt and water excretion than the juxtamedullary nephrons. We use diuretics here as an adjunct to the treatment mentioned above. Potassium must be monitored to avoid possible digitalis toxicity. If the patient has renal failure, peritoneal dialysis against hypertonic glucose is a rapid and effective treatment for pulmonary edema.

Tense Ascites

Patients with tense ascites pose a difficult problem. If one removes ascitic fluid by paracentesis, there is a tendency for continued leakage of fluid through the needle tract, protein loss, electrolyte shifts, and reaccumulation of ascitic fluid at the expense of plasma volume. There is evidence that removal of small amounts (less than 1000 ml.) of ascitic fluid reduces intraperitoneal and portal pressure, reverses compression of the inferior vena cava, and increases GFR.[7]

We prefer a pharmacologic paracentesis, using potent diuretics in single, spaced doses. This is accomplished by use of the same basic protocol elaborated earlier for the treatment of refractory edema. The patient is given either 100 mg. of ethacrynic acid or 160 mg. of furosemide, and electrolyte replacement solution is given after each liter of urine output as described previously. In most cases this emergency therapy is followed up with the regular protocol for treatment of massive ascites, but the immediate goal is to relieve acute respiratory distress due to the tenseness of the ascitic mass.

Outpatient Use of Diuretics

We have devoted most of this article to discussion of large doses of potent diuretics given to hospitalized patients because of the frequency and severity of problems attendant thereto. By far the bulk of diuretics is administered to clinic and office patients for treatment of chronic ECF overload and hypertension. Most of these patients respond well to the thiazide diuretics; only the more resistant subject should require a more potent diuretic. We prefer to use hydrochlorothiazide ordered generically because of the reduced cost to the patient. There is no real clinical advantage to be gained by using thiazides which have greater milligram for milligram potency but no greater therapeutic efficacy. The claims for greater urine sodium to potassium excretion ratios are of little clinical consequence.

What about volume and electrolyte control in outpatients? Basically, the same rules obtain as for inpatients. It remains essential to follow body weight. Many patients can be taught to record not only their weight but also their urinary output. No one really knows the electrolyte replacement requirements of patients on long-term diuretic therapy. We generally encourage our patients to drink orange juice and eat bananas and prunes when they are on low doses of diuretic. We advise moderate sodium restriction in cooperation with a dietitian. Most of these patients do not require additional medicinal potassium. Patients on higher doses generally receive supplements of 20 to 60 mEq. of potassium chloride daily, depending on their individual requirements. We know of no reliable method for predicting potassium losses in such cases and must treat each patient individually.

REFERENCES

1. Bricker, N. S.: The control of sodium excretion with normal and reduced nephron populations: The preeminence of third factor (Editorial). Amer. J. Med., 43:313–321, 1967.
2. Dewardener, H. E., Mills, I. H., Clapham, W. F., and Hayter, C. J.: Studies on efferent mechanism of sodium diuresis which follows administration of intravenous saline in dogs. Clin. Sci., 21:249, 1961.
3. Edelman, I. S., Leibman, J., O'Meara, M. P., and Birkenfeld, L. W.: Interrelations between serum sodium concentration, serum osmolarity and total exchangeable sodium, total exchangeable potassium and total body water. J. Clin. Invest., 37:1236–1256, 1958.
4. Eknoyan, G., Martinez-Maldonado, M., Yium, J. J., and Suki, W. M.: Combined ascitic-fluid and furosemide infusion in management of ascites. New Eng. J. Med., 282:713–717, 1970.
5. Goodman, B., Cohen, J. A., Levitt, M. F., and Kahn, M.: Renal concentration in the normal dog: Effect of an acute reduction in salt excretion. Amer. J. Physiol., 206:1123, 1964.
6. Kassirer, J. P., Berkman, P. M., Lawrenz, D. R., and Schwartz, W. B.: Critical role of chloride in the correction of hypokalemic alkalosis in man. Amer. J. Med., 38:172, 1965.
7. Knauer, C. M., and Lowe, H. M.: Hemodynamics in the cirrhotic patient during paracentesis. New Eng. J. Med., 276:491–496, 1967.
8. Lieberman, F. L., and Reynolds, T. B.: The use of ethacrynic acid in patients with cirrhosis and ascites. Gastroenterology, 49:531–538, 1965.
9. Muldowney, F. P., and Williams, R. T.: Clinical disturbances in serum sodium and potassium in relation to alteration in total exchangeable sodium, exchangeable potassium and total body water: The value of muscle biopsy analysis in diagnosis and management. Amer. J. Med., 35:768, 780, 1963.
10. Olesen, K. H.: Intravascular interstitial and intracellular phase changes during acute furosemide or ethacrynic acid diuresis. Israel J. Med. Sci., 5:942–946, 1969.
11. Puschett, J. G., and Goldberg, M.: The acute effects of furosemide on acid and electrolyte excretion in man. J. Lab. Clin. Med., 71:666–677, 1968.
12. Rector, F. C., Jr., Van Giesen, G., Kiil, F., and Seldin, D. W.: Influence of expansion of extracellular volume on tubular reabsorption of sodium independent of changes in glomerular filtration rate and aldosterone activity. J. Clin. Invest., 43:341, 1964.
13. Shear, L., Bonkowsky, H. L., and Gabuzda, G. J.: Renal tubular acidosis in cirrhosis: A determinant of susceptibility to recurrent hepatic precoma. New Eng. J. Med., 280:1–7, 1969.

14. Shear, L., Ching, S., and Gabuzda, G. J.: Compartmentalization of ascites and edema in patients with hepatic cirrhosis. New Eng. J. Med., 282:1391–1396, 1970.
15. Sherlock, S., Senewiratne, B., Scott, A., and Walker, J. G.: Complications of diuretic therapy in hepatic cirrhosis. Lancet, 1:1049, 1966.
16. Slone, D., Jick, H., Lewis, G. P., Shapiro, S., and Miettinen, O. S.: Intravenously given ethacrynic acid and gastrointestinal bleeding. J.A.M.A., 209:1668–1671, 1969.
17. Smith, H. W.: The Kidney: Structure and Function in Health and Disease. New York, Oxford, 1951.
18. Stein, R. M., Levitt, B. H., Goldstein, M. H., Porush, J. G., Eisner, G. M., and Levitt, M. F.: Effects of salt restriction on the renal concentrating operation in normal, hydropenic man. J. Clin. Invest., 41:2101, 1962.
19. Zatuchni, J.: The diuretic effects of intravenously administered ethacrynic acid. Amer. J. Med. Sci., 252:162–170, 1966.

Department of Medicine
University of Miami School of Medicine
P. O. Box 875, Biscayne Annex
Miami, Florida   33152

Therapeutic Considerations in Selected Forms of Acute and Chronic Liver Disease

Arvey I. Rogers, M.D.[*]

This paper will explore some of the therapeutic advances being made in certain forms of acute and chronic liver disease. A certain degree of caution should be exercised in interpreting the real significance of much of the data presented, insofar as there are too few well-controlled studies available from which to derive such data. Continued emphasis is being placed on the need for such studies, but it is likely to be some time before any find their place in the already voluminous literature.[2] The paucity of such ideal studies should not cause us to "pay inadequate tribute to the unceasing quantity of investigation and the subtle, though immediately non-miraculous advances which are coalescing—as in most vigorous scientific endeavor—almost imperceptibly."[7] It is to some of these advances that consideration will be given in this article.

Diagnostic aspects of both acute and chronic disturbances of hepatic structure and function will be considered together, as it is felt that such consideration will enhance an appreciation of the role of any given therapeutic approach. Emphasis will be placed on the following forms of liver disease: acute, uncomplicated viral hepatitis; fulminant hepatic failure; chronic hepatitis and alcoholic hepatitis. Brief consideration will be given to hepatic coma, the pruritus of biliary cirrhosis, and aspects of nutrition in cirrhosis. Therapeutic aspects of portal hypertension, ascites, and esophageal varices have been emphasized in recent issues of the *Medical Clinics of North America* and will not be considered in this article.

HEPATIC COMA, PRURITUS, AND MALABSORPTION

An excellent review of therapeutic aspects of hepatic coma has been published recently by Conn.[3] One advance has been recorded in the

---

[*]Associate Professor of Medicine, University of Miami School of Medicine; Chief, Gastroenterology, Veterans Administration Hospital, Miami, Florida

treatment of hepatic coma. Lactulose, a synthetic disaccharide for which there exists no intestinal brush border disaccharidase, has been used with benefit in such patients.[1,4] The nonhydrolyzed disaccharide undergoes fermentation by intestinal bacteria, resulting in the production of lactic acid and a lowering of intestinal pH. The increased availability of hydrogen ion results in an equilibrium shift for $NH_4^+ \leftrightarrow NH_3 \uparrow$ in the direction of the nondiffusible ionized form (NH_4^+). Increasing quantities of the freely diffusible, non-ionic NH_3 are trapped within the gut lumen. Blood ammonia levels are thereby reduced, and it is presumably through this effect that the lactulose exerts its therapeutic benefit. Large doses of the disaccharide may produce diarrhea. Its major advantages over the popularly employed orally or rectally administered antibiotic, neomycin, is that ototoxicity and nephrotoxicity have not attended its use to date. Available commercially in Europe, where it is widely used as a laxative, this product should be approved for marketing in this country in the near future.

A recent article by Schaffner[8] summarizes the use of cholestyramine (Cuemid, Questran) in controlling the pruritus of biliary cirrhosis. This orally administered anion-exchange resin binds bile acids in the gut lumen, exchanging Cl^- in the process. The binding process interrupts the ileal enterohepatic circulation of bile acids and effectively reduces the circulating bile acid pool and serum bile acid levels. It is through this effect that pruritus is thought to be controlled. An initial dose of 4.0 gm. is administered in water, fruit juice, or applesauce before each meal; it takes 5 to 10 days to reduce the bile acid pool, after which time the dose may be reduced to as low as 4.0 gm. per day and maintained at that level in order to control the distressing pruritus. Malabsorption may be encountered with large doses of the medication; hypercalcemia is a rare complication, as are right upper abdominal quadrant calcifications. Serum bilirubin levels may decrease in patients taking cholestyramine, possibly by interfering with the reabsorption of lithocholic acid which may be hepatotoxic and lead to increased cholestasis when hydroxylation to dihydroxy and trihydroxy bile acid forms does not take place.

Fat malabsorption with caloric loss with or without diarrhea may occur in patients with cirrhosis.[6] The isocaloric substitution of medium-chain triglycerides (MCT) for dietary long-chain lipids may suffice to correct the absorptive defect. Lipids with 8 to 10-carbon chains do not require micellarization by conjugated bile acids prior to their entrance into the absorbing unit of the small intestine. They may be administered in Portagen (Mead Johnson) made up to 30 calories per ounce, or as the pure oil at 7.0 calories per gm. One possible disadvantage to the use of Portagen is that it contains lactose; if there is an associated lactose deficit, diarrhea may be exaggerated.[5]

UNCOMPLICATED ACUTE "VIRAL" HEPATITIS

The usual questions asked concerning therapeutic aspects of viral hepatitis are:

Is it necessary to hospitalize the patient?
What is the best treatment for the disease?
How frequently should laboratory tests be obtained?
When is it safe to discharge the patient?
How should the patient be followed after discharge?

Hospitalization?

I do not feel that hospitalization is essential for all patients with viral hepatitis.[15] If home care is decided upon, the physician must be certain of the diagnosis and feel that he is not faced with a problem patient who may require hospitalization for diagnosis, therapy, or both. Toxic hepatic damage usually requires liver biopsy for confirmation. Deepening of jaundice after 14 days of illness should alert the physician to the possibility of more severe disease. High-risk patients should be hospitalized; these include (1) elderly patients with serum hepatitis complicating blood transfusion; (2) postmenopausal women with suspected active chronic hepatitis; and (3) patients with any history of associated metabolic or systemic disorders.

Treatment?

Despite the observation that there are no properly controlled studies to demonstrate any major benefits of traditionally applied therapeutic modalities as bed rest, limited activity, high-calorie, high-protein diets, or multivitamins, these remain among the therapeutic mainstays in this infectious disease associated with a diffuse hepatic cellular inflammatory response. While strenuous exercise is logically to be avoided in any illness which physically disables a patient, a recent study by Repsher and Freebern[12] concerning physical activity in acute viral hepatitis adds further support to the observations published by Chalmers et al.[10] in 1955 which demonstrated that exercise did not alter the course of acute viral hepatitis or provoke a greater incidence of relapse. Both of these studies would tend to militate against the necessity for enforced or prolonged bed rest in the young patient with mild viral hepatitis who otherwise feels well.

There is no justification for utilizing *steroids* in any form in uncomplicated acute viral hepatitis. The apparent advantage of the predictable steroid-associated accelerated decline in serum bilirubin level is outweighed by the high incidence of presumably steroid-related complications and the relapse rate upon steroid withdrawal. A recently published fortuitously controlled study of steroid therapy in Scandinavian patients with acute viral hepatitis underlined the deleterious effects of steroid therapy and demonstrated no distinct therapeutic advantages related to steroid usage.[9]

Patients receiving steroid therapy had a greater incidence of disease-associated gastrointestinal hemorrhage and septic complications. There was a high hepatitis relapse rate on steroid withdrawal. The use of steroids neither reduced nor increased the incidence of developing chronic hepatitis.

The responsible physician's need to "do something" for the patient with hepatitis who is recovering slowly or who has prolonged jaundice should be tempered by the fact that some patients just require longer than others to recover, and that steroid therapy cannot be used without an attendant risk of complication or relapse on withdrawal of the drug.

When in doubt as to the diagnosis, it is always advisable to eliminate all drugs being administered the patient prior to the onset of his illness. Drugs which may mimic viral hepatitis are:[14] isoniazid, halothane, indomethacin, phenylbutazone, 6-mercaptopurine, and acetohexamide.

I prefer to eliminate all medications when treating a patient with hepatitis, maintaining only those essential to the patient's well-being. When it is felt that a medication should be continued, it is worthwhile to review its metabolism, with regard to its dependency on the liver for activation as well as degradation; adjustment of dosage may become necessary to achieve the desired therapeutic goal or to reduce the risk of side-effects and toxicity reactions. Sedatives in particular should be avoided, as "overdoses" may mimic hepatic encephalopathy, a serious occurrence in viral hepatitis.

Frequency of Laboratory Tests

There is no data available to determine how often one should perform liver function tests during a bout of acute viral hepatitis. Obviously, how often blood is obtained and analyzed does not appear to affect the patient's outcome. Furthermore, one would logically expect that any significant deterioration of hepatocellular function would be accompanied by a clearly worsening clinical course. The anicteric patient will feel better as he recovers; the jaundiced patient characteristically becomes less jaundiced when recovery is imminent. Once the diagnosis of viral hepatitis has been established by the characteristic history and physical findings in conjunction with significant elevation of SGOT or SGPT (usually >500 U) with or without jaundice, and perhaps a biopsy of the liver, all that is probably necessary in order to follow the patient adequately is prothrombin time. The prothrombin time typically becomes increasingly prolonged when deterioration is imminent; this test of hepatic function has been proved to correlate most closely with the development of stupor or coma in the course of vital hepatitis.[13]

It is probably unnecessary to obtain blood tests (usually bilirubin, SGOT or SGPT, prothrombin time) more frequently than twice weekly. In the face of apparent clinical improvement, less frequent laboratory tests would appear justified.

Timing of Discharge From Hospital or Home Care

An even more important question is: When can you safely discharge a patient with vital hepatitis? No data establishes definitive criteria to provide an answer. I send people home when I feel they are distinctly improved or progressively improving; they should be free of fever, anorexia, nausea, or vomiting. At this time, usually 10 days to 3 weeks following hospitalization, the SGOT is less than 200 units and the bilirubin is less than 3.0 mg. per 100 ml. The prothrombin time should be no more than 1 or 2 seconds off a control value. The patient should be returning to a social setting which will encourage reasonable rest, abstinence from alcohol, and a nutritious diet.

Follow-Up After Discharge From Hospital or Home Care

Follow-up examination should be carried out within 6 weeks of discharge and should include the standard laboratory tests (an SGOT or SGPT and fractional bilirubin are all that is absolutely essential). If the SGOT is less than 100 units and the total bilirubin less than 2.0 mg. per 100 ml., it is likely that the patient is recovering normally. If, on the other hand, liver function tests have worsened since discharge, whether or not the patient is ill, it becomes necessary to follow the patient more closely. Rehospitalization is rarely necessary; relapses should be identified easily and can be treated at home. An atypical course following the initial episode of viral hepatitis, whether it be an enlarging or persistently tender liver, the appearance of stigmata of chronic hepatic disease, or sustained abnormalities of hepatic function may suggest the advisability of hospitalization and liver biopsy to establish a diagnosis and dictate a therapeutic approach. Generally, most patients with viral hepatitis have recovered completely clinically, chemically, and histologically within 4 months of the acute episode. Minor abnormalities of liver function, such as minimally elevated SGPT and flocculation tests, may persist up to a year without significance.[11]

FULMINANT HEPATIC FAILURE

Etiology

Viral hepatitis is implicated most often in the etiology of this syndrome. Lacking definitive proof of a virus infection, however, this is no more than a presumed cause. Other factors have been implicated in the syndrome. Halothane accounted for 20 per cent of the 318 cases of fulminant hepatic failure reported from 98 centers to the Fulminant Hepatic Failure Surveillance Study being carried out by Dr. Charles Trey of Boston City Hospital.[17] Table 1 summarizes the provocative factors in these 318 patients.

Because of the widespread use of halothane as an anesthetic agent and its probable implication in fulminant hepatic failure syndromes, it is important to review certain characteristics of halothane-associated hepatic necrosis: (1) There have usually been multiple anesthetic exposures within 60 days; 77 per cent of those patients reported by Trey had

Table 1. *Causes of Fulminant Hepatic Failure (Hepatic Coma, Stages I to IV)* in 318 Patients*

| | AGE OF PATIENT | | | | |
CAUSE	0–14	15–44	45–64	65+	TOTAL
Infectious hepatitis	26	55	22	6	109
Serum hepatitis	5	58	20	9	92
Halothane	2	18	35	9	64
Drugs	–	8	6	–	14
Other	9	16	11	3	39

*As defined by Sherlock.

multiple exposures. (2) Hepatic necrosis occurred as an unexpected event, complicating low-risk operations. (3) Jaundice occurred from 3 to 6 days following surgery in 60 per cent of patients; 30 per cent develop jaundice within 9 to 14 days. (4) Unexplained postoperative fever occurred in 70 per cent of affected patients. The occurrence of unexplained fever, jaundice, high SGOT activity, or eosinophilia in the postoperative period of a patient who has previously received halothane should contraindicate its subsequent usage.[20, 23]

Diagnosis

It is usually not difficult to recognize fulminant hepatic failure. There has generally been some type of exposure. The patient is jaundiced; mental changes progress rapidly from euphoria and confusion through drowsiness to frank coma. Typically, the sudden severe impairment in hepatic structure and function is associated with deepening jaundice, a decreasing liver size, fetor hepaticus, and hepatic coma. On rare occasions, fulminant hepatic failure may occur so rapidly that icterus is absent at its outset; psychosis and meningoencephalitis should be considered in the differential diagnosis of the anicteric neuropsychiatric disorder. There are no pathognomonic laboratory tests, although blood ammonia level is usually elevated and serum prothrombin time invariably prolonged and unresponsive to vitamin K therapy. The level of the SGOT does not correlate with extent or severity of hepatic damage. Hypoglycemia may complicate the syndrome. Serum albumin usually falls within several days of its onset.

Treatment

The main objective of therapy in fulminant hepatic failure is to prolong life long enough to allow hepatic regeneration to take place. Scrupulous, intensive care by medical and nursing staff is an absolute necessity. An adequate airway should be maintained. Nasogastric intubation and aspiration are suggested to enable early detection of gastrointestinal bleeding, to minimize gastric dilatation, and to provide an added route for administering medications and nutrition. If ascites is present, the fluid should be studied to exclude infection, hemorrhage, or pancreatitis.

The standard approaches utilized in the treatment of hepatic coma are employed. Protein is restricted and enemas are given to reduce fecal mass and flora and gut ammonia content; neomycin is given orally (4.0 gm. per day) and rectally (1 or 2.0 gm. per 100 ml. solution). Glucose is administered as a source of calories in order to minimize gluconeogenesis from tissue protein.

Every attempt must be made to recognize and eliminate precipitating or aggravating factors. "Excess" dietary protein, gastrointestinal bleeding, sedatives, infection, certain ammonia-producing diuretics, electrolyte imbalance, and azotemia are among these provocative factors.

Massive doses of steroids have been administered with variable results (1000 mg. cortisone or its equivalent per day).[18] Adequately controlled studies are difficult to achieve, but the difference in survival figures for those patients receiving steroids is not so clear-cut as to justify their routine application. Metabolic consequences and side-effects of steroid administration often weigh against therapeutic advantages.

Mortality rate varies with etiology, but overall survival is less than 25 per cent; 1 of 20 patients over age 45 in Stage IV hepatic coma can be expected to survive. Three of 10 patients under age 45 in Stage IV hepatic coma will survive.[17]

The high mortality rate in patients with fulminant hepatic failure, even with the application of many varieties of therapy, has given way to the development of newer approaches. Hemodialysis, peritoneal dialysis, exchange transfusion, cross-circulation with a donor, ex vivo liver perfusion with the same or a different species, and heterotopic liver transplants all have as their basic purpose sustaining life until regeneration dominates over degeneration of the patient's hepatic parenchymal cells.

Exchange transfusion has been the most widely employed of the newer approaches.[16, 21, 22] Deleterious substances may be removed and substances "essential" to hepatic recuperation donated in the process. The critical need for blood coagulation factors may justify exchange transfusion in the presence of severe bleeding. Repeated exchanges can be employed to effect or sustain improvement. Methods for exchange transfusion have been described elsewhere.[20, 21]

An extensive review of the literature, which was published in 1970 by Rivera et al., revealed that of 47 patients treated by exchange transfusion (the majority received steroids), survival was 34 per cent.[19] This was in contrast to an overall recovery of 19.2 per cent in 263 patients treated conventionally. It is of interest that 147 of these 263 patients received steroids; recovery in this subgroup was 25.1 per cent.[19]

Data presented in the Third Progress Report of the Fulminant Hepatic Failure Surveillance Study, albeit tentative and based on strictly uncontrolled studies, allow certain conclusions to be drawn regarding the effects of exchange transfusion and other newer therapeutic modalities in fulminant hepatic failure.[17] The relevant material is summarized in Table 2.

Few dispute the necessity for a well-controlled cooperative prospective study to answer the many questions surrounding the use of exchange transfusions in fulminant hepatic failure. Those with the widest personal experience in the application of the technique and those who have critically evaluated the pertinent literature find some justification

Table 2. *Results of Therapy in 284 Patients With Fulminant Hepatic Failure (Stage IV Hepatic Coma)*

THERAPY	PATIENTS TREATED	PATIENTS DYING	PER CENT SURVIVING
Conservative	28	26	7.1
Steroids	73	65	11.0
Total (no procedure)	101	91	9.9
Exchange transfusion	42	32	23.8
Exchange and steroids	105	78	25.7
Other procedures	36	33	8.3
Total (with procedure)	183	143	21.8

for the use of exchange transfusion and steroids in the patient with extensive hepatic necrosis and liver failure.

It seems most reasonable to suggest that at least one hospital capable of serving a reasonably designated geographic area should be equipped with the equipment and personnel to treat fulminant hepatic failure by exchange transfusion. The actual exchange technique is not difficult but does require a knowledge of the procedure. Hazards related to mismatching of blood, late serum hepatitis, and unexplained aplastic anemia should be known to those who employ exchange transfusion procedures.

CHRONIC HEPATITIS

Abnormalities of hepatic function persisting 6 to 12 months after a bout of apparent viral hepatitis suggest the need to ascertain the nature of concomitant hepatic histopathology. Several categories can apply in such instances: (1) no pathologic diagnosis, (2) acute viral hepatitis, (3) chronic hepatitis, and (4) postnecrotic cirrhosis with or without active necrosis. Category 3 may be further subdivided into chronic persistent hepatitis and chronic aggressive (active) hepatitis, as suggested by DeGroote et al.[26] The relative value of this classification has been questioned recently by Geale et al.,[27] but it appears to have clinical relevance as emphasized by Becker et al.,[25] who demonstrated the benign course of 20 patients with chronic persistent hepatitis.

At an early stage the differentiation of the forms of chronic hepatitis can be made only by liver biopsy employing reticulin stains of supporting framework. Scheuer[31] has given extensive representations of histopathologic alterations in the two forms of chronic hepatitis. Figures 1 and 2 illustrate changes demonstrable by reticulin staining procedures. The major differential features appear to be the extent of piecemeal necrosis (cell erosion at lobular periphery associated with plasma cell and lymphocytic infiltrate); the formation and proliferation of periportal fibrous septa; and the disruption of lobular architecture as evidenced by collapse and condensation of reticulin framework. These findings characterize active chronic aggressive hepatitis.

Although it is not definitively established, it appears that chronic *persistent* hepatitis is a non-progressive benign disease with less severe clinical manifestations.[25] In sharp contrast, the *aggressive* form of the disease appears to be just that, and probably represents one stage in the inexorable progression to postnecrotic cirrhosis. The aggressive form is more frequently associated with clinical stigmata of chronic, progressive, active hepatic disease and endocrine and systemic manifestations. A "partial" list of such clinical findings in 86 affected patients reported by Mistilis and Blackburn[28] is presented in Table 3.

Abnormal tissue and serologic antibody reactions, such as false positive reactions for syphilis, LE cell phenomena, antinuclear factors, and smooth muscle antibodies, are not uncommonly observed in chronic active (aggressive) hepatitis. Their basis is unknown but may be of some value in differentiating this form of liver disease from infectious hepati-

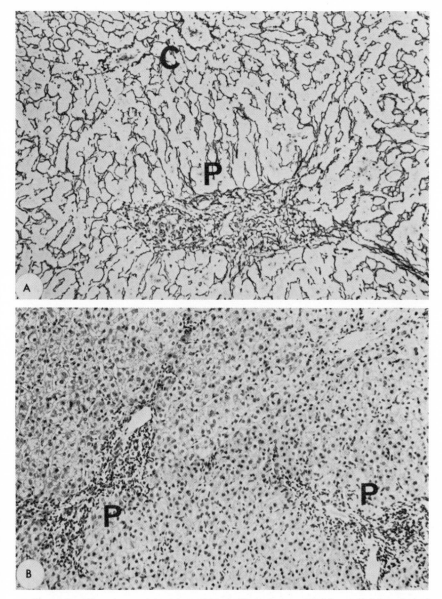

Figure 1. *Chronic persistent hepatitis. A,* Short septa extend from slightly enlarged portal tract (P). Central veins (C) are unaffected, and lobular architecture is preserved. Needle biopsy, reticulin, × 135. *B,* There is inflammatory infiltration of the portal tracts (P) but with little piecemeal necrosis. Needle biopsy, hematoxylin and eosin, × 125. (Figures 1 and 2 from Scheuer, P.: Liver Biopsy Interpretation. Baltimore, Williams and Wilkins, 1968. Reproduced with permission.)

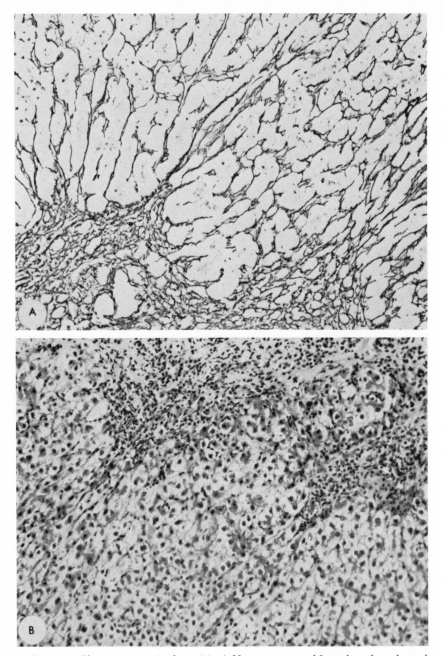

Figure 2. *Chronic aggressive hepatitis.* A, Many septa extend from the enlarged portal tract (above) into the lobule, and architecture is distorted. Needle biopsy, reticulin, × 145. B, Area similar to that in A, from the same biopsy. Liver cells are swollen and rounded in the zone of piecemeal necrosis next to the fibrous tissue. Needle biopsy, hematoxylin and eosin, × 150.

Table 3. *Clinical Features of Chronic Active Hepatitis*

FEATURE	FREQUENCY
Recurrent "hepatitis"	Frequent
Episodic jaundice	60%
Prolonged (1–2 years) cholestasis	25%
Hepatic coma	30%
Portal hypertension	40%
Amenorrhea	38%
Acne	21%
Diarrhea	28% (chronic)
Ulcerative colitis	10–15%
Skin lesions	20%
Polyarthralgias	18% (recurrent)

tis, alcoholic liver disease, drug-induced hepatitis, and extrahepatic biliary obstruction and biliary cirrhosis.[28]

Etiology

The etiology of chronic hepatitis is not known. A *persistent viral infection* independent from an autoimmune process, and an *autoimmune process*, possibly, though not necessarily, related to a preceding viral infection of the liver, constitute the main theoretical etiologic considerations. Apparent "viral" hepatitis has occurred in 30 per cent of affected patients. Large group surveys for Australia antigen have revealed positive titers in up to 25 per cent of patients with chronic hepatitis.[33] In a recent paper, Boyer and Klatskin reported that serum hepatitis predominated over infectious hepatitis as apparent causes in 52 patients studied with subacute hepatic necrosis (active chronic hepatitis).[25a] One would suspect that had Australia antigen assays been carried out by these authors, the incidence of positive results would have been high in view of the known close correlation between serum hepatitis infection and a positive titer for Australia antigen.[30a] These observations suggest the possibility that a persistent viral infection may be responsible for chronic hepatitis.

Further observations of possible relevance to obtaining assays for HAA (hepatitis-associated antigen) are as follows: (1) In one reported series, 90 per cent of patients with HAA-positive hepatitis had a more prolonged hospital course, with SGOT values remaining above 100 units until after the eighth week; this was contrasted with HAA-negative cases in whom SGOT values were less than 100 by the fifth week of illness.[25c] (2) Unusually long persistence of HAA indicates progression to chronic hepatitis, whether symptoms subside or laboratory tests return to normal.[31a]

Application of HAA assays to serum from patients with chronic hepatitis has disclosed that there are "HAA-positive" and "HAA-negative" types. The latter patient category is generally female, is more likely to have positive LE cell tests, circulating smooth muscle antibodies, and other lupus-like features. Those patients with chronic hepatitis and circulating HAA are predominantly male, usually give a history of antecedent acute hepatitis with a strong parenteral exposure, and have a low incidence of LE cells and circulating antibodies.[31a]

Mackay's autoimmune "markers" in chronic hepatitis (called "lupoid" hepatitis by Mackay and Wood[27b] are: (1) circulating auto-antibodies such as LE cells, smooth muscle antibodies; (2) evidence of multisystem involvement; (3) association of other diseases felt to have an autoimmune basis such as thyroiditis, nephritis and colitis; (4) the hepatic plasmacytic and lymphocytic infiltrate; and (5) the often favorable response to steroid and antimetabolite immune suppressive therapy.[27b] These are employed as evidence for the autoimmune basis of the disease. No pathogenetic significance can be assigned the circulating autoantibodies; therefore, evidence for autoimmunity as a perpetuating factor is inconclusive. As well, the dosage of antimetabolite drugs commonly employed therapeutically (6-mercaptopurine or azathioprine) may not suppress immune responses but have been shown to exert antiviral effects.

To summarize etiologic considerations, it is likely that there are two varieties of active chronic (aggressive) hepatitis as distinguished by the presence (positive) or absence (negative) of the hepatitis-associated antigen (HAA). That associated with persistent HAA may be a sequel to "viral" hepatitis; that without HAA may represent one manifestation of a spontaneously occurring immunologic disorder affecting many other body tissues. We need to learn more of the etiologic and pathogenic significance of HAA, its immunologic competence, and the presence of HAA antigen-antibody complexes in serum and tissue of patients with certain varieties of active chronic hepatitis.

Aspects of Therapy

Considerable controversy abounds regarding whether, when, and what treatment to apply in patients with active chronic hepatitis. The recognition of the histopathologic category, persistent hepatitis, is important in that in light of a correlated benign clinical course with no progression, there appears to be no need to apply "specific" therapy to this form of disease.

The ill individual with apparent chronic *aggressive* (active) hepatitis, however, poses a therapeutic dilemma. The cumulative 5 year survival of untreated patients was shown to be 65 per cent by Mistilis et al.[29] Patients with the poorest prognosis were those with a hepatitis-like onset, persistent cholestasis, prolonged jaundice, associated colitis, episodes of hepatic coma, ascites, or extensive necrosis on liver biopsy. The fact that these patients are sick the majority of the time and do not lead normal lives raises serious considerations regarding therapy. Numerous anti-inflammatory drugs have been utilized. Corticosteroids, 6-mercaptopurine, and azathioprine (Imuran) have demonstrated the best results. When the disease is most active, in its early stages, these drugs appear to effect improved survival over non-treated patients.[29] The best results, therefore, are apt to be recorded in the sickest patients, the ones in greatest need of treatment.

Table 4. *Chemotherapy in Chronic Active Hepatitis*

DRUG*	INITIAL DOSAGE	MAINTENANCE
Prednisone	40–60 mg. per day	5–20 mg. per day
Azathioprine (Imuran)	1.0–2.0 mg. per kg. per day	Same
6-mercaptopurine (Puri-nethol)	0.5–1.5 mg. per kg. per day	Same

*Mistilis has proposed that a combination of prednisone and azathioprine or 6-mercapto-purine be employed in patients ill with overt jaundice.

The decision to treat a patient is a serious one, especially in view of the serious side-effects and toxicity of the pharmacologic anti-inflammatory (sometimes immunosuppressive) agents commonly employed, and the need for chronic, continuous treatment.

It is to be realized, as well, that patients with chronic active hepatitis are very sensitive to these drugs; low doses may cause serious hematologic, cholestatic, or hepatotoxic effects as well as unpleasant cosmetic effects. Suggested dosage regimens are outlined in Table 4.

At periodic intervals, an effort should be made to determine whether the medications are, in fact, favorably affecting the course of the illness. Attempts should be made to withdraw drugs gradually every 6 months; this is often impossible, however, as clinical and chemical relapses are commonly provoked by such an effort.

Most available evidence reveals that treatment, in any form, neither halts the histologic progression of chronic active (aggressive) hepatitis nor alters significantly the long-term prognosis. Data on both of these important points is being accumulated throughout the world at the present time. Table 5 summarizes the results of four long-term studies concerned with the effects of chemotherapy on the course of active chronic hepatitis.

Table 5. *Results of Chemotherapy in Patients with Active Chronic Hepatitis*

SERIES	NO. OF PATIENTS	THERAPY		PER CENT SURVIVAL (YRS.)		
		Yes	No	5 years	10 years	15+ years
Bearn (1956)[24]	23	–	X	65	50+	20+
Willcox (1961)[31]	33	–	X	40	<20	<20
Mistilis (1968)[29]	139	50	–	80	80	60
		–	89	68	55	55
Page (1969)[30]	21	X	–	80	60	30+
Cook (1970)[25b]	49	22	–	86	–	–
		–	27	44	–	–

ALCOHOLIC HEPATITIS

There are at least three histopathologic consequences of alcohol ingestion on the human liver. They are seen with the greatest frequency, severity, and clinical presentation in undernourished alocholics who have consumed large quantities of alochol for long periods of time. While minimal fatty changes can be demonstrated to occur following the ingestion of moderate quantities of alcohol over a short period of time in nonalcoholic, well-nourished volunteers,[49] more extensive fat accumulation characterizes the fatty liver of the alcoholic with liver disease.[46] When there is necrosis of liver cells, (with or without fat), acute inflammation, and Mallory bodies (alcoholic hyaline), these changes are diagnosed as *alcoholic hepatitis*.[40, 42] Micronodular (Laennec's, portal) cirrhosis is well known to all. The possible pathogenetic interrelationships of these three pathologic entities are illustrated in Figure 3.

Differential Diagnosis

It may be very difficult to differentiate alcoholic hepatitis from fatty liver on strictly clinical grounds alone.[35, 40] In general, jaundice, spider angiomata, splenomegaly, ascites, and coma are encountered with greater frequency in alcoholic hepatitis; as an expected correlate, a greater number of patients with alcoholic hepatitis have more severely abnormal liver function tests (BSP, bilirubin, SGOT, alkaline phosphatase and prothrombin time). In entertaining the diagnosis of alcoholic hepatitis, there should be a positive history for alcohol ingestion and poor diet; there should be no contact with hepatitis or blood products or any identifiable infectious prodrome; toxin history should be negative. An interesting disparity between the transaminase levels has been observed more frequently than can be attributed to chance alone; the SGOT usually exceeds the SGPT significantly, with both values being under 300 units.

Alcoholic hepatitis may present with significant jaundice, fever, and right upper quadrant abdominal pain and tenderness in 25 to 30 per cent of affected patients. When this clinical constellation is accompanied by an elevated alkaline phosphatase level and significant leukocytosis (> 15,000 per cu. mm.), it is easy to appreciate the serious consideration that must be given to an acute complicated cholecystitis, ascending cholangitis, or multiple liver abscesses in differential diagnosis. It may also present as a nonseptic surgical obstructive jaundice.[34, 51]

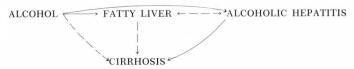

Figure 3.   Possible pathogenetic interrelationships of fatty liver, alcoholic hepatitis, and cirrhosis. Solid arrows represent demonstrated relationships and interrupted arrows speculative ones.

The following important points are helpful in arriving at the correct diagnosis.

1. Fever in alcoholic hepatitis[50] is
   Rarely associated with chills
   Usually intermittent
   Usually < 103° F.
   Does not respond to antibiotics alone
   Associated with severe hepatic damage
2. Patients with alcoholic hepatitis and fever are usually not as "toxic" as those with septic fever.
3. Liver is diffusely tender in alcoholic hepatitis.
4. Liver biopsy can be diagnostic (but it cannot always be performed).

Every effort must be made to exclude a surgically correctible lesion, but this is often impossible short of exploratory laparotomy. When there is significant coexistent deterioration of hepatic function, it is reasonable to err on the side of a nonoperative approach and employ systemic antibiotics in addition to other therapeutic measures, and observe the patient; high doses of intravenous tetracyclines are best avoided, however, because of their hepatotoxic properties secondary to interference with hepatocellular protein synthesis.

The diagnosis of alcoholic hepatitis is dependent upon histopathologic confirmation. Liver biopsy may not be able to be performed in the very ill individual with encephalopathy, significant ascites, prolonged prothrombin time (<50 per cent of normal), and depressed platelet count (<50,000 per cu. mm.). In these instances, however, the diagnosis is usually obvious.

Treatment

Popular therapeutic approaches are listed in Table 6. It is of interest to note that continued moderate alcohol ingestion coupled with a nutritious diet may not delay ultimate healing of alcoholic liver injury;[37] despite this observation, abstinence from alcohol should be urged. At least 1 to 2 gm. of protein per kg. are important for recovery from alcohol-induced liver injury. Lipotropic agents are not of consistent additional value in the patient on a good diet. Multiple vitamin deficiencies exist in alcoholic nutritional hepatic disease; in addition to thiamine (which may be associated with peripheral neuropathy), folate, pyridoxine, and nicotinic acid are deficient and should be replaced.[36, 44, 47] Enforced bed rest is not essential.

It is to be emphasized that no absolute proof exists that there are any

Table 6. *Therapeutic Approaches in Alcoholic Hepatitis*

Abstinence from alcohol
Bed rest (?)
Vitamins (thiamine, B_6, folate)
High protein, normal fat diet
Androgenic steroids
Corticosteroids
Treatment of secondary complications (ascites, hemorrhage)

Table 7. *Therapeutic Efficacy of Prednisone in Alcoholic Hepatitis**

| | PATIENT CATEGORY† | | | |
| | VERY ILL‡ | | MILDLY TO MODERATELY ILL | |
	No Prednisone	Prednisone	No Prednisone	Prednisone
Died	5	1	—	—
Alive	—	7	10	11

*Courtesy of Dr. Harold Fallon, Chapel Hill, North Carolina
†All had biopsies of the liver with 7 days of admission
‡Clinical stigmata of hepatic coma or pre-coma

major advantages to employing androgens or corticosteroids (in any form). Nilevar at 40 mg. per day has been demonstrated to mobilize hepatic fat and improve indocyanine green clearance (5 mg. per kg.), but studies were not controlled.[45, 46] One study by Fenster[38] in 1961 concluded that short-term androgen therapy was not efficacious in alcoholic liver disease.

A controlled study published in abstracted form by Hellman, Temko, and Fallon[43] suggested that prednisone, 40 mg. per day for one month, did not improve clinical or histologic recovery in patients with alcoholic hepatitis who were mildly or moderately ill. Subsequent to that report, which included a total of 25 patients, 9 more patients have been added, including several seriously ill patients with hepatic encephalopathy. The data, as yet unpublished, suggests that prednisone therapy significantly altered the mortality in the sickest patients (Table 7). One important factor that could account for these striking differences related to prednisone administration is related to the appetite-stimulating properties of steroids. In the sickest group of patients, those receiving steroids consumed an average daily caloric intake of 1600, contrasted with 400 in the nonsteroid treated groups. Studies employing forced feeding are now in progress to assess more carefully the role of steroids and the factor of controlled nutrition.

Comment

The mortality of alcoholic hepatitis varies proportionately with the severity of the clinical presentation. The usual rate quoted is from 4 to 8 per cent (although higher figures can be found), with patients dying from hepatic coma, gastrointestinal bleeding, renal failure, sepsis, or unexplained causes. A serum bilirubin exceeding 5 mg. per 100 ml. and rising after 6 days of hospitalization, azotemia, leukocytosis, and prothrombin time prolonged more than 4 seconds seriously alter prognosis.[41] Dramatic progression of alcoholic hepatitis to histologically demonstrable cirrhosis can be seen in patients during treatment and in those who continue to imbibe. Galambos et al.[39] obtained follow-up histologic studies (3.5 ± 2.1 years) of the livers of 65 of 69 patients with disease diagnosed as alcoholic hepatitis. Cirrhosis was present in 33 livers; alcoholic hepatitis persisted for 1 to 7 years without progression in 27; 5 returned to normal. Progression to cirrhosis was related to alcoholic hepatitis and not steatosis alone.

REFERENCES

HEPATIC COMA, PRURITUS, AND MALABSORPTION

1. Bircher, J., Muller, J. Guggenheim, P., and Haemmerli, U. P.: Treatment of chronic portal-systemic encephalopathy with lactulose. Lancet, 1:890–892, 1966.
2. Chalmers, T. C.: A challenge to clinical investigators. Gastroenterol., 57:631–635, 1969.
3. Conn, H. O.: A rational program for the management of hepatic coma. Gastroenterol., 57:715–723, 1969.
4. Elkington, S. G., Floch, M. H., and Conn, H. O.: Lactulose in the control of portasystemic encephalopathy. New Eng. J. Med., 281:408–412, 1968.
5. Holt, P. R.: Medium chain triglycerides. A useful adjunct in nutritional therapy. Gastroenterol., 53:961–966, 1967.
6. Linscheer, W. G., Patterson, J. F., Moore, E. W., Clermont, R. J., Robins, S. J., and Chalmers, T. C.: Medium and long chain fat absorption in patients with cirrhosis. J. Clin. Invest., 45:1317–1325, 1966.
7. Schaffner, F.: Treatment of liver disease. Modern Treatment, 6:121, 1969.
8. Schaffner, F.: Treatment of primary biliary cirrhosis. Modern Treatment, 6:205–214, 1969.

UNCOMPLICATED VIRAL HEPATITIS

9. Blum, A. L., Stutz, R., Haemmerli, U. P., Schmid, P., and Grady, A.: A fortuitously controlled study of steroid therapy in acute viral hepatitis. Amer. J. Med., 47:82–92, 93–100, 1969.
10. Chalmers, T. C., Eckhardt, R. D., Reynolds, W. E., Cigarroa, J. Q., Deane, N., Reifenstein, R. W., Smith, C. W., and Davidson, C. J.: The treatment of acute infectious hepatitis. J. Clin. Invest., 34:1163, 1955.
11. Reisler, D. M., Strong, W. B., and Mosley, J. W.: Transaminase levels in the post convalescent phase of infectious hepatitis. J.A.M.A., 202:37, 1967.
12. Repsher, L. H., and Freebern, R. K.: Effects of early and vigorous exercise on recovery from infectious hepatitis. New Eng. J. Med., 281:1393–1396, 1969.
13. Ritt, D. J., Whelan, G., Werner, D. J., Eigenbrodt, E. H., Schenker, S., and Combes, B.: Acute hepatic necrosis with stupor and coma. Medicine, 48:151, 1969.
14. Schaffner, F., and Raisfeld, I. H.: Drugs and the liver. In Stollerman, G. H., ed.: Advances in Internal Medicine. Year Book Medical Publishers, Inc., 1969, vol. 15, pp. 221–247.
15. Tisdale, W. A.: When to hospitalize the hepatitis patient. Hospital Practice, October 1967, p. 35.

FULMINANT HEPATIC FAILURE

16. Berger, R. L., Liversage, R. M., Chalmers, T. C., Graham, J. H., McGoldrick, D. N., and Stohlman, F.: Exchange transfusion in the treatment of fulminating hepatitis. New Eng. J. Med., 274:497, 1966.
17. Fulminant Hepatic Failure Surveillance Study. Third Progress Report, October, 1969. Charles Trey, M.D., Chairman, Boston City Hospital, Boston, Mass.
18. Katz, R., Velasco, M., Klinger, J., and Alessandri, H.: Corticosteroids in treatment of acute hepatic coma. Gastroenterol., 42:258, 1962.
19. Rivera, R. A., Slaughter, R. L., and Boyce, H. W.: Exchange transfusion in the treatment of patients with acute hepatitis in coma. Amer. J. Dig. Dis., 15:588, 1970.
20. Trey, C.: Management of fulminant hepatic failure. In Popper, H., and Schaffner, F., eds.: Progress in Liver Diseases. Grune and Stratton, New York, 1970, vol. 3, pp. 282–298.
21. Trey, C., Burns, D. G., and Saunders, S. J.: Treatment of hepatic coma by exchange blood transfusion. New Eng. J. Med., 274:473, 1966.
22. Trey, C., King, N., and Garcia, F.: Exchange transfusion in massive hepatic necrosis. (Abstract.) Gastroenterol., 54:171, 1968.
23. Trey, C., Lipworth, C., Chalmers, T. C., Davidson, C. S., Gottlieb, L. S., Papper, H., and Saunders, S. J.: Fulminant hepatic failure, presumable contribution of halothane. New Eng. J. Med., 279:798, 1968.

CHRONIC HEPATITIS

24. Bearn, A. G., et al.: Problem of chronic liver disease in young women. Amer. J. Med., 31:3, 1956.
25. Becker, M. D., Scheuer, P. J., Baptista, A., and Sherlock, S.: Prognosis of chronic persistent hepatitis. Lancet, 1:53–56, 1970.
25a. Boyer, J. L., and Klatskin, G.: Pattern of necrosis in acute viral hepatitis. New Eng. J. Med., 283:1063, 1970.
25b. Cook, G. C., et al.: Quart. J. Med., 1970 (in press).
25c. Cossart, Y. E., and Vahrman, J.: Studies of Australia-SH antigen in sporadic viral hepatitis in London. Brit. Med. J., 1:403, 1970.

26. DeGroote, L. J., Gedigk, P., Popper, H., Scheuer, P. J., Thaler, H., Desmet, V. J., Krob, G., Poulsen, H., Schmid, M., Uehlinger, F., and Wepler, W.: A classification of chronic hepatitis. Lancet, 2:626–628, 1968.

27. Geale, M. G., Schoenfeld, L. J., and Summerskill, W. H. J.: Classification and treatment of chronic active liver disease. Gastroenterol., 55:724–729, 1968.

27a. Mackay, I. R.: The problem of persisting destructive disease of the liver. Gastroenterol., 40:617–627, 1961.

27b. Mackay, I. R., and Wood, I. J.: Autoimmunity in liver disease. In Popper, H., and Schaffner, F. (eds.): Progress in Liver Disease. New York, Grune and Stratton, 1961.

28. Mistilis, S. P., and Blackburn, C. R. B.: Active chronic hepatitis. Amer. J. Med., 48:484–495, 1970.

29. Mistilis, S. P., Skyring, A. P., and Blackburn, C. R. B.: Natural history of active chronic hepatitis. Aust. Ann. Med., 17:214, 277, 1968.

30. Page, A. R., et al.: Long-term results of therapy in patients with chronic liver disease associated with hypergammaglobulinemia. Amer. J. Med., 47:765, 1969.

30a. Prince, A. M., et al.: Immunologic distinction between infectious and serum hepatitis. New Eng. J. Med., 282:987–991, 1970.

31. Scheuer, P. J.: Liver Biopsy Interpretation. Baltimore, Williams and Wilkins, 1968.

31a. Sholman, N. R.: Hepatitis-associated antigen. Amer. J. Med., 49:669–692, 1970.

32. Willcox, R. G., and Isselbacher, K. J.: Chronic liver disease in young people. Amer. J. Med., 30:185, 1961.

33. Wright, R., McCollum, R. W., and Klatskin, G.: Australia antigen in acute and chronic liver disease. Lancet, 2:117–121, 1969.

ALCOHOLIC HEPATITIS

34. Ballard, H., Bernstein, M., and Farrar, J. T.: Fatty liver presenting as obstructive jaundice. Amer. J. Med., 30:196, 1961.

35. Bradus, S., et al.: Hepatic function and serum enzyme levels in association with fatty metamorphosis of the liver. Amer. J. Med. Sci., 246:69, 1963.

36. Eckhardt, R. D., et al.: Effect of protein starvation and of protein feeding on the clinical course, liver function and liver histochemistry of three patients with active fatty alcoholic cirrhosis. J. Clin. Invest., 29:227, 1950.

37. Erenoglu, E., Edriera, J. G., and Patek, A. J.: Observations on patients with Laennec's cirrhosis receiving alcohol while on controlled diets. Ann. Int. Med., 60:814, 1964.

38. Fenster, T.: The non-efficacy of short-term anabolic steroid therapy in alcoholic liver disease. Ann. Int. Med., 65:738, 1966.

39. Galambos, J. T., Alexander, J. F., and Lischner, M. W.: Prognosis of acute alcoholic hepatitis. Gastroenterol., 58:1025, 1970.

40. Green, J., Mistilis, S., and Schiff, L.: Acute alcoholic hepatitis. Arch. Int. Med., 112:67, 1963.

41. Hardison, W. B., and Lee, F. I.: Prognosis in acute liver disease of the alcoholic patient. New Eng. J. Med., 275:61, 1966.

42. Havinasuta, V., Chomet, B., Ishak, K., and Zimmerman, H. J.: Steatonecrosis – mallory body type. Medicine, 46:141, 1967.

43. Hellman, R. M., Temko, M. H., and Fallon, H. J.: Alcoholic hepatitis: Natural history and evaluation of therapy. Clin. Res., 17:26, 1969.

44. Leevy, C. M.: Clinical diagnosis, evaluation and treatment of liver disease in alcoholics. Fed. Proc., 26:1474, 1967.

45. Leevy, C. M.: Fatty liver: A study of 270 patients with biopsy-proven fatty liver and a review of the literature. Medicine, 41:249, 1962.

46. Mendenhall, C. L.: Anabolic steroid therapy as an adjunct to diet in alcoholic hepatic steatosis. Amer. J. Dig. Dis., 13:783, 1968.

47. Post, J., et al.: The effects of diet and choline on fatty infiltration of the human liver. Gastroenterol., 20:403, 1952.

48. Powell, W. J., and Klatskin, G.: Duration of survival in patients with Laennec's cirrhosis. Influence of alcohol withdrawal and possible effects of recent changes in general management of the disease. Amer. J. Med., 44:406, 1968.

49. Rubin, G., and Lieber, C. S.: Alcohol-induced hepatic injury in non-alcoholic volunteers. New Eng. J. Med., 278:869, 1968.

50. Tisdale, W. A., and Klatskin, G.: The fever of Laennec's cirrhosis. Yale J. Biol. Med., 32:94, 1961.

51. Weinstein, B. R., Kern, R. J., and Zimmerman, H. J.: Obstructive jaundice as a complication of pancreatitis. Ann. Int. Med., 58:245, 1963.

University of Miami
School of Medicine
P.O. Box 875, Biscayne Annex
Miami, Florida 33152

Management of the Obese Patient

Jonathan J. Braunstein, M.D.[*]

Obesity is the most common nutritional disorder confronting the physician in this country today. It has been estimated that approximately 30 per cent of our adult population is more than 20 per cent overweight. There is evidence that the obesity is associated with an increase in morbidity and mortality which can be lessened by weight reduction.[13] It is because of the prevalence and health risks associated with obesity that the management of the obese patient should be of interest to all physicians.

Unfortunately, the results of the treatment of the obese patient are often discouraging; not only does the obese patient often fail to lose weight but when therapy is initially successful the patient frequently relapses to his former state within a short time. Perhaps because of these poor results, physicians have become discouraged with the management of the obese patient and, occasionally, in the place of rational medical therapy, less reputable forms of therapy have sprung up.

This paper will review some general concepts with regard to the management of the obese patient, including: diagnosis, underlying causes, complications, and therapeutic programs for weight reduction. It is only by such a systematic approach to the management of each obese patient that a better understanding of this complex condition and better therapy will result.

DIAGNOSIS OF OBESITY

The diagnosis of obesity is generally made on simple inspection of the patient. There are instances clinically and for research purposes when a more exact qualitative and quantitative definition of the obese state is necessary. It is important to keep in mind that body weight is contributed to by all of the body tissues (water, muscle, other fat-free protoplasm, skeleton, and adipose tissue) and that an alteration of any of these can influence the total body weight.

Obesity is the excessive accumulation of body fat or adipose tissue which is usually associated, but not synonymous, with the overweight

[*]Assistant Professor of Medicine, University of Miami School of Medicine

state. For example, there are the well known situations in which the excessive accumulation of fluid (as in the edematous states) or muscle tissue (as in the muscular athlete) result in an abnormal increase in weight without excess adipose tissue or obesity being present. For usual purposes, however, excess weight in the adult is a reflection of the deposition of excess adipose tissue.

The diagnosis of obesity is, therefore, made by weighing the patient and comparing the actual weight to an ideal or desirable weight as determined from weight tables in which body proportions, height, and sex are taken into consideration. A body weight greater than 20 per cent of the ideal or desirable weight is felt to represent a significant degree of obesity. More exact measurement of the degree of obesity can be made by determining the skin-fold thickness in certain body areas using a specially designed caliper. This method is based on the fact that the subcutaneous fat deposits reflect the overall body content of adipose tissue.[9]

The greater the degree of obesity, the more serious the condition, both in terms of associated morbidity and mortality, and in terms of difficulty in treatment. The prognosis for the very overweight patient is much poorer than for the mildly obese individual.

THE UNDERLYING CAUSES OF OBESITY

Obesity is a very complex disorder in which multiple causative factors are potentially operative in any given patient (Fig. 1). It is only by a careful and comprehensive evaluation of the individual patient that the particular causes present in a given situation can be determined.

The fundamental metabolic disturbance in the obese patient is a

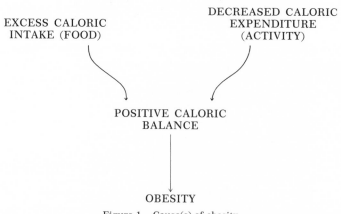

UNDERLYING FACTORS:

Genetic, metabolic, psychological, social, environmental, underlying disease

EXCESS CALORIC
INTAKE (FOOD)

DECREASED CALORIC
EXPENDITURE
(ACTIVITY)

POSITIVE CALORIC
BALANCE

OBESITY

Figure 1.   Cause(s) of obesity.

positive caloric or energy balance in which the calories ingested exceed those expended by the patient at some time during his life. This is generally the result of both excessive caloric intake in the diet and decreased caloric expenditure in the form of physical activity in the usual obese patient. The excessive caloric intake of obese patients has been greatly emphasized and rightly so, but it has become increasingly evident that reduction in physical activity also plays a significant role in the positive caloric balance.[5]

The underlying factors responsible for this positive caloric or energy balance are multiple and differ from patient to patient. These should be sought for and determined in each case, if possible, for the correction of these underlying pathogenetic factors would form the most rational approach to the correction of the caloric imbalance. These underlying factors include genetic, metabolic, psychological, social, and environmental factors.

Obesity is properly thought of not as a disease but as a symptom or sign of positive caloric balance; as such, it requires that a careful search be made for the underlying causative factors (genetic, metabolic, psychological, social, and environmental) which can lead to a positive caloric balance.

The vast majority of obese patients do not have an underlying disease to account for their overweight state. Conditions such as hypothyroidism, hyperadrenalcorticism, hypogonadism, insulinoma, and hypothalamic disease may be associated with obesity, but these are unusual and account for less than 1 per cent of all obese patients. Nevertheless, a consideration of these secondary causes of obesity should be given, if only because therapy in these instances would be, of course, directed toward the underlying disease.

As noted, most patients with obesity have idiopathic or primary obesity, in that no underlying disease can be demonstrated to be present. However, a good deal of evidence has been accumulated to support the role of genetic, metabolic, psychological, social, and environmental factors in the pathogenesis of the condition. For example, Mayer has presented data to support the importance of genetic factors in obesity,[14] and it is generally felt that obesity starting in childhood is a much more difficult problem in management and carries a poorer prognosis than adult-onset obesity. Recent literature summarized by Bortz[7] shows numerous studies in which significant metabolic differences between obese and lean subjects have been shown to exist, but whether these differences are a reflection of the primary or causative factors in obesity or they are merely secondary phenomena resulting from the obese state has yet to be determined.

The psychological factors in obesity are as complex as the condition itself and have been the subject of many papers. Suffice it to say that some obese patients have deep seated psychological dysfunction and, in these individuals, the prognosis for weight reduction is poor, compared with the more psychologically adjusted patients. The social and environmental factors influencing caloric intake and caloric output in our modern affluent society are so obvious that they hardly need mentioning. The social emphasis in recent years of the cosmetic attractiveness of leanness in this country has tended to offset these otherwise strong socioeconomic factors leading to obesity.

COMPLICATIONS OF OBESITY

Obesity is associated with certain medical complications which form the basis of the increased morbidity and mortality attributed to the overweight state. The more severe the obesity, the more prominent are these complications. First, as mentioned above, there are numerous metabolic abnormalities which characterize the obese patient when compared with the lean individual (Table 1). It is probable that many of these are the result of the obesity, as they may remit with weight reduction and correction of the obese state.[3]

There are a number of diseases which are clinically associated with obesity: diabetes mellitus, atherosclerosis, cholelithiasis, and hypertensive cardiovascular disease. In addition, there is the cardiopulmonary syndrome associated with extreme degree of obesity, the Pickwickian syndrome.

Obese patients are said to be more accident prone and have a higher rate of complications following surgical procedures than lean patients. There are a number of medical conditions in which the obese state plays an aggravating role and in which weight reduction is a major therapeutic goal: spine and hip joint disease, congestive heart failure, etc.

The psychologic and social effects of the overweight state may also be considered important complications of obesity in that they may interfere with the overall adaptation of the individual. In summary, it would be fair to state that a significant degree of obesity carries with it a risk to health, certainly enough to warrant an attempt at prevention and therapy.

THERAPEUTIC APPROACH

As may be inferred from the preceding discussion, the management of the obese patient begins with a thorough general medical evaluation, one in which the underlying causative factors and complications of obesity are carefully considered. A critical part of this evaluation is a

Table 1. *Metabolic Abnormalities in Obesity*

Increased fat utilization
Decreased glucose utilization
Increased blood levels of glucose, amino acids, triglycerides, and cholesterol
Increased plasma free fatty acid level and turnover rate (fed state)
Increased insulin secretion and plasma level
Insulin resistance
Increased cortisol secretion and turnover rate
Decreased growth hormone secretory responsiveness

---

detailed dietary history and assessment of the physical activity pattern of the patient, present and past. Other historical information includes the age of onset of the obesity (childhood or adult) and the psychologic makeup of the individual, as these aspects form important therapeutic and prognostic guides. The degree of motivation of the patient to reduce weight is a key factor to assess, as this will ultimately form the basis of the success or failure of any therapeutic plan. As in most chronic ills, an important part of any therapeutic program is patient education with regard to certain of the basic concepts of the illness. The patient's understanding is necessary for good motivation and cooperation. This education is a continuing process and built on at subsequent visits.

Finally, the physician must be fully aware that the management of the obese patient will require prolonged therapy with close and frequent follow-up visits, and that relapses may occur as in any chronic illness. He must realize that his understanding and guidance are strong factors in the success of any program. Assistance for the physician may come from the dietician and, when indicated, from the psychiatrist or psychologist.

The basic concept underlying all therapy for obesity is the production of a negative caloric or energy balance, so that the patient is forced to burn his excess body fat as a source of energy (Fig. 2). This can be accomplished by a reduction of caloric intake in the diet or an increase in caloric expenditure in the form of physical activity. In most instances, a combination of these is most effective. The production of a negative caloric balance by these means will result in a loss of adipose tissue in the obese patient which will be reflected by a loss of weight.

It is important to emphasize once again that total body weight is contributed to by all the body tissues and that body water content is particularly prone to fluctuations quite apart, at times, from calorie balance. These day to day fluctuations in body water may initially mask a reduction in adipose tissue weight resulting from a negative caloric balance, but over a longer period of observation, an overall weight loss will occur in response to a negative caloric balance. The physician and his patient must thoroughly understand these basic concepts to avoid the discouragement that sometimes occurs with a patient who faithfully follows a therapeutic program which produces a negative caloric balance, but despite this fails to lose weight, or even gains weight owing to fluid retention. To emphasize again, this is usually a transient phenomenon which will correct itself over a period of time.

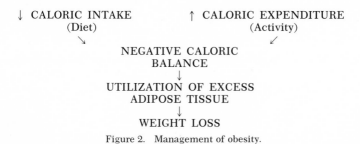

Figure 2.   Management of obesity.

Dietary Management

The basic concept of the dietary management of obesity is the production of a negative caloric balance by providing in the diet fewer calories than are utilized by the patient. In addition to the quantitative caloric aspects, the qualitative aspects of the diet are also important: protein, carbohydrate, fat, salt, and vitamin content.

In general, there are several degrees of calorie restriction that may be used in dietary therapy (Table 2).

1. "Common sense" reduction in calories. Here, no specific count of calories is made, but the patient merely eliminates or reduces from his usual diet, on a "common sense" basis, obviously high caloric foods, particularly those high in carbohydrate and fat content. While not a quantitatively exact diet, this is a rational approach to therapy in which the patient learns to eat fewer calories in a diet which is familiar and usual for him. This may be effective in weight reduction for the mildly overweight person whose obesity began in middle or late life.

2. 1000 calorie deficit. In this diet the number of calories required by the patient for daily living (basal caloric requirement plus the calories necessary for daily activity) is determined, and 1000 calories subtracted from this figure. For an active young man this may represent a reducing diet of 1500 to 2000 total calories a day or more, and for a woman, from 1200 to 1500 total calories. In this diet, there is a deficit of 1000 calories a day or 7000 calories per week, resulting in a theoretical weight loss of about 2 pounds during this time provided that the activity pattern is unchanged. A weight loss of 1 to 2 pounds a week is an ideal rate of reduction, and avoids the weakness that sometimes occurs with more rapid loss of weight.

3. 1000 to 1200 calorie diet. This is just a stricter reduction in calories than in (2), and while it is quite satisfactory and effective for the middle-aged or elderly patient who is relatively inactive, it may not be as acceptable to the active young working patient, because the weakness which sometimes occurs with this diet may prevent necessary daily activities from being carried out.

4. Intermittent fasting. In this form of therapy of total caloric restriction popularized by Duncan,[10] the patient is fasted for 1 to 2 days a week, or for a 7 to 14 day period while in a hospital under the supervision of a physician experienced in this therapy. A period longer than 7 to 14 days should not be used, and even this period of fasting should be reserved for the severely and intractably obese patient for whom the other more conservative programs have not been successful. It should be noted, however, that the fast is well tolerated and accepted by the patient, who

Table 2. *Dietary Therapy. Control of Calorie Intake*

1. "Common sense" reduction
2. 1000 calorie deficit
3. 1000 to 1200 calorie total
4. Fasting

is actually anorexic and euphoric during the absolute fast and does have the great psychological advantage of the rapid induction of weight loss.

The fact that most of this weight loss is, in fact, water and lean body tissue rather than adipose tissue, as several studies have indicated,[1, 2, 6] is important to recognize, and certainly detracts from the physiologic effectiveness of the diet. Also, side-effects do occur, some serious, and there are definite contraindications to the use of this therapy (pregnancy, labile diabetes, liver disease, etc.).

As regards the qualitative aspects of the diet, the following are important points for the physician to keep in mind.

The composition of the diet should be planned to allow sufficient protein content (at least 1 gm. per kg. of body weight in the adult), and adequate carbohydrate content; finally, the amount of fat is added to make up the desired final caloric content. The different foods (i.e., protein, carbohydrate, and fat) are completely interchangeable on the basis of 4 calories per gram of protein and carbohydrate and 9 calories per gram of fat, and with the exception of the points listed below there is no advantage in terms of weight reduction in altering the usual distribution of calories in the diet.

It has been observed that carbohydrate ingestion is associated with the retention of salt and water to a greater degree than with protein or fat, and that a sodium diuresis may occur with carbohydrate restriction.[4] Also, protein is said to have a "high satiety value" and does have a higher specific dynamic action than the other foods. From these points, it might be argued that a diet somewhat higher in protein and lower in carbohydrate would be more effective in inducing weight loss. In the practical planning of meals, the diabetic exchange lists may be of great help to the physician and patient in the conversion of calories to actual food equivalents in the diet.

The spacing of meals has been shown to affect the metabolic influence of the diet on body composition in animal experiments.[8] If animals that usually feed by continuous nibbling during the day are forced to ingest the same number of calories in one or two large meals they will become obese, despite the fact that the number of calories ingested is the same in both instances. This has not been demonstrated to occur in patients, and the rate of weight loss is the same whether the reducing diet is consumed in three meals a day or six small frequent feedings, provided that the total number of calories is the same.

Activity

Activity is a very important part of any therapeutic program for the obese patient. As previously noted, studies have shown that obese children and adults are less active than their lean counterparts and that this inactivity does play a significant role in their positive caloric or energy balance. Further, because a good deal of energy is expended in moving the heavier obese body, a significant loss of energy can be induced by encouraging increased physical activity in the obese patient. This increase in activity can be in the form of brisk walking or engaging in sports such as swimming, golf, or tennis, but it should be emphasized that any program of activity should begin with a small increase over the usual activity pattern and a gradual progressive increase to the desired amount. The activity should be a regular, habitual event, occurring daily at the same time.

Salt and Water Metabolism

It is well known that obese patients following a reducing diet will gain and lose weight on an irregular basis, at times having no apparent relation to caloric balance. This forms the basis of the frequent complaint of the patient who faithfully follows the reducing diet but despite this either fails to lose or actually gains weight. These discrepancies are due to gains or losses of salt and water and are related to the metabolism of sodium in the obese patient.

The tendency to sodium retention in the obese patient can be dealt with by the physician in several ways. First, the restriction of sodium in the diet and reduction in carbohydrate intake may result in sodium and water diuresis and weight loss. Secondly, if necessary, a diuretic agent may be used to promote this diuresis and weight loss. The influence of sodium and water metabolism on the response to dietary therapy in the obese individual is emphasized again, principally because of the psychological effect on the patient. In terms of the goal of therapy, the loss of excess adipose tissue, these fluctuations in weight due to fluid gains and losses have no real importance. What is important in the therapy of obesity is the reduction of excess adipose tissue and weight loss due to this.

Miscellaneous Therapy

Little will be said here about the role of drugs in the therapy of obesity, because they certainly play a secondary role in management. The anorexigenic agents (derivatives of amphetamine) do have a temporary appetite-suppressing effect, but this effect abates over several weeks as tolerance to the drugs develops. While they can be helpful in some patients in curbing the appetite, they are not usually major determinants in the success or failure of any program. Also, they have side-effects which may be quite significant, particularly in the obese patient.

Diuretic agents have been alluded to previously and may be of psychological value in promoting a salt and water diuresis with resulting weight loss in a patient who has failed to lose weight while following the calorically restricted diet. It would be much better, however, first to attempt dietary sodium restriction for this effect before prescribing a drug. Tranquilizing agents have been used to aid an emotional patient in coping with anxiety that may promote excessive eating or anxiety associated with dietary restriction, but frequent visits to a supportive and understanding physician may be more effective than a drug in these instances. Needless to say, the thyroid analogues have no role in the therapy of obesity unless, of course, the patient is hypothyroid.

Surgery for obesity, in the form of intestinal shunt operations, has been performed with a resulting loss of weight. This is obviously a drastic form of therapy with significant morbidity and possible mortality, and one yet to be evaluated adequately. It should be limited to those medical centers in which there is experience and in which studies are being undertaken to evaluate its effectiveness, and to those patients with extreme degrees of obesity, intractable to medical therapy, in whom obesity is a serious hazard to health.

EFFECT OF MANAGEMENT AND ROLE OF THE PHYSICIAN

The goal in the management of the obese patient is the loss of excess adipose tissue and the return of body weight to the level desirable for that patient. The real effectiveness of any therapeutic program for obesity, however, should be measured with regard to the long-term maintenance of any weight reduction and not the achievement of a temporary loss of weight, followed, all too often, by a relapse in a short time to the former state of obesity.

Regardless of the form of therapy used in obesity, the results of treatment have been relatively poor, particularly as regards the long-term maintenance of weight reduction. The effectiveness of self-help groups (TOPS, Weight Watchers) appears to be as good as the record of many physicians in dealing with this problem.

Although the overall prognosis for successful management is not good, certain general guidelines can be used to predict the response of the individual patient (Table 3). Those patients whose obesity had its onset in childhood, those with extreme degrees of obesity, those with serious psychological problems, and those who are poorly motivated in terms of following a therapeutic program will generally not respond well to therapy; those with the onset of obesity of middle and late life, those with mild degrees of obesity, those in whom no significant emotional problems exist, and those who have good motivation are more likely to lose weight and maintain the reduced weight as a result of management.

In any case, the role of the physician should be that of helping the patient to achieve weight reduction with a therapeutic program in keeping with the magnitude of the medical problem. Although the effects of obesity have been emphasized, there are those physicians who are not so convinced of the ill effects of mild to moderate degrees of obesity.[12]

In the vast majority of instances, this means that simple and conservative management, consisting of mild to moderate caloric restriction coupled with increased physical activity, will suffice; extreme forms of therapy such as extended periods of fasting and surgery have no place in the management of the usual mildly to moderately obese patient.

Table 3. *Management of Obesity. Prognostic Factors*

Age of onset
Emotional state of patient
Degree and duration of obesity
Motivation of patient
Past history of response to therapy

As emphasized by a recent editorial,[11] the physician must always keep a clear perspective in the management of the obese patient. We would like to correct a potentially harmful condition but certainly not by accepting a risk of injury to the patient out of proportion to the original medical problem.

SUMMARY

The management of the obese patient is the commonest and one of the most difficult nutritional problems confronting the physician in clinical practice. Obesity is associated with an increased risk of morbidity and mortality which warrants therapeutic attempts at weight reduction.

The fundamental cause of obesity is a positive caloric or energy balance occurring at some time in the patient's life, with the resultant deposition of excess adipose tissue; but the underlying factors leading to this imbalance are complex and differ from patient to patient. The starting point in the management of the obese patient is a thorough medical evaluation, in which an attempt is made to define these underlying causes and, if possible, to correct them.

Management of the overweight patient consists of dietary restriction of calories and a program of increased physical activity in an effort to induce a negative caloric balance with resultant weight loss. Proper attention should be given to fluctuations in salt and water metabolism, which are often the cause of weight changes apparently unexplained by caloric balance. Above all, the physician must exercise discretion in the treatment of the obese patient, avoiding drastic therapeutic programs in the management of the usual mild to moderately overweight patient.

As in many chronic illnesses, the results of the treatment of obesity are often discouraging with frequent relapses even if initial weight reduction is successful. The physician must be prepared for long-term treatment with frequent follow-up visits, in which his role as a supportive and understanding figure will be a major factor in the success of any program.

REFERENCES

1. Ball, M. F., Canary, J. J., and Kyle, L. H.: Comparative effects of caloric restriction and total starvation on body composition in obesity. Ann. Intern. Med., 67:60, 1967.
2. Benoit, F. L., Martin, R. L., and Watten, R. H.: Changes in body composition during weight reduction in obesity. Balance studies comparing effects of fasting and a ketogenic diet. Ann. Intern. Med., 63:604, 1965.
3. Berkowitz, D.: Metabolic changes associated with obesity before and after weight reduction. J.A.M.A., 187:103, 1964.
4. Bloom, N. L., and Azar, G. J.: Similarities of carbohydrate deficiency and fasting. I. Weight loss, electrolyte excretion and fatigue. Arch. Intern. Med., 112:333, 1963.
5. Bloom, W. L., and Eidex, M. F.: Inactivity as a major factor in adult obesity. Metabolism, 16:679, 1967.
6. Bolinger, R. E., Lukert, B. P., Brown, R. W., Gurvara, L., and Steinberg, R.: Metabolic balance of obese subjects during fasting. Arch. Intern. Med., 118:3, 1966.
7. Bortz, W. M.: Metabolic consequences of obesity. Ann. Intern. Med., 71:833, 1969.

  8. Cohn, C. J., and Joseph, D.: Role of rate of ingestion of diet on regulation of intermediary metabolism (meal eating vs. nibbling). Metabolism, 9:492, 1960.
  9. Cook, G. H., Bennett, C. A., Norwood, W. D., and Mahaffey, J. A.: Evaluation of skin-fold measurements and weight chart to measure body fat. J.A.M.A., 198:157, 1966.
 10. Duncan, G. G., Jenson, W. K., Fraser, R. I., and Cristofori, F. C.: Correction and control of intractable obesity. Practical application of intermittent periods of total fasting. J.A.M.A., 181:99, 1962.
 11. Editorial: Drastic cures for obesity. Lancet, 1:1094, 1970.
 12. Hollifield, G., and Parson, W.: Corpulence, calories and confusion. In Ingelfinger, F. J., Relman, A. S., and Finland, M., eds.: Controversy in Internal Medicine. Philadelphia, W. B. Saunders, 1966, p. 443.
 13. Marks, H. H.: Influence of obesity on morbidity and mortality. Bull. New York Acad. Med., 36:296, 1960.
 14. Mayer, J.: Genetic factors in human obesity: Ann. N.Y. Acad. Sci., 131:412, 1965.

Department of Medicine
University of Miami School of Medicine
P. O. Box 875, Biscayne Annex
Miami, Florida   33152

A Clinical Approach to the Hyperlipidemias

Lee A. Bricker, M.D.[*]

Atherosclerosis is an ubiquitous affliction of Western society. It has numerous causes, and much about it remains poorly understood. Among the predisposing factors, such as heredity, diet, lack of exercise, stress, and hypertension, the question of the various hyperlipidemias stands out prominently.[36, 61] Many believe that these entities represent situations in which specific therapy may help prevent or forestall atherosclerotic catastrophes.[2, 17, 18, 19, 20, 21, 31, 42, 62]

A clinical approach to the hyperlipidemias can be derived from three resources easily available to the practicing physician. These are: (1) a complete history and physical examination, (2) a chemical determination of the cholesterol and the fasting triglyceride concentration in plasma, and (3) direct observation of a refrigerated sample of the patient's fasting plasma. The terminology in common use is defined in Table 1. This table illustrates that a useful classification of the hyperlipidemias can be based solely on whether the plasma is lactescent or clear. Clear plasma can reliably be equated with normal or only very slightly elevated triglyceride concentrations. Plasma lactescence, almost invariably a reflection of elevated triglyceride (fat), does not occur unless plasma triglyceride concentrations are in excess of 400 mg. per 100 ml. In contrast, the plasma cholesterol level can be strikingly elevated while the plasma remains clear.

The upper limit of normal for plasma cholesterol in our laboratory, as in most others, is 250 mg. per 100 ml. This level applies primarily to middle-aged individuals, and is set appropriately lower in younger individuals.[26] We do not regard fasting plasma triglyceride levels as "abnormal" in a physiological sense until concentrations of 250 to 300 mg. per 100 ml. are encountered. While levels between 190 and 250 mg. per 100 ml. are perhaps *statistically* abnormal,[26] there is no evidence that a fasting plasma triglyceride in this range represents in itself any risk or danger to the individual, or that drug therapy or severe dietary restrictions are needed.[64]

*Assistant Professor of Medicine, University of Miami School of Medicine; Attending Physician, Jackson Memorial Hospital and University of Miami Hospital

Table 1. *Terminology in Plasma Lipid Disorders*

Lactescent = lipemic = milky (always due to triglyceride)
Triglyceride = fat
Hyperlipemia = hypertriglyceridemia
Hyper*lipid*emia
    1. Includes both hyperlipemia and hypercholesterolemia with clear plasma
    2. Is the same as *hyperlipoproteinemia*

Plasma triglyceride can be conveniently divided into two major forms: (1) exogenous triglyceride, carried in the postabsorptive state in the form of large, bulky but extremely light lipoprotein complexes (chylomicrons), and (2) endogenous triglyceride, manufactured in the liver, and carried in more dense, smaller lipoproteins. Though heavier than chylomicrons, these endogenous (hepatic) triglyceride particles are nonetheless referred to (on the basis of their behavior in an ultracentrifuge) as "very low density lipoproteins."

HYPERLIPIDEMIA WITH CLEAR PLASMA

In an individual with hyperlipidemia and clear plasma, the elevated lipid is, in all likelihood, cholesterol. Hypercholesterolemia occurs in very few conditions, and its differential diagnosis is limited. The plasma cholesterol is commonly elevated only in myxedema, obstructive liver disease, primary hypercholesterolemia, and sometimes in hepatoma.

Myxedema

Thyroid insufficiency is often accompanied by hypercholesterolemia. Moreover, hypercholesterolemia may be present before other signs of thyroid deficiency are evident. Rarely, triglyceride levels may also be elevated. In any case, tests of thyroid function are prudent in an individual who presents with an unexplained elevation of plasma cholesterol on a screening test. The mechanism of this elevation is not completely clear.[65]

Obstructive Liver Disease

The obstructive liver diseases are associated with hypercholesterolemia (largely unesterified)[57] and very distinctive physical findings, including jaundice, and, in long-standing cases, tendinous and cutaneous xanthomas, and xanthelasmas. Although this entity does not usually cause any difficulties in the differential diagnosis of hypercholesterolemia, an occasional young patient may be free of jaundice and yet have malignant xanthomatosis. History, elevated alkaline phosphatase, bilirubin levels, and the uniquely enormous cholesterol levels help to distinguish this problem from primary hypercholesterolemia.

Hepatoma

Many patients with hepatoma have hypercholesterolemia. This entity, while rare in the United States, is frequent in other parts of the

Table 2. *Clinical Features of Primary Familial Hypercholesterolemia*

Family history of coronary artery disease
Coronary artery disease
Xanthomas, tendinous
Xanthelasmas
Arteriosclerosis obliterans (unusual)
Corneal arcus
Elevated plasma cholesterol levels

---

world. It is likely that the hepatoma itself synthesizes and releases the cholesterol that accumulates in the plasma.[16] Moreover, the normal feedback system for regulation of cholesterol synthesis appears to be deleted in these patients.[9, 60]

Primary Familial Hypercholesterolemia

This entity is transmitted as a genetic autosomal dominant trait, and presents in either a heterozygous, mild form, or in a more unusual and more severe homozygous form. Primary familial hypercholesterolemia, particularly when present in the homozygous form, is not a difficult process to recognize. There is often a family history of severe atherosclerosis and myocardial infarction. Such patients may manifest tendinous and planar xanthomas, and xanthelasmas, and myocardial infarction may be seen as early as the late teens or early twenties. Table 2 lists the major findings. Figure 1 illustrates Achilles tendon xanthomas in a patient with this disease, and Figure 2 shows similar findings on the tendons of the dorsum of the hand. These findings, however, may be absent.

The major laboratory abnormality accompanying the disease is a marked elevation of the plasma cholesterol, with clear plasma.[31] The protein-bound iodine and bilirubin concentrations are normal.

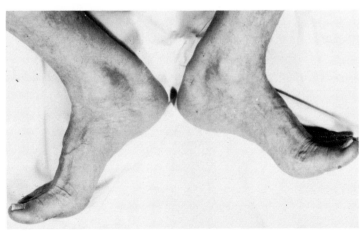

Figure 1. Grossly visible xanthomas of the Achilles tendons of a patient with primary familial hypercholesterolemia. Smaller lesions of this kind are often easily palpated, even when not visible.

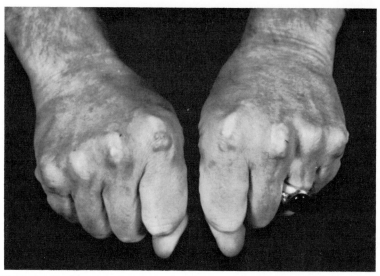

Figure 2.   Tendinous xanthomas on the extensor surfaces of the hands of a patient with primary familial hypercholesterolemia.

In milder cases, therapy with diet alone may suffice. About 30 to 40 per cent of the diet should be in the form of fat, largely polyunsaturated[43, 53] (Table 3). Polyunsaturated fats may act by enhancing fecal excretion of cholesterol[49] or by redistributing body cholesterol from plasma into the tissues.[10, 30] Many patients, particularly those with homozygous disease, will not respond well to this regimen. Drug therapy, though often also unsatisfactory, may sometimes significantly lower the plasma cholesterol levels (Table 4). Whether the successful lowering of plasma cholesterol has any beneficial effect on the progress of the patient's vascular disease remains unknown. However, disappearance of xanthelasmas or other physical manifestations of the disease may occur, and occasionally, the severity of angina pectoris may also lessen. One drug of choice is aluminum nicotinate (Nicalex) usually in doses of 3 gm. per day, and increasing to tolerance as needed. Diarrhea and flushing

Table 3.   *Polyunsaturated to Saturated Fat Ratios in Common Foods*

FOOD	RATIO OF POLYUNSATURATED TO SATURATED FAT
Milk	1:30
Butter	1:20
Egg yolk	1:4
Beef	1:20
Chicken	1:1
Salmon	3:1
Trout	2:1
Tuna	2:1
Walnuts	9:1
Corn oil	5:1

Table 4. *Drugs Used in Treatment of Primary Hypercholesterolemia*

AGENT	DOSE	SIDE EFFECTS
Aluminum nicotinate (Nicalex)	1 tablet QID to 4 tablets QID	Glucose intolerance, flushing, diarrhea, gastric hyperacidity
Dextro-thyroxine (Choloxin)	1.0 to 2.0 mg./day increased to 4.0 to 8.0 mg./day; 0.1 mg./kg. in children, to 4.0 mg. maximum	Precipitation of angina pectoris; clinical hyperthyroidism; potentiation of antiprothrombin anticoagulants; precipitation of cardiac arrhythmias, particularly during surgery
Cholestyramine (Questran)	4 gm. QID	Binds fat-soluble vitamins, requires vitamin A
Clofibrate	Not effective	

are occasional side-effects. Dextro-thyroxin, in daily doses up to 8 mg. may also be useful alone or in combination. However, at effective doses it may also worsen angina pectoris. Another valuable antihypercholesterolemic agent is cholestyramine, a resin which binds bile salts and cholesterol in the intestine and prevents their absorption.[33]

Clofibrate (Atromid-S) has proved to be of little value in treating hypercholesterolemia.[23, 42] Surgical by-pass of the terminal ileum is similarly unlikely to be of lasting value in primary familial hypercholesterolemia, and if used at all, should be reserved for desperate situations, in our opinion. This view is not shared by a number of other workers.

HYPERLIPIDEMIA WITH CLOUDY PLASMA (HYPERLIPEMIA)

The following is a discussion of the causes of hyperlipemia in man.

Nephrotic Syndrome

The nephrotic syndrome is a well-known cause of hyperlipemia in man.[7, 52] The reasons for this hyperlipidemic response are not understood. Recent studies suggest that hepatic synthesis of new albumin, initiated by reduced colloid oncotic pressure, is also associated with enhanced lipoprotein synthesis.[3, 8, 46, 47, 55, 56] Unlike albumin, which is subjected to massive loss through diseased glomerular membranes, the relatively water-insoluble lipoprotein is not excreted and accumulates in the plasma.

Zieve's Syndrome

This is an acute hyperlipemia occurring in alcohol addicts and may be associated with a hemolytic anemia. It is usually seen with a fatty liver.[14, 68] The hyperlipemia is often intense, disappearing rapidly after the patient has abandoned alcohol. A somewhat related entity has been studied by Kudzma and Schonfeld, in which alcohol induces an intense endogenous hypertriglyceridemia in certain susceptible individuals.[40]

Oral Contraceptives

The oral contraceptive agents have been observed to be associated with the formation of abnormal amounts of endogenous triglyceride.[35, 69]

Transient or long-standing mild elevations of triglyceride are quite common in women taking contraceptives,[4] but it is unusual for the levels to become high enough so that plasma lactescence is noted.

Dysproteinemias

In particular, multiple myeloma, lymphoma, and systemic lupus erythematosus may be associated with hyperlipemia.[44, 58] Apparently, an abnormal immunoglobin associated with the dysproteinemia binds heparin so that it cannot activate lipoprotein lipase.[28] This inactive enzyme is then unable to break down chylomicron triglyceride, which accumulates in the plasma.

Pancreatitis

Pancreatitis is rarely associated with hyperlipemia. Greenberger et al.[29] studied this association and concluded that primary hyperlipemia often pre-exists in these patients. Other workers have implicated the pancreatitis itself as the major causative factor.[39] Still other workers have suggested that the insulin insufficiency in glucose intolerance of pancreatitis is responsible for the hyperlipemia.[5, 38] The precise mechanism(s) therefore remain controversial.

Glycogen Storage Diseases

Von Gierke's disease (glucose-6-phosphatase deficiency, Type I), Forbes-Cori disease (debranching enzyme deficiency, Type III), and Hers' disease (phosphorylase deficiency, Type VI), are often associated with marked hyperlipemia. In the latter two types, survival to adult life is usual, and such patients therefore may seek the advice of a physician other than a pediatrician. The hyperlipemias of Type I and Type III are unique in that they are associated with hypoglycemia. The combination of hyperlipemia and hypoglycemia is so unusual as to be highly suggestive of glycogen storage disease.[24]

The Primary Hyperlipemias

Three major forms of primary hyperlipemia are known.[1, 45]

FAT-INDUCED HYPERLIPEMIA. Fat-induced hyperlipemia is an uncommon disease. It usually manifests itself clinically in the first or second decade of life, but is not known to predispose to atherosclerosis.[42] The patient frequently will consult a physician because of a "skin rash" (Fig. 3), an eruptive form of xanthomatosis involving the elbows, thighs, back, and buttocks. These lesions are approximately 2 mm. in diameter, tend to be yellowish, and rest upon a small erythematous base. Approximately 50 per cent of these patients have hepatosplenomegaly at some time in their disease.

Repeated bouts of severe abdominal pain is a second major complaint. Many patients in this group undergo fruitless abdominal exploration, sometimes repeatedly. These patients have extremely lactescent plasma. Triglyceride levels may reach or exceed 10,000 mg. per 100 ml. The plasma cholesterol may reach levels as high as 1,500 mg. per 100 ml., with no primary reason.

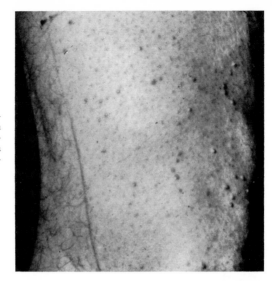

Figure 3. Eruptive xanthomas on the thigh of a patient with fat-induced hyperlipemia. The lesions are identical to "xanthoma diabeticorum" occurring in patients with diabetic lipemia.

An additional physical finding is the presence of lipemia retinalis. Figure 4 illustrates the optic fundus of one such patient, with the characteristic "cream of tomato soup" appearance in the color of the vessels, represented in the black and white photograph as a lighter hue. This is the result of a large amount of chylomicron fat (triglyceride) in suspension in the circulating blood.[37] When lipemia retinalis is fully developed, the plasma triglyceride level is generally in excess of 3500 mg. per 100 ml.

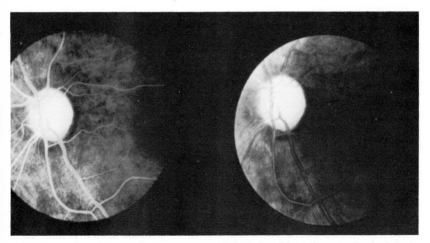

Figure 4. Lipemia retinalis in a patient with fat-induced hyperlipemia. On the left, the blood vessels in the optic fundus are very light in color, due to excessive circulating triglyceride. When lipemia retinalis is fully developed, plasma triglyceride concentration is generally in excess of 3500 mg. per 100 ml. At the right is shown the response in the retinal vessels to 48 hours of a low-fat diet. Triglyceride levels have returned to nearly normal levels and the colors of the blood vessels are normal. Courtesy of Bascom Palmer Eye Institute.

The primary defect in fat-induced hyperlipemia is apparently a congenital absence of the enzyme, lipoprotein lipase.[32, 34, 63] The lipoprotein lipase acts by removing fatty acids from the glycerol backbone of the triglyceride molecule; when the enzyme is absent, the triglyceride remains intact for abnormally long periods of time and accumulates in the plasma. Under ordinary circumstances, the fatty acids mobilized by lipoprotein lipase are either consumed as metabolic fuel by muscle and other tissue, or are reconverted to fat and stored in adipose depots. Figure 5 illustrates normal fat metabolism, and the defects apparent in fat-induced hyperlipemia.

Figure 6 attempts to depict the value of simple inspection of the fasting plasma in the diagnosis of this hyperlipemia. If the collected plasma is separated from the red cells and allowed to stand overnight in the refrigerator, chylomicron fat will float to the top of the tube. In contrast, endogenous (hepatic) fat particles will not float, but rather will remain in homogeneous suspension (see section below). This simple refrigerator test, then, allows an accurate and reliable diagnosis of hyperlipidemia with chylomicronemia. The diagnosis of fat-induced hyperlipemia per se, while usually readily suspected from the patient's age,

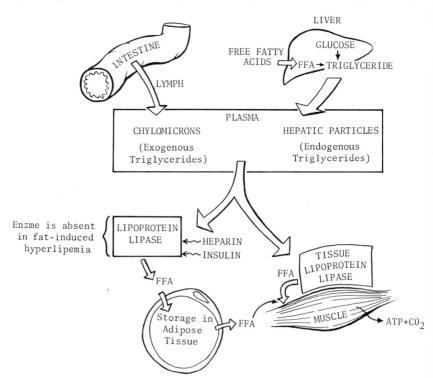

Figure 5. Fat metabolism. Two major sources of plasma triglyceride are dietary (producing chylomicrons) and hepatic (endogenous). The triglyceride is broken down by lipoprotein lipase (activated by insulin and heparin) to glycerol and free fatty acids, which, in turn, are either stored as newly synthesized triglyceride or burned as fuel. In fat-induced hyperlipemia, where lipoprotein lipase is absent, triglycerides, particularly chylomicrons, are metabolized extremely slowly and accumulate in plasma.

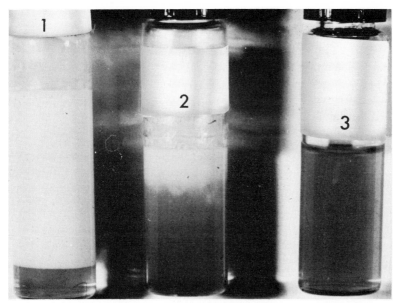

Figure 6.   Tubes of plasma sequentially obtained from a patient with fat-induced hyperlipemia. Left, on admission, plasma triglyceride 9722 mg. per 100 ml., cholesterol 1269 mg.
per 100 ml.; middle, after 36 hours on a low-fat diet, plasma triglyceride 488 mg. per 100 ml.,
cholesterol 716 mg. per 100 ml.; right, after 6 months on dietary therapy, plasma triglyceride
192 mg. per 100 ml., cholesterol 202 mg. per 100 ml.

history, physical findings, and inspection of the fasting plasma, is easily
confirmed clinically by simply observing the brisk disappearance of
chylomicron fat from the fasting plasma after 48 hours on a low fat diet
(less than 30 gm. of fat per day, mostly polyunsaturated). Figure 6 also
sequentially illustrates the effect of a low-fat diet on the plasma lipids of
a patient with fat-induced hyperlipemia.

CARBOHYDRATE-INDUCED HYPERLIPEMIA.   This disease tends to be
familial, and in contrast to fat-induced hyperlipemia, has its onset
generally in middle-life.[1] The remarkable findings on physical examination consist of conjunctival microxanthomas, tuberous xanthomas
(with a predilection for the elbows but occurring elsewhere as well)
(Fig. 8), and xanthelasmas. A clear-cut association of this disease with
premature atherosclerosis has long been suspected but remains statistically unproved.[17, 18, 20, 62] The hyperlipemia appears to be due to an
overproduction of endogenous (hepatic) triglyceride from dietary sugar.
A small number of patients with this disease may present with cholesterol elevations as well.[13]

Therapy for the disease consists of caloric restriction to obtain a
normal body weight and specific restriction of carbohydrates, particularly
simple sugars. A generous amount of fat (60 to 70 per cent of total
calories), largely polyunsaturated, substitutes for carbohydrate in the
diet (Table 3).[41, 67] This diet will usually result in a marked lowering of
the plasma triglyceride and cholesterol levels.[1, 50] Figure 7 shows the
plasma from a patient with this disorder. The plasma lactescence is

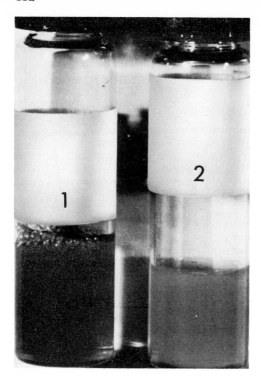

Figure 7. Tubes of plasma sequentially obtained from a patient with carbohydrate-induced hyperlipemia. At the left, on a high-fat diet, the plasma is clear, and the plasma triglyceride level is 251 mg. per 100 ml. At the right, on a low-fat diet, the plasma is homogenously lactescent and plasma triglyceride is 475 mg. per 100 ml.

homogenously distributed (hepatic triglyceride) in contrast to fat-induced hyperlipemia (Figure 6). Also shown is the lack of improvement on a low-fat diet, and the favorable response to a high-fat, low-carbohydrate diet.

Carbohydrate-induced hyperlipemia may mimic diabetes mellitus. The glucose tolerance test may be markedly abnormal and glycosuria may be present, often in the presence of demonstrable hyperinsulinism.[12, 22, 54] It is reasonable to suppose that a considerable number of these patients are being treated as diabetics, with low-fat diets being used in conjunction with oral hypoglycemic agents. This diagnostic pitfall can be avoided simply by examining a refrigerated sample of the fasting plasma in such patients. A persistent homogeneous distribution of lactescence throughout the plasma assures the physician that the lactescence is due to an overproduction of hepatic triglyceride rather than to unmetabolized dietary chylomicrons as seen in the typical diabetic lipemias (see below).[13] It is also unlikely that the well-regulated diabetic patient will manifest any plasma lactescence. Figure 9 illustrates the metabolic defect in carbohydrate-induced hyperlipemia, and Table 5 summarizes and contrasts the findings in carbohydrate-induced and fat-induced hyperlipemias.

MIXED (METABOLIC) HYPERLIPEMIA. Another group of patients appear to have a mixture of fat-induced and carbohydrate-induced hyperlipemias. The physical findings in the disease may mimic those of

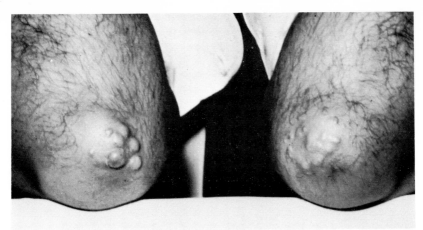

Figure 8. Tuberous xanthomas of the elbows in a man with carbohydrate-induced hyperlipemia. These lesions responded completely to a diet high in polyunsaturated fats.

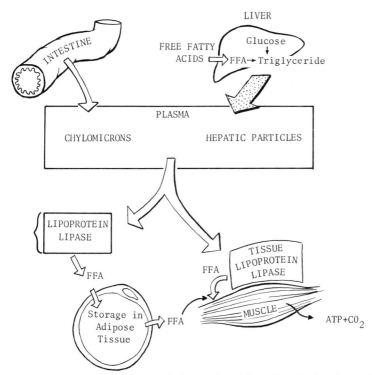

Figure 9. Fat metabolism in carbohydrate-induced hyperlipemia. An abnormal out-pouring of hepatic particles occurs in response to dietary carbohydrate, particularly simple sugars, leading to hyperlipemia.

Table 5. *Fat-Induced vs. Carbohydrate-Induced Hyperlipemia*

	FAT-INDUCED	CARBOHYDRATE-INDUCED
Usual age of onset	Childhood	Middle age
Pancreatitis	50 per cent	Rare
Xanthelasmas	No	Yes
Xanthomas	Mainly eruptive	Mainly tuberous and tendinous
Lipemia retinalis	Often present	Rare
Triglyceride level	2,000 to 15,000 mg. per 100 ml.	300 to 1000 mg. per 100 ml.
Appearance of fat in plasma	Floats (creamy)	Homogeneously suspended (milky)
Predisposition to atherosclerosis	None known	Suspect

either entity separately, or may show features of both together. Lipemia retinalis may be present, and attacks of abdominal pain (often associated with serum amylase elevations) may occur; and eruptive xanthomas are frequently seen. Further, tuberous xanthomas, xanthelasmas, and tendinous xanthomas may also be observed. The refrigerated fasting plasma may show both chylomicron fat and homogeneously distributed endogenous triglyceride, separately or in combination. A high-fat diet persistently induces hyperchylomicronemia in the fasting state,[10] and a low-fat diet induces homogeneous fasting hyperlipemia. Even when accompanied by return of the body weight to normal, therapy is not entirely successful.[42, 62, 66]

We have found that a diet containing 30 per cent carbohydrate, 40 per cent protein, and 30 per cent fat (largely polyunsaturated) is often efficacious. While fasting lactescence is not always eliminated by such a diet, it is usually reduced to a reasonably low level, with fasting triglyceride levels between 400 and 600 mg. per 100 ml. Other centers have reported beneficial effects in this condition with clofibrate (Atromid-S) and progestational hormones.[27, 66]

A form of mixed hyperlipemia may also be seen as a complication of carbohydrate-induced hyperlipemia.[26] In our experience, this is the most common form of mixed hyperlipemia. In these patients, conventional therapy with an augmented polyunsaturated fat diet does not clear the hyperlipemia but rather converts it to a hyperchylomicronemia, such as is seen in fat-induced hyperlipemia. We have found, however, that weight reduction frequently simplifies the clinical picture and changes the nature of the hyperlipemia to a more conventional and pure form of carbohydrate inducibility. Under these circumstances, the high-fat diet no longer induces fasting hyperchylomicronemia. Such patients, in our experience, then respond in a fashion typical of other carbohydrate-induced patients with further weight loss and a conventional high fat diet clearing the hyperlipemia completely.

The Diabetic Lipemias

Hyperlipemia and hyperglycemia can be interrelated.[41, 59] The diabetic lipemias occur in association with marked hyperglycemia. They are quite unusual, and are seen primarily in patients manifesting acute ketoacidosis or chronic, poorly regulated diabetes mellitus. They have been suspected, but never proved, to be related to the atherosclerotic complications of diabetes.[51] There is reason to believe that insulin, like heparin, is an activator of the enzyme lipoprotein lipase.[6] Accordingly, in some patients with severe insulin deprivation, hyperchylomicronemia may develop. Such patients may present with lipemia retinalis and with elevated plasma levels of fasting triglycerides similar to those seen in genetically-determined fat-induced hyperlipemia. The patient with insulin insufficiency may develop an even more congruent picture of fat-induced hyperlipemia,[11] complete with the eruptive xanthomas as shown in Figure 3. This particular skin lesion, when it occurs in conjunction with *diabetic* hyperchylomicronemia, however, is referred to as "xanthoma diabeticorum." Despite the apparent similarity of diabetic hyperchylomicronemia and fat-induced hyperlipemia, it is quite clear that the patient with diabetes requires adequate insulin replacement rather than a low-fat diet. With this therapy, the hyperlipemia and its complications will disappear.

The patient with adult onset diabetes mellitus and the patient with familial carbohydrate-induced hyperlipemia may appear clinically similar.[12, 15] While observation of the fasting plasma for lactescence is useful in distinguishing most of these patients, the problem may be confounded by the occasional patient with true genetic diabetes mellitus who manifests a diabetic lipemia consisting of fasting, homogeneously lactescent plasma. One can speculate that in such a patient an unusual sensitivity to *endogenous* hyperglycemia results in stimulation of brisk endogenous hepatic triglyceride production. This induced hyperlipemia would aggravate the hyperglycemia, with the hyperlipemia and hyperglycemia tending to "feed" on each other. Such a patient should then be controlled with a low-carbohydrate diet, augmented polyunsaturated fats, and meticulous control of the hyperglycemia with oral agents or insulin. The majority of patients manifesting diabetic endogenous hyperlipemia, however, are easily treated by simply providing adequate insulin replacement.

SPECIAL TECHNIQUES

In many centers, the techniques of lipoprotein electrophoresis and analytical ultracentrifugation are available. The various lipoprotein classes (chylomicrons, very low density lipoproteins carrying hepatic triglyceride, and low density lipoproteins carrying primarily cholesterol) have different electrophoretic mobilities, and can be separated and displayed in this fashion. Furthermore, since they have different flotation properties and densities, one can separate them with an analytical ultracentrifuge.

Fredrickson and Lees, and others, have studied extensively the electrophoretic properties of these lipoproteins.[25, 26] They have noted, for example, that dietary chylomicrons, which separate and float to the top of the tube of plasma, do not migrate in an electrophoretic field.

Consequently, when one performs an electrophoretic analysis of the fasting plasma of a patient with hyperchylomicronemia, a dense band remains at the origin. This is the Type I pattern of Fredrickson and Lees, and is compatible with fat-induced hyperlipemia or the hyperchylomicronemias of diabetes or other etiologies.

The lipoproteins with the least degree of mobility (next to the completely immobile chylomicrons themselves) are the betalipoproteins, which carry primarily cholesterol. When the clear plasma of the hypercholesterolemic patient is studied with electrophoresis, the pattern will reveal a beta band likely to be more dense than normal. This pattern is compatible with primary familial hypercholesterolemia, myxedema with hypercholesterolemia, and obstructive liver disease. This is the Type II pattern of Fredrickson and Lees.

Similarly, the plasma lipoprotein electrophoresis from the patient with carbohydrate-inducible (endogenous) hyperlipemia (increased synthesis of very low density lipoprotein triglyceride) may show an increased density of the pre-beta band. These endogenous triglyceride-carrying lipoproteins with a greater electrophoretic mobility than the cholesterol-carrying beta lipoproteins, migrate just ahead of them, and, accordingly, are referred to as pre-beta. An abnormally dense pre-beta band, then, is the electrophoretic hallmark of Type IV disease.

A rare genetic variant of this disease is the so-called Type III disease of Fredrickson and Lees.[48] In this entity, both the pre-beta band and the beta band are abnormally dense, and the two may run together on electrophoresis (the broad beta pattern). Ultracentrifugation of the plasma of such a patient will yield a fraction which floats to the top of the tube. When this floating fraction is subjected to electrophoresis it will migrate with the beta fraction. This disease, known electrophoretically as broad beta disease, therefore, is sometimes also called "floating-beta" disease.

Finally, the mixed lipemias, manifesting both augmented endogenous triglyceride and chylomicrons, would therefore combine the electrophoretic patterns of both Types I and IV, and are thereby referred to as the Type V pattern. None of these patterns, taken alone, is specific for any single disease entity.

The judgment that an electrophoretic band is abnormal must be made carefully. That densitometric measurements of lipoprotein bands are strictly proportional to the concentrations of lipoprotein present has never been shown. In the absence of established "linearity" of lipoprotein staining, then, the electrophoretic patterns can serve mainly as adjunct to confirm that which may be more readily deduced by simpler techniques.

CONCLUSIONS

The hyperlipidemias are common diseases. They have major implications in the lives of many of our patients. While primary hypercholesterolemia remains discouraging to treat, the hyperlipemias quite often lend themselves to successful therapy. It clearly behooves the physician to know which of these entities he is dealing with, because the therapies for them are so markedly different from each other. Quite often, with the selection of appropriate dietary therapy, the rewards are great. Furthermore, rational diagnostic decisions about these patients can be made by the physician in his office, using nothing more than a history, a physical examination, chemical determinations of the plasma cholesterol and fasting triglyceride, and simple inspection of the fasting plasma.

ACKNOWLEDGMENTS

I acknowledge with pleasure the conversations and clinical consultations with Dr. Marvin D. Siperstein during my years of postdoctoral fellowship with him. Many of the illustrations in this report are from his collection and are used with his permission. They were made by the Medical Illustrations Department of the University of Texas Southwestern Medical School, Dallas.

REFERENCES

1. Ahrens, E. H., Hirsch, J., Oette, K., Farquhar, J. W., and Stein, Y.: Carbohydrate-induced and fat-induced lipemias. Trans. Assoc. Amer. Phys., 74:134, 1961.
2. Albrink, M. J.: Triglycerides, lipoproteins and coronary artery disease. Arch. Intern. Med., 109:345, 1962.
3. Allen, J. C., Baxter, J. H., and Goodman, H. C.: Effects of dextran, polyvinylpyrrolidone, and gamma globulin on the hyperlipidemia of experimental nephrosis. J. Clin. Invest., 40:499, 1961.
4. Aurell, M., Cramér, K., and Rybo, G.: Serum lipids and lipoproteins during long-term administration of oral contraceptive. Lancet, 1:291, 1966.
5. Bagdade, J. D.: Diabetic lipaemia complicating acute pancreatitis. Lancet, 2:1041, 1969.
6. Bagdade, J. D., Porte, D., and Bierman, E. L.: Diabetic lipemia: A form of acquired fat-induced lipemia. New Eng. J. Med., 276:427, 1967.
7. Baxter, J. H.: Hyperlipoproteinemia in nephrosis. Arch. Intern. Med., 109:742, 1962.
8. Baxter, J. H., Goodman, H. C., and Allen, J. C.: Effects of infusions of serum albumin on serum lipids and lipoproteins in nephrosis. J. Clin. Invest., 40:490, 1961.
9. Bhattathiry, E. P. M., and Siperstein, M. D.: Feedback control of cholesterol synthesis in man. J. Clin. Invest., 42:1613, 1963.
10. Bieberdorf, F. A., and Wilson, J. D.: Studies on the mechanism of action of unsaturated fats on cholesterol metabolism in the rabbit. J. Clin. Invest., 44:1834, 1965.
11. Bierman, E. L., Amaral, J. A., and Belknap, B. H.: Hyperlipemia and diabetes mellitus. Diabetes, 15:675, 1966.
12. Bierman, E. L., and Porte, D., Jr.: Carbohydrate intolerance and lipemia. Ann. Intern. Med., 68:926, 1968.
13. Bierman, E. L., Porte, D., Jr., O'Hara, D. D., Schwartz, M., and Wood, F. C., Jr.: Characterization of fat particles in plasma of hyperlipemic subjects maintained on fat-free, high carbohydrate diets. J. Clin. Invest., 44:261, 1965.
14. Blass, J. P., and Dean, H. M.: The relation of hyperlipemia to hemolytic anemia in an alcoholic patient. Amer. J. Med., 40:283, 1966.
15. Bricker, L. A., and Mintz, D. H.: Insulin-independent diabetes mellitus. MED. CLIN. N. AMER., 55:295, 1971.
16. Bricker, L. A., Morris, H. P., and Siperstein, M.D.: Loss of the cholesterol feedback system in the intact, hepatoma-bearing rat. (Submitted for publication.)
17. Brown, D. F., and Doyle, J. T.: Pre-beta lipoproteinemia: Its bearing on the dietary management of serum lipid disorders as related to ischemic heart disease. Amer. J. Clin. Nutr., 20:324, 1967.
18. Brown, D. F., Kinch, S. H., and Doyle, J. T.: Serum triglycerides in health and in ischemic heart disease. New Eng. J. Med., 273:947, 1965.
19. Cornfeld, J.: Joint dependence of risk of coronary heart disease on serum cholesterol and systolic blood pressure: A discriminant function analysis. Fed. Proc., 21(Suppl. 11):58, 1962.
20. Dayton, S., Chapman, J. M., Pearce, M. L., and Popják, G. J.: Cholesterol, atherosclerosis, ischemic heart disease, and stroke. UCLA Interdepartmental Conference. Ann. Intern. Med., 72:97, 1970.

21. Dayton, S., and Pearce, M. L.: Prevention of coronary heart disease and other complications of atherosclerosis by modified diet. Amer. J. Med., 46:751, 1969.
22. Eden, M. A. M., and Phaure, T. A. J.: Hyperinsulinism and carbohydrate-induced hyperlipoproteinemia. Lancet, 2:264, 1968.
23. Eder, H. A.: Primary hyper- and hypolipidemias. *In* Beeson, P. B., and McDermott, W., eds.: Cecil-Loeb Textbook of Medicine. Philadelphia, W. B. Saunders Co., 13th ed., 1971.
24. Fernandes, J., and Pikaar, N. A.: Hyperlipemia in children with liver glycogen disease. Amer. J. Clin. Nutr., 22:617, 1969.
25. Fredrickson, D. S., and Lees, R. S.: A system for phenotyping hyperlipoproteinemia. Circulation, 31:321, 1965.
26. Fredrickson, D. S., Levy, R. I., and Lees, R. S.: Fat transport in lipoproteins – An integrated approach to mechanisms and disorders. New Eng. J. Med., 276:34, 94, 148, 215, 273, 1967.
27. Glueck, C. J., Brown, W. V., Levy, R. I., Greten, H., and Fredrickson, D. S.: Amelioration of hypertriglyceridemia by progestational drugs in familial Type V hyperlipoproteinemia. Lancet, 1:1290, 1969.
28. Glueck, C. J., Kaplan, A. P., Levy, R. I., Greten, H., Gralnick, H., and Fredrickson, D. S.: A new mechanism of exogenous hyperglyceridemia. Ann. Intern. Med., 71:1051, 1969.
29. Greenberger, N. J., Hatch, F. T., Drummey, G. D., and Isselbacher, K. J.: Pancreatitis and hyperlipemia: A study of serum lipid alterations in 25 patients with acute pancreatitis. Medicine, 45:161, 1966.
30. Grundy, S. M., and Ahrens, E. H., Jr.: The effects of unsaturated dietary fats on absorption, excretion, synthesis, and distribution of cholesterol in man. J. Clin. Invest., 49: 1135, 1970.
31. Harlan, W. R., Graham, J. B., and Estes, E. H.: Familial hypercholesterolemia: A genetic and metabolic study. Medicine, 45:77, 1966.
32. Harlan, W. R., Jr., Winesett, P. S., and Wasserman, A. J.: Tissue lipoprotein lipase in normal individuals and in individuals with exogenous hypertriglyceridemia and the relationship of this enzyme to assimilation of fat. J. Clin. Invest., 46:239, 1967.
33. Hashim, S. A., and Van Itallie, T. B.: Resin therapy for hypercholesterolemia. J.A.M.A., 192:289, 1965.
34. Havel, R. J., and Gordon, R. S., Jr.: Idiopathic hyperlipemia: Metabolic studies in an affected family. J. Clin. Invest., 30:1777, 1960.
35. Hazzard, W. R., Spiger, M. J., Bagdade, J. D., and Bierman, E. L.: Studies on the mechanism of increased plasma triglyceride levels induced by oral contraceptives. New Eng. J. Med., 280:471, 1969.
36. Heinle, R. A., Levy, R. I., Fredrickson, D. S., and Gorlin, R.: Lipid and carbohydrate abnormalities in patients with angiographically documented coronary artery disease. Amer. J. Cardiol., 24:178, 1969.
37. Heyl, A. G.: Intraocular lipemia. Trans. American Ophthal. Soc., 3:54, 1880.
38. Joffe, B. I., Krut, L., Bank, S., Marks, I. N., and Keller, P.: Serum lipid levels in diabetes secondary to chronic pancreatitis. Metabolism, 19:47, 1970.
39. Kessler, J. I., Miller, M., Barza, D., and Mishkin, S.: Hyperlipemia in acute pancreatitis: Metabolic studies in a patient and demonstration of abnormal lipoprotein-triglyceride complexes resistant to the action of lipoprotein lipase. Amer. J. Med., 42:968, 1967.
40. Kudzma, D. J., and Schonfeld, G.: Alcoholic hypertriglyceridemia: Induction by ethanol but not by carbohydrate. J. Lab. Clin. Med. (in press).
41. Kuo, P. T.: Dietary sugar in the production of hyperglyceridemia in patients with hyperlipemia and atherosclerosis. Trans. Assoc. Amer. Phys., 78:97, 1965.
42. Kuo, P. T.: Hyperlipidemia in atherosclerosis: Dietary and drug treatment. MED. CLIN. N. AMER., 54:657, 1970.
43. Kuo, P. T., and Bassett, D. R.: Primary hyperlipidemias and their management. Ann. Intern. Med., 59:495, 1963.
44. Lennard-Jones, J. E.: Myelomatosis with lipaemia and xanthomata. Brit. Med. J., 1:781, 1960.
45. Levy, R. I., and Langer, T.: Mechanisms involved in hyperlipidemia. Modern Treatment, 6:1313, 1969.
46. Marsh, J. B., and Drabkin, D. L.: Experimental reconstruction of metabolic pattern of lipid nephrosis: Key role of hepatic protein synthesis in hyperlipemia. Metabolism, 9:946, 1960.
47. Marsh, J. B., Drabkin, D. L., Braun, G. A., and Parks, J. S.: Factors in the stimulation of protein synthesis by subcellular preparations from rat liver. J. Biol. Chem., 241:4168, 1966.
48. Matthews, R. J.: Type III and IV familial hyperlipoproteinemia: Evidence that these two syndromes are different phenotypic expressions of the same mutant gene(s). Amer. J. Med., 44:188, 1968.
49. Moore, R. B., Anderson, J. T., Taylor, H. L., Keys, A., and Frantz, I. D., Jr.: Effect of dietary fat on the fecal excretion of cholesterol and its degradation products in man. J. Clin. Invest., 47:1517, 1968.

50. Muto, Y., and Gibson, D. M.: Selective dampening of lipogenic enzymes of liver by exogenous polyunsaturated fatty acids. Biochem. Biophys. Res. Commun., 38:9, 1970.
51. New, M. I., Roberts, T. N., Bierman, E. L., and Reader, G. G.: The significance of blood lipid alterations in diabetes mellitus. Diabetes, 12:208, 1963.
52. Page, I. H., Kirk, E., and van Slyke, D. D.: Plasma lipids in chronic hemorrhagic nephritis. J. Clin. Invest., 15:101, 1936.
53. Page, I. H., and Stamler, J.: Diet and coronary heart disease (1). Med. Conc. Cardiovas. Dis., 37:119, 1968.
54. Reaven, G. M., Lerner, R. L., and Stern, M. D.: Role of insulin in endogenous hypertriglyceridemia. J. Clin. Invest., 46:1756, 1967.
55. Rothschild, M. A., Oratz, M., Evans, C. D., and Schreiber, S. S.: Role of hepatic interstitial albumin in regulating albumin synthesis. Amer. J. Physiol., 210:57, 1966.
56. Rothschild, M. A., Oratz, M., Mongelli, J., and Schreiber, S. S.: Effect of albumin concentration on albumin synthesis in the perfused liver. Amer. J. Physiol., 216:1127, 1969.
57. Russ, E. M., Raymunt, J., and Barr, D. P.: Lipoproteins in primary biliary cirrhosis. J. Clin. Invest., 35:133, 1956.
58. Savin, R. C.: Hyperglobulinemic purpura terminating in myeloma, hyperlipemia, and xanthomatosis. Arch. Derm., 92:679, 1965.
59. Siperstein, M.D.: Interrelations of glucose and lipid metabolism. Amer. J. Med., 26:685, 1959.
60. Siperstein, M. D., and Fagan, V. M.: Deletion of the cholesterol-negative feedback system in liver tumors. Cancer Res., 24:1108, 1964.
61. Slack, J.: Risks of ischaemic heart-disease in familial hyperlipoproteinemic states. Lancet, 2:1380, 1969.
62. Stamler, J., et al.: Detection of susceptibility to coronary disease. Bull. N.Y. Acad. Med., 45:1306, 1969.
63. Steiner, G.: Lipoprotein lipase in fat-induced hyperlipemia. New Eng. J. Med., 279:70, 1968.
64. Van Handel, E., and Zilversmit, D. B.: Micromethod for the direct determination of serum triglycerides. J. Lab. Clin. Med., 50:152, 1957.
65. Walton, K. W., Scott, P. J., Dykes, P. W., and Davies, J. W. L.: Alterations of metabolism and turnover of I[131] low density lipoprotein in myxedema and thyrotoxicosis. Clin. Sci., 29:217, 1965.
66. Wessler, S., and Avioli, L. A.: Classification and management of familial hyperlipoproteinemia. J.A.M.A., 207:929, 1969.
67. Wilkinson, C. F., Jr.: Spaced fat feeding: A regime of management for familial hyperlipemia. Ann. Intern. Med., 45:674, 1956.
68. Zieve, L.: Jaundice, hyperlipemia, and hemolytic anemia: A heretofore unrecognized syndrome associated with alcoholic fatty liver and cirrhosis. Ann. Intern. Med., 48:471, 1958.
69. Zorilla, E., Hulse, M., Hernandez, A., and Gershberg, H.: Severe endogenous hypertriglyceridemia during treatment with estrogen and oral contraceptives. J. Clin. Endocrin. Metab., 28:1793, 1968.

Department of Medicine
University of Miami School of Medicine
P. O. Box 875, Biscayne Annex
Miami, Florida   33152

Diagnostic and Therapeutic Aspects of Stable Angina Pectoris

Robert J. Myerburg, M.D.[*]

Angina pectoris occurs as a result of an imbalance between the availability of oxygen to myocardial cells and the metabolic demand for oxygen by myocardial cells. "Availability," in the modern sense, must extend beyond the simple physical delivery of blood to the myocardial cells, and must include the problems of dissociation of oxygen from hemoglobin and the metabolic utilization of the oxygen at a cellular level. Implicit in the supply and demand concept is the clinical mandate that therapy be directed toward balancing the abnormal relationship, either by increasing effective myocardial oxygen delivery or by decreasing metabolic demands. The modern approach to the management of patients having angina pectoris requires an acquaintance with much of the clinical, metabolic, and pathophysiological knowledge accumulated over the past 10 to 15 years. A brief overview of some of this material is presented here. It is intended as a stimulus to the interested physician, rather than as a definitive presentation and synthesis of the newer concepts.

CAUSES OF ANGINA PECTORIS

In the vast majority of patients having angina pectoris, coronary atherosclerosis is the indentifiable pathological lesion limiting oxygen delivery.[40, 66, 74] There is a very strong correlation (> 90 per cent) between angina pectoris and coronary artery disease when the angina is typical in onset, character, response to rest or nitroglycerin, and electrocardiographic findings. The correlation is less strong when any of these factors are atypical, and a significant number of patients have clinical angina pectoris in the absence of obvious coronary disease (Table 1).[40, 49, 52, 66, 74]

Angina may occur in hypertensive patients and abate with control of the hypertensive state. Many hypertensive patients have coexistent coronary artery disease, and it is not clear whether hypertension alone

[*]Assistant Professor of Medicine and Physiology, University of Miami School of Medicine; Chief, Cardiology Section, Miami Veterans Administration Hospital

Table 1. *Causes of Angina Pectoris*

Coronary atherosclerosis
Systemic or pulmonary hypertension
Acquired valvular disease
Congenital heart disease
Arrhythmias (?)
Spasm of coronary arteries (?)
Abnormal oxyhemoglobin dissociation
Abnormal muscle metabolism (?)

may precipitate angina. Pulmonary hypertension may also be accompanied by angina pectoris, as may cor pulmonale in chronic lung disease, pulmonary embolism, and Eisenminger's physiology in congenital lesions. Aortic valve disease, whether predominantly stenotic or regurgitant, may cause angina pectoris. The precise mechanisms are not clearly delineated. Aortic valve lesions frequently become clinically manifest in the age range when coronary artery disease becomes manifest, and the pathologic coexistence of the two states is common. On the other hand, angina does occur in aortic valve disease in the absence of coronary artery disease. The degree of valvular disease is usually severe in such cases. Mitral valve disease, particularly mitral stenosis, may produce angina pectoris. Angina also occurs in cardiomyopathies, of both the obstructive and diffuse types.

Paroxysmal arrhythmias, occurring in the presence of coronary artery disease, may precipitate angina. It is doubtful whether angina pectoris occurs during tachycardias in the absence of coronary artery disease. Spasm of large coronary arteries, with reversal by nitroglycerin, has been shown to occur during coronary arteriography,[35, 66] but pain does not necessarily accompany the spasm. Whether or not spasm of smaller vessels contributes to the production of angina is enigmatic, and therefore the role of spasm alone as a cause of angina pectoris must remain uncertain.

When all the conditions which fail to produce a sufficiently increased effective myocardial blood flow in response to an increased or normal demand for oxygen are excluded from the total group, an interesting patient population remains. The majority of this group are women, and there is normal coronary blood flow and oxygen extraction.[49] Abnormal exercise tests and lactate production during tachycardia (see below) or isoproterenol infusion occur in significant number of these patients. A metabolic failure of oxygen utilization at a cellular level has been proposed in this type of patient,[61] but no firm positive evidence for this type of mechanism is forthcoming as yet. Small vessel disease[46] or cardiomyopathies may also play a role in some patients. It is further noteworthy that abnormalities of carbohydrate metabolism are common in this group.[49] Finally, abnormalities of oxyhemoglobin dissociation have been implicated in myocardial ischemia without coronary artery disease.[19]

CLINICAL FEATURES OF ANGINA PECTORIS

No one has improved upon the clinical description of exertional angina pectoris published by Heberdin in 1772.[42] However, meticulous clinicians and modern clinical researchers have broadened our views of several clinical aspects of the syndrome. Most patients describe the pain of angina pectoris as substernal in location with radiation to the neck, or left shoulder, or left arm and hand, or some combination thereof. However, there are enough patients with variant pain patterns to demand our awareness of their existence (Table 2).

Some patients may experience no chest pain whatever, but rather complain of pain in *either* shoulder or *either* arm or hand. Pain in the back, especially the interscapular area to the left of the spine, may signal the presence of angina. In addition to the well-known anterior cervical and mandibular radiations, pain may also be experienced in the back of the neck, the oropharynx, or the upper jaw.

The common difficulty of differentiating epigastric discomfort of cardiac origin from that of gastrointestinal origin is well-known. It is sometimes impossible to make the distinction, even with the most meticulous history and physical examination. Finally, more difficulties arise when the patient does not experience pain at all, but rather describes a vague discomfort, or dyspnea on exertion.

Transient myocardial ischemia is frequently associated with transient abnormalities of ventricular function,[63, 64] and the description of dyspnea-on-exertion may represent transient acute left ventricular failure rather than an inability on the part of the patient to describe his symptoms accurately.

Angina decubitus, or angina at rest, is quite common, and is a somewhat different clinical situation than stable exertional angina pectoris. This probably represents a more advanced state of the underlying disease process, and may be accompanied by latent congestive heart failure. Progressive exertional angina, "pre-infarctional" angina, and the first attack of angina are all special situations which will not be covered in this discussion.

Valuable information may be obtained when the patient is asked to characterize the dynamics of his symptoms. In classical exertional angina pectoris, patients frequently describe very specific precipitating factors. It is not necessary to review the many well-known activities and environmental conditions which aggravate the symptoms of the angina patient,[54] nor those which relieve the discomfort. However, one potential

Table 2. *Variations in Pain Patterns in Angina Pectoris*

Left or right shoulder	Interscapular Area
Left or right arm	Lower or upper jaw
Fingers	Oropharynx
Anterior or posterior cervical area	Epigastrium
	Dyspnea on exertion

Table 3. *Physical Findings During Angina Pectoris*

Tachycardia	Ischemic bulges, transient
Hypertension	Paradoxically split S_2
S_3 and S_4 gallops	Pulsus alternans
Apical systolic murmur	Findings of underlying disease

trap is worthy of emphasis. Some patients, followed over a long period of time, will report a gradual decrease in angina pectoris attacks. Careful questioning of these patients will reveal that some are actually progressively decreasing their physical activity to avoid angina attacks, and that their exercise tolerance is actually decreasing, indicating progressive angina pectoris. On the other hand, an abrupt true decrease in the frequency of attacks may indicate that a myocardial infarction has occurred.

The physical findings in angina patients are either normal or show only the abnormalities which may be associated with their underlying condition, and are not specific for angina pectoris. However, the examination of a patient *during* an attack of angina pectoris may be quite revealing, especially when there has been some doubt as to the diagnosis (Table 3). It has been clearly demonstrated that tachycardia and hypertension may accompany the pain of angina pectoris.[75] In many instances, the hemodynamic changes precede the onset of the pain. If the patient is experiencing pain or prodromata at the time the physician is at the bedside, it may be helpful to check the pulse and blood pressure during and after the attack. Transient S_3 and S_4 gallops may also occur during an attack,[80] as well as transient palpable ischemic bulges,[14, 82] transient mitral regurgitation due to papillary muscle dysfunction,[10] paradoxical splitting of the second heart sound, and pulsus alternans.

CONFIRMATION OF THE DIAGNOSIS

When the clinical description of angina pectoris, including the response to nitroglycerin, is typical, the only confirmatory procedure that need be done is electrocardiography. The results are not always supportive of the diagnosis of ischemic heart disease, but a negative result does not necessarily rule out the diagnosis. The resting electrocardiogram will be normal in half to two thirds of patients with exertional angina who have not suffered previous myocardial infarctions.[54] Of those who have normal resting electrocardiograms, the yield of positive exercise tests relates to the nature of the test done and the criteria used for interpretation. Perhaps as many as 30 to 50 per cent will have negative double Master's tests, but as the intensity of the exercise is increased (e.g., by ergometry), the yield of positive tests is also increased. The use of multiple leads, as well as recording during exercise, will also increase the yield of positive tests.[5]

Coronary arteriography is an effective way of evaluating the pathological status of the coronary arteries during life. It is safe and relatively simple in trained hands. Typical exertional angina, especially with a positive exercise test, correlates with a positive arteriographic study to the extent of 95 per cent[66] or better. Unless surgery is being contemplated, therefore, it is not necessary to perform coronary arteriography on this group of patients. When the angina is atypical, however, correlation falls to 65 per cent. Angina at rest correlates to the extent of 79 per cent.

A reasonable group of indications for coronary arteriography was recently discussed by Abrams and Adams.[1] Their criteria centered around the atypical patient and the surgical patient. Any patient presenting with one or more atypical features of angina should be considered for coronary arteriography. This includes atypical age (the young patient), atypical pain, typical pain in the absence of electrocardiographic documentation, and electrocardiographic findings in the absence of pain. When a patient with valvular heart disease has angina and is being considered for surgery, coronary arteriograms should be performed since coronary disease will influence the operative risk. Finally, coronary arteriography is necessary to evaluate the nature and distribution of coronary disease when coronary artery surgery is being contemplated, and to evaluate the results of such surgery.

It is sometimes difficult to correlate the arteriographic picture of the coronary arteries with the clinical picture of the patient. Lesions of borderline size, or the absence of lesions in vessels large enough to be resolved by ciné equipment, frequently cause a dilemma. In such settings, a metabolic approach to the evaluation of myocardial oxygenation may be of value. The normally oxygenated myocardium consumes lactate.[12, 60] This is reflected by the fact that the aortic lactate concentration is higher than the coronary sinus lactate concentration in the resting patient with normal coronary blood flow and distribution.[63, 64]

In patients subject to attacks of angina pectoris, however, the production of angina by a tachycardia induced by atrial pacing is usually associated with a marked elevation of the coronary sinus lactate concentration,[63] with little or no change in the aortic concentration. The production of lactate, S-T segment depression, and depression of ventricular function usually precede the onset of pain under these conditions. During exercise-induced angina, the coronary sinus lactate concentration generally remains below the aortic concentration, although both levels rise significantly.[64] Nonetheless, the left ventricular end diastolic pressure rises and the S-T segments are depressed prior to the onset of angina. The failure to demonstrate lactate production by the myocardium during exercise-induced angina may result from metabolic changes induced by the exercise, obscuring the ischemic metabolism of abnormal areas of myocardium.

These metabolic and hemodynamic approaches to the evaluation of the patient with angina are clinically useful in demonstrating abnormalities, other than coronary atherosclerosis, hypertension, and valvular disease, which may result in the angina syndrome. Of current interest is the delineation of syndromes producing angina which may be related to abnormalities of oxyhemoglobin dissociation[19] or primary abnormalities of myocardial metabolism.[61] Angina pectoris occurring in patients having arteriographically normal coronary arteries, and presumably caused by such metabolic abnormalities, could be associated with abnormalities of lactate metabolism by the myocardium.

TREATMENT OF ANGINA PECTORIS

A general consideration enters into the management of all patients who have angina pectoris. This involves the management of precipitating factors. Many patients are able to identify a number of triggering activities or situations, and are able to abort pain by ceasing such activities or taking nitroglycerin prior to the onset of an attack.

The nature of these events may be emotional or physical, and cover a broad range of activities or feelings, but may be quite specific in a given patient. These should be identified by the physician and patient. In some instances, anxiety-preventing agents may be of value. The patient's activities and participation in individual or organized exercise programs must be balanced against his tolerance for such activities.

Physical activity certainly enhances a patient's general feeling of well-being, and may actually improve exercise tolerance. Pushed to the point of producing symptoms, however, exercise becomes a hazard. Serious arrhythmias and transient ventricular function abnormalities may occur.

Tobacco consumption and obesity should be controlled if possible for the well-being of the patient.

Nitrites

The mechanism of the action of the nitrites in the relief of angina pectoris is still not completely understood. The major effect of the nitrites on the vascular system is relaxation of vascular smooth muscle, resulting in vasodilatation in peripheral as well as in coronary beds. However, there has been some discussion as to whether it is the coronary vasodilatation itself, or the fall in systemic blood pressure incident upon decreased peripheral resistance, which is primarily responsible for relief of angina pectoris. A third and more subtle hypothesis suggests an alteration of myocardial metabolism resulting in more effective oxygenation.[44, 50, 67, 68]

Coronary vasodilatation as the mechanism of action of the nitrites is a simple and desirable hypothesis. There is no question that the drugs do have the ability to dilate the coronary vessels directly, and possibly indirectly.[50, 91] Unfortunately, however, several strong arguments have

Table 4. *Treatment of Angina Pectoris*

Management of precipitating factors
Nitroglycerin and long-acting nitrites
Beta-adrenergic blocking agents
Carotid sinus nerve stimulation
Surgical approaches

been raised against the acceptance of this mechanism. The increase in coronary blood flow resulting from the administration of nitrites is only transient,[22, 58] and is exceeded in duration by the fall in systemic blood pressure.[58, 88] After the initial increase in coronary blood flow,[88] there is a tendency for the coronary blood flow to fall.[6, 36, 88]

Counter to this evidence is the widely used suggestion that the regional increase in blood flow in diseased areas or via collateral vessels may not be apparent by our current methods of estimating total coronary blood flow. Some experimental evidence has been accumulated to suggest that nitrites do indeed act primarily on collaterals to areas of decreased blood flow,[23, 24] implying that such increases may not be reflected in total coronary blood flow. However, it is well-known that hypoxia is an extremely powerful stimulus to vasodilatation, and the ability of the vessels in ischemic areas to further dilate must be questioned.[88] The existence of such conflicting arguments leaves the concept of the vasodilator mechanism of action of nitrites in a tenuous position.

The nitrites have a complex systemic effect, triggered primarily by peripheral vasodilatation. Pooling of blood in the systemic circulation,[27, 43, 44, 70, 77] as well as in the pulmonary circulation,[27] results in a decreased venous return with reduction of ventricular volume and diastolic filling pressure.[34, 89] This decreased preload on the ventricle reduces oxygen demand. Moreover, the concomitant decrease in arterial pressure, against which the heart must work, results in a decrease in myocardial wall tension, another major determinant of oxygen demand.[72] Pooling of blood peripherally and decreased arterial pressure result in a reflex tachycardia.[44] The net effect is a somewhat decreased cardiac output.[2, 6, 27, 77]

The onset of an attack of angina pectoris is frequently preceded by or concomitant with an increase in blood pressure or tachycardia or both.[75, 76] Both of these are oxygen-consuming factors. Therefore, it is reasonable to assume that mechanisms which decrease oxygen consumption, such as decreased venous return and decreased arterial pressure as outlined above, should play some role in the mechanism of action of the nitrites. Perhaps this acts in concert with regionally increased oxygen delivery.

The short-acting drug, nitroglycerin, remains the primary nitrite in clinical use. Administered in sublingual doses of 1/400 (0.16 mg.) to 1/150 (0.1 mg.) grain, it affords prompt relief to many patients having angina attacks. The drug has been in use a long time and is well known to the medical profession. However, several points in its use are worthy of emphasis.

The drug does tend to lose potency over a period of time, and this can be confused with loss of effectiveness. The patient who uses nitroglycerin only occasionally should be advised to purchase only small amounts of the drug and replenish his supply every 3 months. Many patients will have relief of attacks with a dose of 1/400 grain (0.16 mg.) of a potent preparation. This dose level may avoid unpleasant side-effects, and should be used when possible instead of the more commonly used 1/200 grain (0.32 mg.)

Nitroglycerin also has some value as a prophylactic drug. Many patients are able to identify accurately the amount of exercise or the situations in which an angina attack is precipitated. These patients should be instructed to try to abort such attacks with the drug prior to the onset of pain.

Finally, in the occasional patient in whom angina is precipitated or intensified by nitroglycerin, it is essential to rule out the presence of idiopathic hypertrophic subaortic stenosis.[8, 11]

A number of preparations of long-acting, orally administered nitrites have been introduced in the hope of providing a means of reducing the frequency and intensity of anginal attacks. The experience with these agents has been debatable at best.[88] Individual patients seem to have some response to these drugs, but their general effectiveness has been disappointing. Isosorbide dinitrate currently seems to be the best of the group. The dose level must be tailored to the individual patient. Treatment is begun with 5 mg. three times a day and the daily dosage increased in 5 mg. increments until a dose of 10 mg. four times daily is achieved, or until headache or postural hypotension force termination of the increments at a lower dosage level. Isosorbide dinitrate and the beta-adrenergic blocking agent, propranolol, may be a combination of particular value.[4, 78]

Beta-Adrenergic Blocking Agents

The use of beta-adrenergic blocking agents in patients with angina pectoris has been studied,[13, 20, 28, 30-33, 38, 41, 48, 69, 84] and results have been encouraging. Official approval of its use for this purpose is still forthcoming.

The determinants of myocardial oxygen demand are multiple, and include the contractile state of the myocardium, myocardial wall tension, and heart rate, as three primary factors.[9, 39, 47, 56, 57, 59, 62, 73, 79, 83] Clinically useful indices of change in myocardial oxygen demand are the tension time index[62, 79] and the simpler but less accurate product of heart rate and blood pressure.[47, 71] When a beta-adrenergic blocking agent is used in doses sufficient to depress the myocardium and thereby decrease myocardial oxygen demand, there is a decrease in heart rate, contractile state of the myocardium, stroke volume, left ventricular dp/dt, and ejection period.[20] Moreover, there is depression of the positive inotropic and chronotropic response to exercise.[16] The net effect, reflected by the change in tension-time index, is a decrease in cardiac work and oxygen consumption which seems to override the decrease in coronary flow that these drugs cause.[90]

The dose level of propranolol, when used for the treatment of angina pectoris, is variable. Maximum effect may be achieved with as little as 10 mg. orally four times daily when the drug is used in combination with a nitrite.[4, 78] On the other hand, it may be necessary to approach the range of 200 to 400 mg. daily in some patients.[29] The usual cautions in the use of beta-adrenergic blocking agents must be observed in these patients.[85] These include the problem of congestive heart failure, bradycardia, worsening of asthma and pulmonary hypertension, and intensification of hypoglycemic tendencies.

Other Drugs

Angina may be aggravated by mild or latent congestive heart failure. Angina decubitus is particularly likely to be associated with left ventricular failure. A careful search for heart failure should be made in all patients having angina decubitus or intractable exertional angina. A trial of digitalis is often rewarding in these settings.

The emotional responses to stresses of daily life commonly precipitate angina attacks in the vulnerable patient. The anxiety-preventing agents may be used to dull the intensity and decrease the frequency of such emotional responses. Their use will not be uniformly successful, and they should not be considered routine therapy.

The production of hypothyroidism in troublesome cases of angina pectoris[45, 53, 65] is not used as often today as in the past. However, the procedure is still of value in selected cases. Radioactive iodine is the method of choice.

Carotid Sinus Nerve Stimulation

Carotid sinus massage and the Valsalva maneuver may abort attacks of angina pectoris.[51] Because of this clinical observation, carotid sinus nerve stimulation, using a surgically implanted radiofrequency stimulator, has been a recent approach to the management of angina pectoris.[7, 21, 55] Bipolar electrodes are attached to both carotid sinus nerves and connected to a receiving unit implanted subcutaneously. An external induction coil attached to a battery-powered signal generator is used by the patient to activate the stimulator when he experiences or anticipates an attack of angina. Carotid sinus nerve stimulation reflexly causes peripheral arteriolar vasodilatation, thereby decreasing blood pressure and myocardial wall tension. It also decreases heart rate and depresses the contractile state of the myocardium. These three major determinants of oxygen demand are depressed during stimulation to a combined degree probably not achieved with nitrites or with beta-adrenergic blocking agents.[55]

The role of carotid sinus nerve stimulation in the management of angina pectoris is difficult to assess. Obviously, the risk of general anaesthesia in these patients is significant, and therefore it should not be considered in patients whose angina is controllable by means of drug therapy. Patients whose lesions are amenable to some of the newer coronary artery surgery techniques (see below) might also be excluded from consideration in centers where adequate surgical facilities and personnel are available. Thus we are left with a group of patients who have uncontrollable angina, and whose lesions are not amenable to direct surgery, in whom carotid sinus nerve stimulation might be used.

Surgery

Internal mammary artery implants for myocardial revascularization have been given extensive trials.[3, 25, 26, 37, 87] While it is clear that a functioning implant can decrease lactate production in ischemic areas,[37] indicating a return to aerobic metabolism, present data does not demonstrate a change in the natural history of the disease as a result of the procedure. Only 54 per cent of patients in one series having postoperative visualization studies[26] showed run-off from the implant into previously existing coronary vessels. While perhaps 70 per cent or more of the patients undergoing the procedure show symptomatic improvement,[3] it must be remembered that 60 per cent of those having a sham procedure[15] showed improvement by placebo effect. In view of these facts, the 5 to 10 per cent mortality of the procedure and the 10 per cent myocardial infarction rate[25] seem a high price to pay.

Two new surgical procedures, however, seem promising. The vein graft by-pass procedures, in which one or more saphenous vein grafts are interposed between the aorta and coronary arteries distal to segmental obstructions, provide immediate revascularization. The mortality rate is less than 5 per cent,[18] and the early results of the effectiveness of the procedure look promising. A procedure similar in concept, employing an internal mammary artery to coronary artery by-pass, is also being tried.[17] This may be used in combination with saphenous vein graft by-pass.

The other new procedure being investigated is gas endarterectomy.[81, 86] While the value of by-pass techniques is limited to segmental lesions, gas endarterectomy can be used in more diffuse lesions of the right coronary artery. Carbon dioxide is used to establish the natural plane of cleavage between the atherosclerotic core and the remainder of the vessel. By so doing, the high subsequent thrombosis rate, seen with earlier endarterectomy techniques, might be avoided. Gas endarterectomy provides immediate revascularization to ischemic areas, as do the bypass techniques.

REFERENCES

1. Abrams, H. L., and Adams, D. F.: The coronary arteriogram: Structural and functional aspects. New Eng. J. Med., *281*:1276, 1969.
2. Afonso, S., Rowe, G. G., Lowe, W. C., and Crumpton, C. W.: Systemic and coronary hemodynamic effects of isosorbide dinitrate. Amer. J. Med., *246*:584, 1963.
3. Anonymous: Coronary Surgery Surveyed. J.A.M.A., *206*:1010, 1968.
4. Aranow, W. S., and Kaplan, M. A.: Propranolol with isosorbide dinitrate versus placebo in angina pectoris. New Eng. J. Med., *280*:847, 1969.
5. Bellet, S., and Muller, O. F.: The electrocardiogram during exercise: Its value in the diagnosis of angina pectoris. Circulation, *32*:477, 1965.
6. Brachfeld, N., Bozer, J., and Gorlin, R.: Action of nitroglycerin on the coronary circulation in normal and in mild cardiac subjects. Circulation, *19*:697, 1959.
7. Braunwald, E., Epstein, S. E., Glick, G., Wechsler, A. S., and Braunwald, N. S.: Relief of angina pectoris by electrical stimulation of the carotid-sinus nerves. New Eng. J. Med., 277:1279, 1969.
8. Braunwald, E., Lambrew, C. T., Rockoff, S. D., Ross, J., Jr., and Morrow, A. G.: Idiopathic hypertrophic subaortic stenosis: Description of the disease based upon an analysis of 64 patients. Circulation, 29(Suppl. IV):1, 1964.
9. Britman, N. A., and Levine, H. J.: Contractile element work: A major determinant of myocardial oxygen consumption. J. Clin. Invest., *43*:1397, 1964.
10. Cheng, T. O.: Some new observations on the syndrome of papillary muscle dysfunction. Amer. J. Med., 47:924, 1969.
11. Cohen, L. S., and Braunwald, E.: Amelioration of angina pectoris in idiopathic hypertrophic subaortic stenosis with beta-adrenergic blockage. Circulation, 35:847, 1967.
12. Cohen, L. S., Elliott, W. C., Klein, M. D., and Gorlin, R.: Coronary heart disease: Clinical, cinearteriographic and metabolic correlations. Amer. J. Cardiol., *17*:153, 1966.
13. Conn, R. D., and Bruce, R. A.: The efficiency of beta-adrenergic blockade in angina pectoris. Clin. Res., *15*:92, 1967.

14. Dimond, E. G.: Precordial vibrations: Clinical clues from palpitation. Circulation, 30:284, 1964.
15. Dimond, E. G., Kittle, C. F., and Crockett, J. E.: Comparison of internal mammary artery ligation and sham operation for angina pectoris. Amer. J. Cardiol., 5:483, 1960.
16. Dwyer, E. M., Jr., Wiemer, L., and Cox, J. W.: Effects of beta-adrenergic blockade (propranolol) on left ventricular hemodynamics and the electrocardiogram during exercise-induced angina pectoris. Circulation, 38:250, 1968.
17. Edwards, W. S., Jones, W. B., Dean, H. D., and Kerr, A. R.: Direct surgery for coronary artery disease. Technique for left anterior descending coronary artery bypass. J.A.M.A., 211:1182, 1970.
18. Effler, D. B., Favaloro, R. G., and Groves, L. K.: Coronary artery surgery utilizing saphenous vein graft techniques. J. Thor. Cardiovasc. Surg., 59:147, 1970.
19. Eliot, R. S., and Bratt, G. T.: Paradox of myocardial ischemia and necrosis in young women with normal coronary arteriograms: Relationship to anomalous hemoglobin-oxygen dissociation. Amer. J. Cardiol., 21:98, 1968.
20. Elliott, W. C., and Stone, J. M.: Beta-adrenergic blocking agents for the treatment of angina pectoris. Prog. Cardiovasc. Dis., 12:83, 1969.
21. Epstein, S. E., Beiser, G. D., Goldstein, R. E., et al.: Treatment of angina pectoris by electrical stimulation of the carotid-sinus nerves. New Eng. J. Med., 280:971, 1969.
22. Essex, H. E., Wigria, R., Herrick, J. F., and Mann, F. C.: The effect of certain drugs on the coronary blood flow of the trained dog. Amer. Heart J., 19:554, 1940.
23. Fam, W. M., and McGregor, M.: Effect of coronary vasodilator drugs on retrograde flow in area of chronic myocardial ischemia. Circulation Res., 15:355, 1964.
24. Fam, W. M., and McGregor, M.: Effect of nitroglycerin and dipyridamole on regional coronary resistance. Circulation Res., 22:649, 1968.
25. Favaloro, R. G., Effler, D. B., Groves, L. K., Sones, F. M., and Fergusson, D. J. G.: Myocardial revascularization by internal mammary artery implant procedures: Clinical experience. J. Thorac. Cardiovasc. Surg., 54:359, 1967.
26. Fergusson, D. J., Shirey, E. K., Sheldon, W. C., Effler, D. B., and Sones, F. M., Jr.: Left internal mammary artery implant. Postoperative assessment. Circulation, 37(Suppl. II):24, 1968.
27. Ferrer, M. I., Bradley, S. E., Wheeler, H. O., Enson, Y., Preisig, R., Brickner, P. W., Conroy, R. J., and Harvey, R. M.: Some effects of nitroglycerin upon the splanchnic, pulmonary and systemic circulations. Circulation, 33:357, 1966.
28. Fitzgerald, J. D., and Grant, R. E. H.: The treatment of angina pectoris by propranolol (Inderal). Cardiologia, 49:49, 1966.
29. Frieden, J.: Propranolol as an antiarrhythmic agent. Amer. Heart J., 74:283, 1967.
30. Gillam, P. M. S., and Prichard, B. N. C.: Use of propranolol in angina pectoris. Brit. Med. J., 2:337, 1965.
31. Gillam, P. M. S., and Prichard, B. N. C.: Propranolol in the therapy of angina pectoris. Amer. J. Cardiol., 18:366, 1966.
32. Ginelly, R. E., Goldman, R. H., Treister, B., and Harrison, D. C.: Propranolol in patients with angina pectoris. Ann. Intern. Med., 67:1216, 1967.
33. Ginn, W. M., and Orgain, E. S.: Propranolol hydrochloride in the treatment of angina pectoris. J.A.M.A., 198:1214, 1966.
34. Goldberg, L. I.: Pharmacology of cardiovascular drugs. In: Hurst, J. W., and Logue, R. B., eds.: The Heart. New York, McGraw-Hill, 2nd ed., 1970, ch. 101.
35. Gorlin, R.: Pathophysiology of cardiac pain. Circulation, 32:138, 1965.
36. Gorlin, R., Brachfeld, N., MacLeod, C., and Bopp, P.: Effects of nitroglycerin on coronary circulation in patients with coronary artery disease or increased left ventricular work. Circulation, 19:705, 1959.
37. Gorlin, R., and Taylor, W. J. Selective revascularization of the myocardium by internal-mammary-artery implant. New Eng. J. Med., 275:283, 1966.
38. Grandjean, T., Hamer, N. J., Sowton, G. E., and Melendez, L.: The effect of propranolol (Inderal) on effort tolerance in angina pectoris. Cardiologia, 49:57, 1966.
39. Graham, T. P., Jr., Covell, J. W., Sonnenblick, E. H., Ross, J., Jr., and Braunwald, E.: Control of myocardial oxygen consumption: Relative influence of contractile state and tension development. J. Clin. Invest., 47:375, 1968.
40. Hale, G., Dexter, D., Jefferson, K., and Leatham, A.: Value of coronary arteriography in the investigation of ischemic heart disease. Brit. Heart J., 28:40, 1966.
41. Hamer, J., Grandjean, T., Melendez, L., and Sowton, G. E.: Effect of propranolol (Inderal) in angina pectoris: Preliminary report. Brit. Med. J., 2:720, 1964.
42. Heberden, W.: Some account of a disorder of the heart. M. Tr. Roy. Coll. Phys., 2:59, 1772.
43. Hirshleifer, I.: A pharmacodynamic approach to the evaluation of nitrites in the treatment of angina pectors. Amer. J. Cardiol., 5:66, 1960.
44. Honig, C. R., Tenny, S. M., and Gabel, P. V.: The mechanism of cardiovascular action of nitroglycerine. Amer. J. Med., 29:910, 1960.

45. Jaffe, H. L., and Corday, E.: The radioactive iodine treatment of angina pectoris. Prog. Cardiovasc. Dis., 3:108, 1960.
46. James, T. N.: Pathology of small coronary arteries. Amer. J. Cardiol., 20:679, 1967.
47. Katz, L. N., and Feinberg, H.: Relation of cardiac effort to myocardial oxygen consumption and coronary flow. Circulation Res., 6:656, 1958.
48. Keelan, P.: Double-blind trail of propranolol (Inderal) in angina pectoris. Brit. Med. J., 1:897, 1965.
49. Kemp, H. G., Elliott, W. C., and Gorlin, R.: The anginal syndrome with normal coronary arteriography. Trans. Assoc. Amer. Physicians, 80:59, 1967.
50. Krantz, J. C., Jr., Carr, C. J., and Bryant, H. H.: Alkyl nitrites: XIV. The effect of nitrites and nitrates on arterial adenosine triphosphatase. J. Pharmacol. Exper. Therap., 102:16, 1951.
51. Levine, H. J., McIntyre, K. M., and Glovsky, M. M.: Relief of angina pectoris by Valsalva maneuver. New Eng. J. Med., 275:487, 1966.
52. Likoff, W., Segal, B. L., and Kasparian, H.: Paradox of normal selective coronary arteriograms in patients considered to have unmistakable coronary heart disease. New Eng. J. Med., 276:1063, 1967.
53. Logue, B.: Treatment of intractable angina pectoris. Circulation, 22:1151, 1960.
54. Logue, R. B., and Hurst, J. W.: Clinical recognition of coronary atherosclerotic heart disease and its complications. In: Hurst, J. W., and Logue, R. B.: The Heart. New York, McGraw-Hill, 1970.
55. Mason, D. T., Spann, J. F., Zelis, R., and Amsterdam, E.: Physiologic approaches to the treatment of angina pectoris. New Eng. J. Med., 281:1225, 1969.
56. McDonald, R. H.: Developed tension: A major determinant of myocardial oxygen consumption. Amer. J. Physiol., 201:351, 1966.
57. McDonald, R. H., Jr., Taylor, R. R., and Cingolani, H. E.: Measurement of myocardial developed tension and its relation to oxygen consumption. Amer. J. Physiol., 211:667, 1966.
58. Melville, K. I., Gillis, R. A., and Sekelj, P.: Coronary flow, blood pressure, heart rate dose-response changes after nitroglycerin administration. Canad. J. Pharmacol., 43:9, 1965.
59. Monroe, R. G., and French, G. N.: Left ventricular pressure-volume relationships and myocardial oxygen consumption in the isolated heart. Circulation Res., 9:362, 1961.
60. Neill, W. A.: Myocardial hypoxia and anaerobic metabolism in coronary heart disease. Amer. J. Cardiol., 22:507, 1968.
61. Neill, W. A., Kassebaum, D. G., and Judkins, M. P.: Myocardial hypoxia as the basis for angina pectoris in a patient with normal coronary arteriograms. New Eng. J. Med., 279:789, 1968.
62. Neill, W. A., Levine, H. J., Wagman, R. J., and Gorlin, R.: Left ventricular oxygen utilization in intact dogs: Effects of systemic hemodynamic factors. Circulation Res., 12:163, 1963.
63. Parker, J. O., Chiong, M. A., West, R. O., and Case, R. B.: Sequential alterations in myocardial lactate metabolism, S-T segments, and left ventricular function during angina induced by atrial pacing. Circulation, 40:113, 1969.
64. Parker, J. O., West, R. O., Case, R. B., and Chiong, M. A.: Temporal relationships of myocardial lactate metabolism, left ventricular function, and S-T segment depression during angina precipitated by exercise. Circulation, 40:97, 1969.
65. Paul, O.: Intractable angina. Progr. Cardiovas. Dis., 6:212, 1963.
66. Proudfit, W. L., Shirey, E. K., and Sones, F. M.: Selective cine coronary arteriography: Correlation with clinical findings in 1000 patients. Circulation, 33:901, 1966.
67. Raab, W., and Lepeschkin, E.: Antiadrenergic effects of nitroglycerin on the heart. Circulation, 1:733, 1950.
68. Raab, W., Van Lith, P., Lepeschkin, E., and Herrlich, H. C.: Catecholamine-induced myocardial hypoxia in the presence of impaired coronary dilatability independent of external cardiac work. Amer. J. Cardiol., 9:455, 1962.
69. Rabkin, R., Stables, D. P., Levine, N. W., and Suzman, M. M.: The prophylactic value of propranolol in angina pectoris. Amer. J. Cardiol., 18:370, 1966.
70. Robin, E., Cowan, C., Puri, P., Ganguly, S., Deboyrie, E., Martinez, M., Stock, T., and Bing, R. J.: A comparative study of nitroglycerin and propranolol. Circulation, 36:175, 1967.
71. Robinson, B. F.: Relation of heart rate and systolic pressure to the onset of pain in angina pectoris. Circulation, 35:1075, 1967.
72. Rodbard, S., Williams, C. B., Rodbard, D., and Berglund, E.: Myocardial tension and oxygen uptake. Circulation Res., 14:139, 1964.
73. Rodbard, S., Williams, F., and Williams, C.: The spherical dynamics of the heart (Myocardial tension, oxygen consumption, coronary blood flow and efficiency). Amer. Heart J., 57:348, 1959.
74. Ross, R. S., and Friesinger, C. G.: Coronary arteriography. Amer. Heart J., 72:437, 1966.

75. Roughgarden, J.: Circulatory changes associated with spontaneous angina pectoris. Amer. J. Med., *41*:947, 1966.
76. Roughgarden, J. W., and Newman, E. V.: Circulatory changes during the pain of angina pectoris: 1772–1965 – A critical review. Amer. J. Med., *41*:935, 1966.
77. Rowe, G. G., Chelius, C. J., Afonso, S., Gurtner, H. P., and Crumpton, C. W.: Systemic and coronary hemodynamic effects of erythrol tetranitrate. J. Clin. Invest., *40*:1217, 1961.
78. Russek, H. I.: Propranolol and isosorbide dinitrate synergism in angina pectoris. Amer. J. Cardiol., *21*:44, 1968.
79. Sarnoff, S. J., Braunwald, E., Welch, G. H., Case, R. B., Stainsby, W. N., and Macruz, R.: Hemodynamic determinants of oxygen consumption of the heart with special reference to the tension-time index. Amer. J. Physiol., *192*:148, 1958.
80. Sawayama, T., Marumto, S., Nicki, I., and Matsura, T.: The clinical usefulness of the amyl nitrite inhalation test in the assessment of the third and atrial heart sounds in ischemic heart disease. Amer. Heart J., *76*:746, 1968.
81. Sawyer, P. N., Kaplitt, M., Sobel, S., Karlson, K. E., Studkey, J., Wechsler, B. M., Summers, D. N., and Dennis, C.: Experimental and clinical experience with coronary gas endarterectomy. Arch. Surg., *95*:736, 1967.
82. Skinner, N. S., Leibeskind, R. S., Phillips, H. L., and Harrison, T. R.: Angina pectoris: Effects of exertion and nitrites on precardial movements. Amer. Heart J., *61*:250, 1961.
83. Sonnenblick, E. H., Ross, J., Jr., and Braunwald, E.: Oxygen consumption of the heart: Newer concepts of its multifactoral determination. Amer. J. Cardiol., *22*:328, 1968.
84. Srivastava, S. C., Dewar, H. A., and Newell, D. J.: Double-blind trial of propranolol (Inderal) in angina of effort. Brit. Med. J., *2*:724, 1964.
85. Stephen, S. A.: Unwanted effects of propranolol. Amer. J. Cardiol., *18*:463, 1966.
86. Urschel, H. C., Jr., Razzuk, M. A., Miller, E. R., Alvares, J. F., and Paulson, D. L.: Vein bypass graft and carbon dioxide gas endarterectomy for coronary artery occlusive disease. J.A.M.A., *210*:1725, 1969.
87. Vineberg, A., and Walker, J.: Six months to six years' experience with coronary artery insufficiency treated by internal mammary artery implantation. Amer. Heart J., *54*:851, 1957.
88. Weisse, A. B., and Regan, T. J.: The current status of nitrites in the treatment of coronary artery disease. Progr. Cardiovas. Dis., *12*:72, 1969.
89. Williams, J. F., Jr., Glick, G., and Braunwald, E.: Studies on cardiac dimensions in intact unanesthetized man. V. Effects of nitroglycerin. Circulation, *32*:767, 1965.
90. Witsitt, L. S., and Lucchesi, B. R.: Effects of propranolol and its stereoisomers upon coronary vascular resistance. Circulation Res., *21*:305, 1967.
91. Wolf, M. M., and Berne, R. M.: Coronary vasodilator properties of purine and pyrimidine derivatives. Circulation Res., *4*:343, 1956.

Miami Veterans Administration Hospital
Miami, Florida 33125

Treatment of Arrhythmias: Basic Considerations

Kenneth C. Lasseter, M.D.*

The current understanding of the mechanisms by which pharmacologic agents produce beneficial effects in disorders of cardiac rhythm is based largely on relatively recent studies of the effects of these agents on the electrical activity of single cardiac fibers. In the intact organism, the beneficial effects of the drug may not only be due to such direct actions, but also mediated through indirect mechanisms such as the autonomic nervous system. Although it is likely that there are other mechanisms yet to be elucidated, the rational therapeutic approach to cardiac arrhythmias requires an understanding of this information and the similarities and differences in the action of the various antiarrhythmic agents. To facilitate such a discussion, a brief review of the electrophysiology of single cardiac fibers will be presented as it pertains to the normal and abnormal generation and propagation of the wave of excitation through the myocardium.

ELECTROPHYSIOLOGY OF THE CARDIAC CELL

If a single cell of a cardiac fiber is impaled with a glass microelectrode such that the potential difference between the interior and exterior of the cell can be recorded, a potential difference of approximately 90 mV., inside negative, is recorded (Fig. 1). This resting membrane potential (RMP) is maintained by the active metabolic activity of the cell and is directly related by the Nernst equation to the ratio of intracellular to extracellular potassium concentration (for review see Hoffman and Cranefield[18]). The resting membrane potential of atrial and ventricular muscle fibers normally remains stable until the depolarization of adjacent cells by the normal spread of excitation. However, the cells of the sinoatrial node and most specialized conducting tissues undergo slow spontaneous depolarization during diastole, until the threshold potential is reached and the self-generative spike depolarization (phase 0) of the action potential (AP) is initiated.

---

*Postdoctoral Fellow, Department of Pharmacology

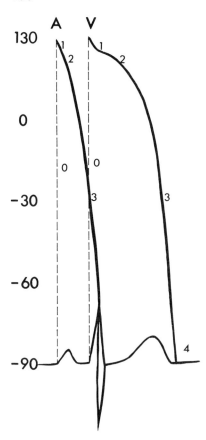

Figure 1. Diagram of atrial (A) and ventricular (V) action potential superimposed on the electrocardiogram. Dashed lines mark upstroke of action potentials. Numbers at the left designate transmembrane potential in millivolts. Phases of action potentials are designated by numbers 0 to 4 (see text). Resting membrane potential of both fibers is approximately −90 mV. Note that the duration of the ventricular action potential corresponds to the QRS complex, S-T segment, and T wave. (*From* Surawizz, B., and Lasseter, K. C.: Prog. Cardiovasc. Dis., *13*:26, 1970. Reproduced with permission.)

The dominant pacemaker of the heart is normally the sinoatrial node because the rate of spontaneous (phase 4) depolarization is more rapid than that of other tissues. Such phase 4 depolarization is probably due to a slow, time-dependent decay of potassium conductance.[34] The sudden spike depolarization of phase 0 of the action potential is due to a decrease in sodium permeability with a rapid influx of sodium ion into the cell.[11] This depolarization spreads through adjacent fibers and down the specialized conducting system to produce the "wave of excitation" normally responsible for the initiation of orderly contraction of all myocardial fibers.

The conduction velocity of this wave of excitation is dependent largely on the maximum upstroke velocity of phase 0 of the action potential in the fibers involved, which is in turn dependent on the resting membrane potential. The upstroke velocity and conduction velocity of most of the specialized conducting fibers is considerably faster than that of the atrial or ventricular muscle fibers, accounting in part for the normal spread of excitation. This spread of depolarization is recognized in the body surface electrocardiogram (ECG) as the P wave for atrial fibers and the QRS complex for the depolarization of ventricular muscle fibers. Only the interval between atrial and ventricular activation (PR interval) or the sequence of ventricular activation (such as in bundle branch block) reflect the specialized conducting system, since the mass of tissue is not sufficient to produce a deflection in the ECG.

Following depolarization, the process of repolarization is initiated rapidly with phase 1 of the action potential and then more slowly with phase 2 or the plateau of the action potential. This relatively stable period of repolarization is more prolonged in the Purkinje fibers than in the ventricular muscle fibers and is probably due to a balance between inward Na^+ and Ca^{++} currents and outward K^+ current.[26] The rapid phase 3 of repolarization is primarily due to outward K^+ current. The summation of repolarization of the atrial fibers accounts for the T_p wave (usually lost in the QRS complex) and that of ventricular fibers for the ST segment and T wave of the ECG.

During phases 1 and 2 of repolarization in any cardiac fiber, the arrival of a further depolarizing stimulus (either exogenously or endogenously produced) has no significant effect on the time course of repolarization; i.e., the tissue is refractory and cannot be excited. During phase 3 of repolarization the tissue begins to recover excitability, initially with local graded responses and then with a fully propagated depolarization or premature action potential. The interval from the basic spike depolarization until the earliest possible propagated premature action potential is termed the effective refractory period (ERP) and has considerable importance in the action of antiarrhythmic drugs.

It is apparent that the effective refractory period can be altered either by changes in the action potential duration or by changes in the level of repolarization necessary to produce a propagated response. Both of these mechanisms are commonly encountered with most antiarrhythmic agents. The level of repolarization necessary to give rise to a propagated premature response may be related to recovery of the sodium ion carrying mechanism. Such recovery is usually described by the relationship between the upstroke velocity of phase 0 of the action potential and the membrane potential at activation. This relationship, first described by Weidman[36] in 1955 as "membrane responsiveness," is affected by many antiarrhythmic agents. A shift of this S-shaped curve down and to the right will produce a decrease in the membrane potential at which an action potential with a given upstroke velocity can arise. If one assumes that some critical recovery of the Na^+ carrying (or Na^+ permeability) mechanism is necessary for the generation and propagation of premature impulses, then such a shift could contribute to the prolongation of the effective refractory period.

When considering the genesis of cardiac arrhythmias only two basic mechanisms are generally acknowledged:

1. Ectopic impulse formation due to accelerated phase 4 depolarization in some part of the specialized conducting system other than sinoatrial nodal tissues. Such ectopic pacemaker activity may be either regular or irregular.

2. Re-entrant type phenomena resulting from disorders in conduc-

tion such that the spread of excitation is blocked (or delayed) in some localized area which can then be activated by depolarization of tissue distal to the block. It is easiest to conceptualize such a phenomenon if one considers the conduction disturbance as "uni-directional," such that after a certain critical time, activation can spread in a retrograde fashion finding tissues that have recovered excitability and produce an ectopic beat.[19] This type of activity can be terminated after a single beat, or a pathway for circus movement producing multiple responses or fibrillation can occur.

QUINIDINE

Quinidine has probably been the most important therapeutic agent in the treatment of cardiac arrhythmias during this century and has often been considered the prototype of the antiarrhythmic agents. The drug decreases automaticity of isolated Purkinje fibers by decreasing the slope of diastolic depolarization.[17, 36] This direct effect also decreases the rate of impulse formation in the sinoatrial node in denervated preparations; however, in the intact organism the anticholinergic effects of the drug usually predominate, resulting in either no charge or slight acceleration of the sinus rate.[20]

In Purkinje fibers, the depression of phase 4 depolarization is seen at concentrations that have essentially no other effect on the action potential configuration. This effect not only tends to suppress automatic rhythms, but also may enhance conduction by allowing the fibers to be activated at a higher (more negative) membrane potential. At slightly higher but still therapeutic concentrations, quinidine decreases the rate of rise of the upstroke of the action potential in all cardiac fibers, and prolongs the action potential duration (APD) in atrial and ventricular fibers by decreasing the slope of phase 3.[14, 17, 21] This effect on the action potential duration is associated with a prolongation of the effective refractory period in the atria and ventricles. In addition, the membrane responsiveness curve is shifted down and to the right,[36] and this may be related to the prolongation of the effective refractory period such that the ratio $\triangle APD/\triangle ERP$ is less than 1.

These effects of quinidine on the electrophysiologic properties of cardiac tissue suggest several possible explanations for the drug's beneficial effects in patients with cardiac arrhythmias. It is apparent that in arrhythmias due to ectopic impulse formation, quinidine may suppress the accelerated phase 4 depolarization and abolish the arrhythmia. This may also be effective in certain re-entrant type arrhythmias, since if the area of delayed conduction is due to phase 4 depolarization, this may allow that area to be activated at a higher membrane potential, enhancing conduction and abolishing the arrhythmia.

Prolongation of the effective refractory period may abolish other re-entrant-type arrhythmias since the "re-entrant pathway" may become refractory at the critical time. Since re-entrant phenomena presuppose some conduction disturbance, the effect of quinidine in depressing the upstroke velocity of the action potential and conduction velocity may be quantitatively greater in this affected area, possibly producing "block" in the retrograde direction and thus abolishing the arrhythmia.

It is immediately apparent, however, that if one extends these observations to more toxic concentrations of quinidine, which depress conduction (and widen the QRS complex significantly) disproportionately with respect to the prolongation of the effective refractory period, the re-entrant pathway may recover excitability prior to the arrival of the "re-entrant activation wave" and favor the establishment of arrhythmias. Hence we have at least one explanation of the mechanism for the well-known phenomenon of arrhythmias in quinidine toxicity.[12, 29]

Even at therapeutic concentrations, quinidine has the undesirable effect of depressing contractility of the myocardium, perhaps by decreasing the permeability of the cell membrane to Ca^{++} during the plateau of the action potential. Quinidine may also produce ventricular ectopic beats, ventricular tachycardia, and ventricular fibrillation, which are not dose-dependent and may occur after the first few doses. These are presumably idiosyncratic reactions.[29]

The cellular mechanisms whereby quinidine produces these several electrophysiologic effects are not certain. The effects on the upstroke of the action potential are presumably due to decreased permeability of the cell membrane to Na^+ during this phase of the action potential. The prolonged duration of the action potential and decreased phase 4 depolarization is presumably due to decreased permeability to potassium ion and the prolonged effective refractory period owing to a combination of these effects with the shift of the membrane responsiveness curve.

PROCAINAMIDE

The effects of procainamide on the electrophysiologic properties of the heart are essentially identical to those of quinidine.[17, 36] Procainamide supresses phase 4 depolarization in Purkinje fibers, decreases the upstroke velocity of the action potential in all types of cardiac fibers, prolongs the action potential duration in ventricular muscle and Purkinje fibers, but prolongs the effective refractory period to a greater degree than the action potential duration. The drug also shifts the "membrane responsiveness" curve to the right and downward. Procainamide does not decrease the rate of spontaneous depolarization in the sinus node but increases the sinus rate apparently through an anticholinergic mechanism similar to that of quinidine.

Procainamide is a shorter acting drug than quinidine, being primarily excreted unchanged or detoxified by plasma esterases. The toxic effects of the drugs on the heart are similar; however, the production of drug-induced systemic lupus erythematosus by procainamide is well recognized. It should be apparent that procainamide and quinidine have similar spectra of usage from their similar electrophysiologic effects. Although some clinicians have favored the use of procainamide for ventricular arrhythmias and quinidine for atrial arrhythmias, the effectiveness of the two drugs appear to be about the same in the treatment of both atrial and ventricular arrhythmias.

LIDOCAINE

This local anesthetic has been used widely in the treatment of acute ventricular arrhythmias, particularly those associated with acute myocardial infarction, cardiac surgery, and digitalis intoxication. Only a few atrial arrhythmias have been responsive to lidocaine. Even if the drug proved effective in larger doses, the intravenous route of administration and the rapid metabolism of the drug would make it of limited usefulness in supraventricular arrhythmias.

The electrophysiologic effects of lidocaine on the heart have recently been reported, and it is apparent that this agent differs significantly from quinidine or procainamide. Lidocaine suppresses both spontaneous and catecholamine-induced phase 4 depolarization in isolated Purkinje fibers at concentrations thought to be comparable to therapeutic concentrations in man (2 to 5 mg. per ml.)[5, 10] At these concentrations the drug has little or no effect on the upstroke velocity of the action potential or on membrane responsiveness, but significantly shortens the action potential duration and effective refractory period of both ventricular muscle and Purkinje fibers. Although this latter effect is opposite to that of quinidine or procainamide, the shortening of the APD is relatively greater than the shortening of the ERP, so that the ratio $\Delta APD/\Delta ERP$ is less than 1, as has been noted for quinidine and procainamide.

This relationship is particularly interesting in that it seems to be one of the few common denominators among all drugs effective against cardiac arrhythmias. It is both fascinating and perplexing that lidocaine, which shares with quinidine and procainamide features of structure thought to be responsible for antiarrhythmic activity, produces the same alteration in this relationship through exactly opposite electrophysiological effects, and with little if any effect on membrane responsiveness. For this reason, it has been suggested that lidocaine may be effective in clinical situations in which quinidine and procainamide are not, and that the reverse may also be true.

Lidocaine shares with other antiarrhythmic agents the undesirable property of depressing myocardial contractility. Nevertheless, the brief duration of the drug's action (due to rapid hepatic metabolism) make this a more desirable agent than longer acting drugs in congestive heart failure. Reports of toxic reactions to lidocaine are restricted primarily to the central nervous system, and include drowsiness, paresthesias, muscle twitching, disorientation, and seizures.

DIPHENYLHYDANTOIN

This drug, long used in the treatment of seizure disorders and structurally related to the barbiturates, has recently been emphasized as an important addition to the armamentarium of antiarrhythmic agents. This is due at least in part to the fact that the electrophysiologic effects of the drug differ significantly from quinidine-like drugs.

Therapeutic concentrations of diphenylhydantoin decrease automaticity of Purkinje fibers by decreasing the slope of diastolic depolarization, but do not affect sinoatrial tissues until considerably higher concentrations are reached.[6, 32] The upstroke velocity of the action potential and the conduction velocity were unchanged by the drug in normal Purkinje fibers.[6] However, in fibers that were partially depolarized and had decreased upstroke velocity of the action potential and conduction velocity, these parameters were increased by the drug, and in such fibers the membrane responsiveness curve was shifted to the left.[6] This obviously striking difference from quinidine or procainamide is supported by observations that diphenylhydantoin enhances atrioventricular conduction in intact animals and in man.[7, 27] Similar to lidocaine, diphenylhydantoin shortens the action potential duration and the effective refractory period in Purkinje fibers and ventricular muscle fibers, but the relative shortening of the effective refractory period is less, so that the ratio $\Delta APD/\Delta ERP$ is less than 1.[5, 10] From these observations, one would predict that diphenylhydantoin is an effective agent in the treatment of cardiac arrhythmias due to either mechanisms of re-entry of ectopic impulse formation.

These different electrophysiologic effects of diphenylhydantoin, compared to those of quinidine or procainamide, suggest that this agent might be effective in some situations in which the latter are ineffective. It also suggests that the drug can be used in combination with quinidine or procainamide without producing the atrioventricular and intraventricular conduction defects that might be induced by higher doses of those drugs alone. The effect of the agents on diastolic depolarization is certainly additive.[16] It has also been suggested that an antiarrhythmic agent, such as diphenylhydantoin, which enhances atrioventricular conduction would be much safer in digitalis-induced arrhythmias than agents which might hinder atrioventricular conduction. Toxic cardiovascular manifestations have been reported after intravenous administration of diphenylhydantoin; however, the mechanisms for such effects are not clear.[8, 13, 28, 33]

PROPRANOLOL

The antiarrhythmic properties of this agent appear to result from a combination of effects: (1) beta-adrenergic receptor blockade, inhibiting adrenergic stimulation of the heart; and (2) direct action on the electrophysiologic properties of the myocardium. The effects produced by the first of these mechanisms can reasonably be predicted from the effects of adrenergic stimulation on the heart. These include increased sinus rate due to accelerated phase 4 depolarization in sinoatrial nodal tissues, accelerated diastolic depolarization in Purkinje fibers, enhanced conduction velocity, and shortening of the effective refractory period. Such adrenergically mediated alterations can lead to the development of tachyarrhythmias which are reversed by beta-blockade.[15] The electrophysiologic effects of beta-blockade are more pronounced in the atrial conductive and nodal tissues than in Purkinje fibers.[30]

In addition to these beta-blocking actions, propranolol exerts direct effects on the electrophysiologic properties of the myocardium. Propranolol decreases the upstroke velocity of the action potential in Purkinje fibers and in ventricular muscle fibers, shortens the action potential duration and effective refractory period in Purkinje fibers (ΔAPD/ΔERP is less than 1), and shifts the membrane responsiveness curve to the right.[9] In addition, propranolol markedly decreases diastolic depolarization in isolated Purkinje fibers, at concentrations which have no other effect on the action potential configuration.[9] It is apparent that these electrophysiologic effects are different than those of any of the previously discussed agents, and are intermediate between those of quinidine and diphenylhydantoin. It is interesting to note that the beta-blocking agent MJ 1999 (Sotolol), thought to possess little direct membrane activity, alters the action potential duration and effective refractory period to produce a ΔAPD/ΔERP ratio greater than 1.[31]

A great deal of clinical investigation has approached the question of which action of propranolol (the beta-blocking or direct) is responsible for the drug's beneficial effects in various arrhythmias. It would appear that in arrhythmias not produced by digitalis, either of these actions can be of importance, depending on the clinical circumstances.[24] Arrhythmias associated with excessive sympathetic activity, such as those precipitated by emotional stress, exercise, or during anesthesia, are largely antagonized by the beta-blocking action, while those not accompanied by excessive sympathetic discharge are controlled by the direct action of the drug. In digitalis-induced tachyarrhythmias (in which propranolol is particularly effective), current evidence suggests that the direct action of the drug is most important since pretreatment with a d-propranolol (with little beta-blocking action) is as effective as dl-propranolol in preventing ouabain-induced arrhythmias in experimental animals.[23, 25]

Unfortunately, propranolol produces deleterious hemodynamic effects that are more pronounced than those of most other antiarrhythmic agents. The drug produces a marked negative inotropic effect on the myocardium which may lead to abrupt decompensation of the failing heart. This may be related to the inhibitory action of the drug on the enzyme adenylcyclase, reducing the formation of cyclic AMP and in turn decreasing the cell membrane permeability to calcium.[22]

BRETYLIUM TOSYLATE

The status of this drug in the antiarrhythmic armamentarium is not entirely clear at the present time. The drug has been shown to spontaneously abolish ventricular fibrillation and to decrease vulnerability to electrically induced ventricular fibrillation in dogs.[2] Clinical studies with the drug are not extensive, but in refractory ventricular fibrillation parenteral bretylium tosylate has allowed successful countershock to sinus rhythm.[3]

The electrophysiologic effects of bretylium on the myocardium have only been sparsely reported. The upstroke velocity of the action potential and the conduction velocity are increased, and the action potential duration and effective refractory period are shortened.[35] It is apparent that these effects are quite different from those of quinidine-like drugs and are similar to those of diphenylhydantoin. Of greater interest is the fact that this drug, unlike any other antiarrhythmic agent, exerts a positive inotropic effect, perhaps by sensitizing the myocardium to endogenous catecholamines.[1] If, indeed, bretylium tosylate does prove to be a useful antiarrhythmic agent, the latter property will be unique and of great value.

PHARMACOLOGIC APPROACH TO ARRHYTHMIAS

The rational therapeutic approach to cardiac arrhythmias is greatly impeded by the lack of ability to classify electrocardiographic entities according to their basic electrophysiologic genesis. Recent techniques promise to yield more information on this pertinent point.[4] In the interim, one can only utilize the best deductive reasoning concerning the probable mechanisms encountered in any given clinical situation, and combine this with what is known about the action of available pharmacologic agents to arrive at the most rational therapeutic program. Fortunately, in many acute situations the procedures of direct-current countershock or electrical overdrive by transvenous pacing, or both, have such broad therapeutic applications that success may be predicted without a thorough evaluation of the mechanisms involved. However, the maintenance of such patients after the acute episode may require a more in-depth analysis.

One source of indirect information concerning problematic arrhythmias is the determination of a pharmacologic profile for any given patient and arrhythmia. This may include determining the response to cholinergic and adrenergic stimulating and blocking agents (for most of which rapid-acting, short-duration drugs are available) and the response to antiarrhythmic agents of basically different actions. One may infer from the responses to these various maneuvers what the probable mechanisms may be and what therapeutic regime is most likely to meet with success. The practical significance of such an approach may actually exceed that which could be achieved on theoretical grounds alone.

REFERENCES

1. Amsterdam, E. A., Spann, J. F., Jr., Mason, D. T., and Zelis, R.: Characterization of the positive inotropic effects of bretylium tosylate; a unique property of antiarrhythmic agent. Amer. J. Cardiol. (in press).
2. Bacaner, M. B.: Quantitative comparison of bretylium with other antifibrillatory drugs. Amer. J. Cardiol., 21:504, 1968.
3. Bacaner, M. B.: Treatment of ventricular fibrillation and other acute arrhythmias with bretylium tosylate. Amer. J. Cardiol., 21:530, 1968.
4. Bigger, J. T., Jr., and Goldreyer, B. N.: The mechanism of supraventricular tachycardia. Circulation, 42:673, 1970.
5. Bigger, J. T., Jr., and Mandel, W. J.: Effect of lidocaine on the electrophysiological properties of ventricular muscle and Purkinje fibers. J. Clin. Invest., 49:63, 1970.
6. Bigger, J. T., Jr., Bassett, A. L., and Hoffman, B. F.: Electrophysiological effects of diphenylhydantoin on canine Purkinje fibers. Circ. Res., 22:221, 1968.
7. Bigger, J. T., Jr., Schmidt, D. H., and Kutt, H.: Relationship between the plasma level of diphenylhydantoin sodium and its cardiac antiarrhythmic effects. Circulation, 38:363, 1968.

8. Conn, R. D.: Diphenylhydantoin sodium in cardiac arrhythmias. New Eng. J. Med., 272: 277, 1965.

9. Davis, L. D., and Tempte, J. V.: Effects of propranolol on the transmembrane potentials of ventricular muscle and Purkinje fibers of the dog. Circ. Res., 22:661, 1968.

10. Davis, L. D., and Tempte, J. V.: Electrophysiological actions of lidocaine on canine ventricular muscle and Purkinje fibers. Circ. Res., 24:639, 1969.

11. Deck, K. A., and Trautwein, W.: Ionic currents in cardiac excitation. Pflueger Arch., 280:63, 1964.

12. Finnegan, T. R. L., and Trounce, J. R.: Depression of the heart by quinidine and its treatment. Brit. Heart J., 16:341, 1954.

13. Gellerman, G. L., and Martinez, C.: Fatal ventricular fibrillation following I.V. sodium diphenylhydantoin therapy. J.A.M.A., 200:337, 1967.

14. Gettes, L. S., Surawicz, B., and Shiue, J. C.: Effect of high potassium, low potassium, and quinidine on QRS duration and ventricular action potential. Amer. J. Physiol., 203:1135, 1962.

15. Gibson, D., and Sowton, E.: The use of beta-adrenergic receptor blocking drugs in dysrythmias. Progr. Cardiovasc. Dis., 12:16, 1969.

16. Helfant, R. H., Scherlag, B. J., and Damato, A. N.: The electrophysiological properties of diphenylhydantoin sodium as compared to procainamide in the normal and digitalis intoxicated heart. Circulation, 36:108, 1967.

17. Hoffman, B. F.: The action of quinidine and procainamide on single fibers of dog ventricle and specialized conducting system. Anais. Acad. Brasil. Cienc., 29:365, 1958.

18. Hoffman, B. F., and Cranefield, P. F.: Electrophysiology of the Heart. New York, McGraw Hill, 1960.

19. Hoffman, B. F., and Cranefield, P. F.: The physiological basis of cardiac arrhythmias. Amer. J. Med., 37:670, 1964.

20. James, T. N., and Nadeau, R. A.: The mechanism of action of quinidine on the sinus node studied by direct perfusion through its artery. Amer. Heart J., 67:804, 1964.

21. Johnson, E.: The effects of quinidine, procainamide and pyrilamine on the membrane resting and action potential of guinea pig ventricular muscle fibers. J. Pharmacol., 117:237, 1956.

22. Levine, R. A., and Vogel, J. A.: Cardiovascular and metabolic effects of adenosine 3,5-monophosphate in vivo. Nature, 207:987, 1965.

23. Lucchesi, B. R., Whitsitt, L. S., and Stickney, J. L.: Antiarrhythmic effects of beta-adrenergic blocking agents. Ann. N.Y. Acad. Sci., 139:940, 1969.

24. Mason, D. T., Spann, J. F., Jr., Zelis, R., and Amsterdam, E. A.: The clinical pharmacology and therapeutic applications of the antiarrhythmic drugs. Clin. Pharm. Therap., 11:460, 1970.

25. Parmely, W. W., and Braunwald, E.: Comparative myodardial depressant and antiarrhythmic properties of d-propranolol, dl-propranolol and quinidine. J. Pharmacol., 158:11, 1967.

26. Reuter, H.: Slow inactivation of currents in cardiac Purkinje fibers. J. Physiol. (Lond.), 197:233, 1968.

27. Rosati, R., Alexander, J. A., Schaal, S. F., and Wallace, A. J.: Influence of diphenylhydantoin on electrophysiological properties of the canine heart. Circ. Res., 21:757, 1967.

28. Rosen, M., Lisak, R., and Rubin, I. L.: Diphenylhydantoin in cardiac arrhythmias. Amer. J. Cardiol., 20:674, 1967.

29. Seltzer, A., and Wray, H.: Quinidine syncope; paroxysmal ventricular fibrillation occurring during treatment of chronic atrial arrhythmias. Circulation, 30:17, 1964.

30. Singer, D. H., Yeh, B. K., Scherlag, B. J., and Hoffman, B. F.: Beta blockade in the specialized conduction system of the heart. Circulation, 29(Suppl. 3):160, 1964.

31. Strauss, H. C., Bigger, J. T., Jr., and Hoffman, B. F.: Electrophysiological and beta receptor blocking effects of MJ1999 on dog and rabbit cardiac tissue. Circ. Res., 26:661, 1970.

32. Straus, H. C., Bigger, J. T., Jr., Bassett, A. L., and Hoffman, B. F.: Actions of diphenylhydantoin on the electrical properties of isolated rabbit and canine atria. Circ. Res., 23:463, 1968.

33. Unger, A. H., and Sklaroff, H. J.: Fatalities following I.V. use of sodium diphenylhydantoin for cardiac arrhythmias. J.A.M.A., 200:335, 1967.

34. Vassalle, M.: Analysis of cardiac pacemaker potential using a "voltage clamp" technique. Amer. J. Physiol., 210:1335, 1966.

35. Watanabe, Y., Josipovic, V., and Dreifus, L.: Electrophysiological mechanisms of bretylium tosylate. Fed. Proc., 28:270, 1969.

36. Weidman, S.: The effects of calcium ions and local anesthetics on electrical properties of Purkinje fibers. J. Physiol. (Lond.), 129:568, 1955.

Department of Pharmacology
University of Miami School of Medicine
P.O. Box 875, Biscayne Annex
Miami, Florida 33152

Airway Obstruction

Jose S. Bocles, M.D.,* and Roberto Llamas, M.D.**

Airway obstruction can be defined simply as obstruction of airflow within the lungs. Emphysema, chronic bronchitis, and asthma are the most common causes of this syndrome, and this presentation will refer exclusively to these clinical entities.

Despite multiple efforts by the American Thoracic Society,[7] the World Health Organization,[8] and the British Medical Research Council Committee,[19] the definition of these diseases is still confusing. This ambiguity stems mainly from a different set of criteria for defining chronic bronchitis and emphysema. Chronic bronchitis, as will be seen later, is defined in clinical terms and hence is relatively easy to recognize during life. Emphysema is mostly defined in anatomical terms and there is no commonly accepted criteria to diagnose it in the living patient.

DEFINITIONS

Chronic bronchitis is defined as chronic excessive production of mucus in the airways, usually associated with cough not due to known specific causes such as bronchiectasis, tuberculosis, etc. This should occur for at least three months in the year for 2 or more successive years. Chronic bronchitis is commoner in men than women, is more prevalent during middle age, and affects about 20 per cent of adult males although most of them are not overly symptomatic.[12]

The bronchial glands are enlarged in bronchitis and there is an increased number of goblet cells. As a result there is excessive secretion of mucus. When the size of the bronchial glands is measured and compared to the size of the bronchial wall, a ratio known as the Reid index is obtained.[28] If this index is high, the patient most likely will have bronchitis.

Emphysema is defined as an anatomic alteration of the lung char-

---

*Clinical Assistant Professor of Medicine, University of Miami School of Medicine, Miami, Florida

**Clinical Assistant Professor of Medicine, University of Miami School of Medicine; Associate Director, Cardiopulmonary Laboratory, Miami Heart Institute, Miami Beach, Florida

acterized by abnormal enlargement of the airspaces distal to the non-respiratory bronchiole, accompanied by destructive changes of the alveolar walls.

Bronchial asthma is a syndrome manifested by paroxysmal dyspnea and wheezing not necessarily related to exertion and usually resulting from a hypersensitivity reaction of the bronchial tree in predisposed individuals. These clinical manifestations are reversible either spontaneously or by proper treatment.

The clinical, physiological, roentgenological, pathological and laboratory features of typical cases of chronic bronchitis, chronic obstructive pulmonary emphysema, and bronchial asthma are summarized in Table 1. We should emphasize that in clinical practice, many of the patients with airway obstruction have combinations of features described in Table 1. This is particularly observed in the chronic bronchitic and emphysematous groups.

ACUTE RESPIRATORY FAILURE IN OBSTRUCTIVE AIRWAY DISEASE

Acute respiratory failure in patients with chronic airway obstruction has become an increasingly recognized medical emergency.

The clinical diagnosis of acute respiratory failure is difficult in many instances. The signs and symptoms of hypoxemia and carbon dioxide retention, such as somnolence, mental confusion, tachycardia, and twitching of extremities, are nonspecific. Correlation between these symptoms and signs and the degree of hypoxemia and hypercarbia is particularly poor in the patients with chronic airway obstruction.[27] Accurate diagnosis of acute ventilatory failure should be established by examination of the level of oxygen, carbon dioxide tension, and pH of the arterial blood. Radial arterial puncture or cannulation are safe and simple procedures for obtaining repeated arterial blood samples.[18, 22]

TREATMENT OF REVERSIBLE FACTORS

The patient with chronic airway obstruction and acute respiratory failure has some reversible factors that should be promptly corrected. These reversible features are: bronchospasm and bronchial narrowing due to edema and retained secretions, pulmonary infection (bronchitis, bronchiolitis, pneumonia), hypoxemia, hypercapnia, and right heart failure.

Management of Hypoxemia

The causes of arterial hypoxemia in patients with chronic airway obstruction and acute respiratory failure are ventilation-perfusion inequalities, underventilation, and right to left shunts.[4, 10]

The level of arterial oxygen tension which constitutes significant hypoxemia is difficult to establish. It is then, advisable, to aim for a normal Po_2 (80 to 100 mm. Hg) during oxygen therapy, although in practice this is not always feasible. Special attention should be paid to those patients whose respiratory control depends mostly on a hypoxic drive. Many of these patients have chronic carbon dioxide retention, and the administration of oxygen in an uncontrolled fashion carries the risk of further carbon dioxide retention and narcosis.

A sound practice is to monitor the response of carbon dioxide to controlled oxygen therapy before higher concentrations are administered. Usually a compromise between a satisfactory level of oxygen tension and a limited elevation of carbon dioxide tension can be achieved. In practice, an arterial oxygen tension of 60 mm. Hg rarely results in significant retention of carbon dioxide.

The method of controlled oxygen therapy described by Campbell is based on the premise that in severely hypoxemic patients, the arterial blood lies in the steep part of the oxygen dissociation curve; hence, a small increase in Po_2 will produce a larger increase in oxygen saturation and content, and a larger amount of oxygen will be delivered to the tissues by blood.[6] Thus, an elevation of arterial oxygen tension from 25 to 40 mm. Hg will increase oxygen saturation from 40 to 70 per cent. These results can be accomplished by increasing the inspired oxygen concentration by 4 to 7 per cent.

Different methods are available at present to provide controlled oxygen therapy and the principle applied is that of high airflow with known concentration of oxygen enrichment. The Ventimask popularized by Campbell produces a fixed concentration of oxygen which depends on the structure of the mask.[6] It is available in three types that deliver concentrations of 24, 28, and 35 per cent depending on the degree of air entrainment. This mask is confortable and cool to wear and the carbon dioxide is washed out by the constant gas flow. Disadvantages of this mask are that it has to be removed to eat or drink, and that the elastic used to hold it very often cuts the patient behind the ears.

Oxygen can also be effectively delivered by a two-pronged cannula which usually is comfortable to the patient.[16]

Management of Bronchospasm

The term "bronchospasm" encompasses not only the abnormal contraction of the bronchial musculature but also edema and inflammation of the bronchial mucosa and the presence of retained secretions.[9] The therapeutic goal should be to decrease airway obstruction by reversing the bronchospasm.

EPINEPHRINE. It is the drug of choice for the severe bronchospasm developed by asthmatics, whereas it is usually ineffective and sometimes hazardous in the other entities discussed here. In acute situations, 0.3 ml. of a 1:1000 aqueous epinephrine solution can be repeated every 10 to 15 minutes up to 1.5 ml. of the solution. Palpitations, nervousness, weakness, insomnia, and tachycardia are the most frequent side-effects, and epinephrine should not be used in patients with significant hypertension, cardiac disease, or hyperthyroidism. Alkalinizing agents should precede it if acidosis is detected, since there appears to be evidence that epinephrine is ineffective when the pH is acid, secondary either to respiratory or metabolic acidosis. We do not advocate the use of the epinephrine oil suspension because of the possible prolonged side-effects.

Table 1. *Characteristics of Patients with Asthma, Chronic Bronchitis and Emphysema*

	ASTHMATIC	BRONCHITIC	EMPHYSEMATOUS
Synonyms	Atopic asthma Allergic asthma	Blue bloater Non-fighter Type B Tussive Wet	Pink puffer Fighter Type A Dyspneic Dry
Family history	Atopic diseases	Unremarkable	Unremarkable
Appearance	Indistinct	Usually obese	Thin or history of weight loss
Age of onset	Usually in childhood	Third decade	Fourth decade
Early and prominent symptoms	Usually preceded by other atopic entities (allergic rhinitis, atopic dermatitis, etc.), spasmodic cough or acute bronchospasms with symptom-free intervals	Productive cough Frequent colds	Dyspnea on exertion
Sputum	Usually mucoid and scanty	Copious, purulent, or muco-purulent	None or scanty mucoid
Physical Examination Chest configuration	Usually unremarkable	Unremarkable	Barrel
Lungs: Tactile fremitus	Normal	Normal	Diminished
Resonance	Normal	Normal	Increased
Breath sounds	Normal	Normal	Diminished
Adventitious sounds	Rhonchi, wheezes (during attacks)	Wheezes	Rare
Right ventricular failure	Absent	Frequent	Rare
Heart, percussion	Normal	Increased	Normal
Peripheral edema	Absent	Frequent	Rare
Cyanosis	Rare	Frequent	Rare

Laboratory Findings			
Electrocardiogram	Normal	Right ventricular hypertrophy	Normal or right axis deviation
Hematocrit	Normal	Elevated	Normal
Chest x-ray:			
Lungs	Usually unremarkable	Increased bronchovascular markings at bases, or normal	Hyperlucent
Diaphragms	Normal	Normal or high	Low, flat
Pulmonary vasculature	Normal	Increased at bases or normal	Diminished at periphery
Hilar regions	Normal	Enlarged	Enlarged
Retrosternal space	Normal	Normal	Increased
Heart	Normal	Enlarged	Small, vertical
Physiological Findings			
Airway obstruction	Variable and reversible	Marked	Marked
Vital capacity	Variable	Decreased	Decreased or normal
Residual volume	Variable	Increased	Markedly increased
Total lung capacity	Variable	Usually normal or slightly decreased	Markedly increased
Diffusion	Normal	Usually normal	Decreased
Ventilation	Usually increased	Decreased	Increased
Blood gases, oxygen	Decreased during paroxysms	Decreased	Normal or slightly decreased
Carbon dioxide	Normal or decreased (rarely increased)	Increased	Normal
Cardiac output	Normal	Normal or increased	Subnormal
Pathology			
Prominent changes	Mucus plugs Curschmann's spirals Charcot Leyden Crystals Eosinophils	Hyperplasia and hypertrophy of bronchial glands	Destructive emphysematous changes
Alveolar walls	No destruction	No destruction	Marked destruction
Pulmonary vessels	Normal	No significant changes	Marked destruction
Right ventricle	Normal	Thickened	Normal

AMINOPHYLLINE. It is a very potent bronchodilator and it also stimulates the respiratory center. It can be administered by the intravenous route, by suppository, or as a retention enema. The dosage should not exceed 2 gm. daily, and if injected undiluted (250 to 500 mg.) intravenously it should be given no faster than 25 mg. per minute because of possible cardiac arrhythmias, especially in hypoxic patients.

CORTICOSTEROIDS. Their anti-inflammatory effects are most effective in diminishing bronchospasms. In acute situations, we prefer the intravenous route, which subsequently might be complemented or replaced by oral administration. The dosage will vary depending on the seriousness of the condition. In general, 300 mg. of hydrocortisone daily, or its equivalent, should be given during the first 2 days. Thereafter, gradual tapering is necessary to prevent relapses. Supplemental potassium and antacids will minimize possible hypokalemia and gastrointestinal bleeding.

OTHER AGENTS. *Iodide preparations* can be used intravenously or orally as expectorants. We have found retention enemas of *ether in oil* quite effective in relieving bronchospasm.

In cases of severe respiratory or metabolic acidosis, among the advocated alkalinizing agents, our choice is sodium bicarbonate solution. Monitoring of the arterial pH will indicate the necessary amount.

RESPIRATORY STIMULANTS. They have been of very limited value in our hands and we have used them only for a very short period of time in patients with carbon dioxide narcosis, until the other therapeutic measures reduced the carbon dioxide levels. There is still controversy about the usefulness of ethamivan and nikethamide.

HANDLING OF SECRETIONS. Secretions retained in the distal airways predispose to patchy atelectasis, ventilation-perfusion inequalities, reduction in lung compliance, and infection. Since secretions are usually abundant, dry, and sticky in patients with acute respiratory failure, and the cough reflex is suppressed, the following measures can be taken to help clear secretions.

Liquefaction of sputum. Hydration of the patient by intravenous infusion and humidification of the inspired gas are usually sufficient to liquify secretions. If the patient has an artificial airway, inspired gas should be continuously humidified to avoid inspissation of secretions in the tracheostomy or endotracheal tube. The value of the so-called mucolytic agents is questionable in acute respiratory failure. These agents may produce significant side-effects, particularly additional bronchospasm in asthmatics.

Stimulation of cough can be accomplished by pharyngeal suction or a plain aerosolized saline solution administered either by an IPPB machine or an ultrasonic nebulizer.

Postural drainage is usually poorly tolerated by the patient in acute respiratory failure. Tilting the head of the bed down is enough, since the bases of the lungs are the areas of the lung that commonly accumulate secretions. Chest tapping may be of additional benefit when abundant secretions are present.

Bronchoscopy. If the above measures fail, bronchoscopy should be considered. Its main value, in the authors' experience, is the productive cough that practically always occurs during and after the procedure. Bronchoscopy is poorly tolerated by hypoxic patients, and cardiac arrhythmias may develop if enough oxygen is not provided during the procedure.

Management of Infection

Pneumonia, bronchitis, and bronchiolitis are commonly the precipitating factors of acute ventilatory failure in patients with chronic airway obstruction. The most common infecting organisms in this group of patients are H. influenzae and D. pneumonia.[11] The type of antibiotics chosen should cover both organisms. H. influenzae is sensitive to streptomycin, ampicillin, and tetracycline. The pneumococcus responds to penicillin, tetracycline and erythromycin.

Since many patients are now being treated with tetracycline on ambulatory basis, it is better to avoid this antibiotic during the acute episode and administer either ampicillin (2 to 4 gm. daily) or sodium cephalothin (6 to 12 gm. daily) or a combination of penicillin and streptomycin. In patients with penicillin allergy, erythromycin or lincomycin can be used. Gram-negative infections frequently develop secondarily in patients with artificial airway and on prolonged positive pressure breathing. Pseudomonas superinfection arising from contaminated mainstream nebulizers has been extensively documented in the literature.[29] Sodium colistimethate (systemically or by aerosol), gentamycin and carbenicillin are the antibiotics presently available against pseudomonas. Their value in completely erradicating pseudomonas pulmonary infection and their efficiency in prolonged usage have still to be established.

Management of Right Heart Failure

Cor pulmonale frequently accompanies chronic bronchitis.[14] Both hypoxia and acidosis, commonly seen in this type of airway obstruction, produce pulmonary hypertension. By correcting the factors responsible for hypoxia and acidosis, right heart failure will improve. Because of significant toxic effects, especially cardiac arrhythmias, and questionable benefits during acute respiratory failure, digitalis preparations should be used cautiously, and after the factors responsible for the heart failure (hypoxia and acidosis) are improved. Diuretics (thiazides, ethacrynic acid, and furosemide) can be used initially, but electrolytes should be carefully monitored. In patients with secondary polycythemia, phlebotomy will also help to alleviate the strain on the right heart.

ESTABLISHMENT OF AN ARTIFICIAL AIRWAY

Hypercarbia is the principal indication for mechanical ventilation. In the emergency situation, any of the self-inflating resuscitation bags is all that is needed to ventilate the patient properly either via an endotracheal tube or a pharyngeal airway. At this point if prolonged respiratory support is foreseen, a decision should be made about type of artificial airway (endotracheal tube vs. tracheostomy) and kind of respirator to be used.

Endotracheal Intubation

If the decision is made to place an endotracheal tube, its diameter should be as large as can safely and readily be passed through the glottis and it should be equipped with an inflatable cuff. The end of the tube should be above the carina. This can be checked very easily by auscultation of the breath sounds in the upper anterior chest. The cuff should be inflated just enough to stop air leakage.

We usually limit the time of endotracheal intubation to about 48 hours; by this time the reversible factors mentioned above have been corrected and the patient can usually be extubated. If further ventilation is necessary, tracheostomy in an operating room under general anesthesia should be considered as an elective procedure.

Management of the Patient Receiving Prolonged Artificial Ventilation

First of all, the patient should be cared for in a special unit where experienced physicians and nurses are at attendance and where diagnostic and therapeutic equipment are available. Respiratory Care Units are now as necessary to treat this patient properly as Coronary Care Units have been for patients with acute myocardial infarction.

Frequent physical examinations, laboratory studies, and roentgenological studies are advised if complications are to be promptly discovered. Specially designed charts to be used by physicians and nurses have been found by the authors to be extremely helpful for both patient care and education of personnel.[2]

Mechanical Ventilatory Aids

Mechanical ventilators are used to increase alveolar ventilation and to decrease the work of breathing. Ventilators can be used as assistors, controllers, or assistor-controllers. The assistor is triggered by the drop in the patient's airway pressure during an inspiratory effort. The controller functions independent of the patient's respirations, and the assistor-controller can either control the patient's breathing automatically or assist him when he breathes on his own.

Types of Respirators

1. Pressure-cycled respirators assist ventilation during inspiration by positive pressure with a passive phase during expiration. Peak inspiratory pressures can be adjusted. The respiratory rate during assisted ventilation is determined by the patient. The main limitation of pressure-cycled respirators is that in some patients they may be unable to deliver the volumes required to maintain effective ventilation.

2. Volume-cycled respirators deliver a predetermined volume even in the presence of high resistance to inflation.

If the patient is to be controlled, the patient's own respiratory efforts must not be allowed to interfere with the respirator. This can be achieved effectively by administering morphine intravenously in small doses every 5 minutes until the desired effect is obtained. The ventilatory requirements of patients requiring artificial ventilation are increased above normal.[25] Nomographs to calculate the needed tidal volume in patients with normal lungs are not reliable when dealing with acute respiratory failure.[26] The only way to maintain a normal carbon dioxide tension is to measure this tension frequently in arterial blood and adjust the volume of the ventilator accordingly.

Maintenance of Gas Exchange

Intrapulmonary right to left shunting and uneven distribution of ventilation are present in the majority of patients receiving artificial ventilation. The large majority of patients will be well oxygenated with concentrations of 30 to 40 per cent. Most modern volume ventilators are equipped with controls to adjust the oxygen concentration desired from 20 to 100 per cent.

While good oxygenation is maintained, gradual lowering of the arterial carbon dioxide tension can be achieved. Precipitous decrease in Pco_2 can be catastrophic by producing ventricular arrhythmias, convulsions, and shock.[30, 33] Once the ideal ventilatory pattern is established, follow-up by repeated arterial blood gas analysis will offer the most reliable information of the patient's progress.

Correction of Acid-Base Abnormalities

During or after the use of controlled or assisted ventilation for the correction of respiratory acidosis, the appearance of an elevated pH is frequently observed. This alkalemia results from the use of diuretics, corticosteroids, and sodium bicarbonate. The acid-base picture produced is that of a hypochloremic and hypokalemic alkalosis. The administration of potassium chloride will both correct the metabolic component produced by potassium deficiency and will provide enough chloride to return bicarbonate in plasma to normal levels.[31]

Weaning From the Respirator

A premature attempt or a delayed decision in weaning the patient from the respirator should be avoided. An attempt should be made as soon as possible, since the respiratory muscles can become weak during prolonged artificial ventilation; but an unjudicious premature separation from the ventilator can produce a recurrence to respiratory failure. Most patients will tolerate weaning off the respirator if the vital capacity is twice the tidal volume or more. Weaning is initiated by taking the patient off the respirator for periods of 5 minutes every half hour, and progressively increasing the off periods as tolerated by the patient.

Humidified oxygen should always be administered to the patient during the off periods, and respiratory support should be provided during the night at the initial phase of the weaning period.

AMBULATORY CARE

PATIENT AND FAMILY EDUCATION.   Extremely helpful to the patient and relatives is a general description of the disease and its complications. Several publications are available to the public. These are very informative and will stimulate further discussion with the physician and assistants.[21, 32]

The reversible components of the disease should be emphasized, as well as the importance of the immediate care when exacerbations occur.

A skillful and understanding physician will greatly relieve the frequent and intense frustration, depression, and despair that these patients display. These emotional factors will probably benefit more from a close patient-physician relationship than from sedatives or tranquilizers.

ENVIRONMENTAL FACTORS. In recent years, intensive public education regarding the harmful effects of smoking has yielded beneficial results. Avoidance of specific irritants (fumes, industrial dusts, cold air) should be emphasized. In cases of atopic asthma, investigation of extrinsic allergens (house dust, pollens, molds, etc.) will help the physician to recommend preventive and therapeutic measures.

ETIOLOGIC FACTORS. Skin tests should be obtained in cases of atopic asthma, and hyposensitization treatments applied. Also, in these patients any possible source of infection, especially sinusitis, should be investigated and treated.

INFLUENZA VACCINATION. Polyvalent influenza virus A and B vaccine should be given every year during the fall.

ANTI-INFECTIVE AGENTS. Broad-spectrum antibiotics, such as ampicillin or tetracycline, should be prescribed to patients with chronic airway obstruction whenever there are signs or symptoms of respiratory tract infection. If no improvement occurs after 3 days, sputum cultures and sensitivities should be done.

Ancillary measures will include strict or partial bed rest, large amounts of oral fluids, and an increase of the amount of bronchodilators that the patient is taking routinely. In case of tenacious bronchial secretions, steam inhalation preceded by aerosolized bronchodilators and postural drainage are extremely helpful. A short-term course of corticosteroids can be used when bronchospasm is a prominent feature.

PROPHYLACTIC ANTIBIOTICS. Some authors advocate systematic prophylactic broad-spectrum antibiotics during the fall and winter months, while others are opposed because of possible secondary infections (pseudomonas, klebsiella) which might be very difficult to control. We justify their use prophylactically in patients with a history of frequent respiratory infections and a significant amount of purulent expectoration (bronchitic type).

BRONCHODILATORS. Most of the commercial oral bronchodilators contain ephedrine, aminophylline, theophylline or derivatives. Ephedrine can produce urinary retention and central nervous system stimulation.

The xanthines, especially aminophylline, frequently lead to gastric irritation.

Adrenergic drugs, such as racemic epinephrine, phenylephrine, and isoproterenol, are excellent aerosol bronchodilators. They are delivered by freon-propelled cartridges, hand-bulb nebulizers, or jet nebulizers actioned by an air compressor or an intermittent positive pressure breathing machine.

Corticosteroids are extremely effective in controlling bronchospasm and should be used when the above described drugs fail. Although the dosage will be tailored according to the characteristics of the patient, we like a short-term course, starting with relatively high doses (40 to 60 mg. of prednisone or the equivalent) the first 2 days, rapidly tapering off in 7 to 10 days.

EXPECTORANTS.   Glycerl guaiacolate and potassium iodide are the most commonly used agents associated with bronchodilators.

MECHANICAL DEVICES.   A hand nebulizer containing isoproterenol, racemic epinephrine, or phenylephrine should be carried by the patient at all times. To accomplish a deep penetration of the aerosolized bronchodilator into the bronchial tree, correct use of the nebulizer is of paramount importance.

For home use, a twin-jet nebulizer actioned by an air compressor or an intermittent positive pressure breathing apparatus is especially indicated in patients with acute bronchospasm or a tendency to carbon dioxide retention, and as a means of reassuring the overanxious patient.

AMBULATORY OXYGEN.   It is especially indicated in the bronchitis group, in which correction of hypoxemia would reduce the pulmonary hypertension and secondary polycythemia.[17]

PHYSICAL THERAPY.   Increasing attention has been given in the recent years to several modalities of physical therapy applied to patients with chronic airway obstruction.[1, 13, 15, 23, 31]

Although no improvement of the pulmonary reserve has been disclosed in controlled studies, there is agreement among the authors directing this therapeutic approach that the majority of patients have a significant subjective improvement. Better tolerance for physical daily activities and an increase in exercise are the usual improvements described by the patients.

Pursed lip breathing during expiration, slowing of respiratory rate especially during expiration, and breathing retraining of the abdominal muscles during both phases of respiration, apparently produce a better emptying of the lungs, reduce the stress of rapid respiratory efforts, and improve the diaphragmatic motion. Graded exercises, mainly walking on a treadmill or riding a bicycle, complemented by additional oxygen, are other maneuvers of this rehabilitation program.[24]

REFERENCES

1. Barach, A. ·L.: Physical exercise in breathless subjects with pulmonary emphysema, including a discussion of cigarette smoking. Dis. Chest, 45:113, 1964.
2. Bendixen, H. H., Egbert, C. D., Hedley-Whyte, J., Laver, M. B., and Pontoppidan, H.: Respiratory Care. St. Louis, C. V. Mosby, 1965.
3. Bocles, J. S.: Status asthmaticus. MED. CLIN. N. AMER., 54:493, 1970.
4. Campbell, E. J. M.: Oxygen Therapy in Diseases of the Chest. Brit. J. Dis. Chest, 58:148, 1964.
5. Campbell, E. J. M.: Respiratory Failure: The relation between oxygen concentration of inspired air and arterial blood. Lancet, 2:10, 1960.
6. Campbell, E. J. M., and Gebbie, T.: Masks and tent for providing controlled oxygen concentrations. Lancet, 1:468, 1966.
7. Chronic Bronchitis, Asthma and Pulmonary Emphysema. A statement by the Committee on Diagnostic Standards for Non-Tuberculous Respiratory Diseases of the American Thoracic Society. Amer. Rev. Resp. Dis., 85:762, 1962.
8. Chronic Cor Pulmonale: Report of an Expert Committee. World Health Organ. Tech. Serv., 213:15, 1961.

9. Cohn, J. E., Carrol, D. G., and Riley, R. L.: Respiratory acidosis in patients with emphysema. Amer. J. Med., *17*:447, 1954.
10. Comroe, J. H., Jr., Forster, R. E., II, DuBois, A. B., Briscoe, W. A., and Carlsen, E.: The Lung. Chicago, Year Book Medical Publishers, 1962.
11. Dowling, H. F., Mellody, M., Lepper, M., and Jackson, G. G.: Bacteriologic studies of the sputum in patients with chronic bronchitis and bronchiectasis. Amer. Rev. Resp. Dis., *81*:329, 1960.
12. Fletcher, C. M.: Some recent advances in the prevention and treatment of chronic bronchitis and related disorders with special reference to the effect of cigarette smoking. Proc. Roy. Soc. Med., *58*:918, 1965.
13. Haas, A., and Cardon, H.: Rehabilitation in chronic obstructive pulmonary disease. Med. Clin. N. Amer., *53*:592, 1969.
14. Harvey, R. M., and Ferrer, M. I.: A clinical consideration of cor pulmonale. Circulation, *21*:236, 1960.
15. Kimbel, P.: Physical therapy for chronic obstructive pulmonary disease patients. Clin. Notes Resp. Dis., Vol. 8, No. 4, Spring, 1970.
16. Kory, R. C., Bergmann, J. C., Sweet, R. D., and Smith, J. R.: Comparative evaluation of oxygen therapy techniques. J.A.M.A., *179*:767, 1962.
17. Levine, B. I., Bigelow, D. B., Hamstra, R. D., et al.: The role of long-term continuous oxygen administration in patients with chronic airway obstruction and hypoxemia. Ann. Int. Med., *66*:369, 1967.
18. Llamas, R., Gupta, S. K., and Baum, G. L.: A simple technique for prolonged arterial cannulation. Anesthesiol., *31*:289, 1969.
19. Medical Research Council Committee Report on the Etiology of Chronic Bronchitis: Definition and Classification of Chronic Bronchitis for Clinical and Epidemiological Purposes. Lancet, *1*:775, 1965.
20. Miller, W. F.: Rehabilitation of patients with chronic obstructive lung disease. Med. Clin. N. Amer., *51*:349, 1967.
21. Petty, T. L., and Nett, L. M.: For those who live and breathe with emphysema and chronic bronchitis. Springfield, Illinois, Charles C Thomas, 1967.
22. Petty, T. L., and Levine, B. L.: The safety and simplicity of the arterial puncture. J.A.M.A., *195*:693, 1966.
23. Physical Adjuncts in the Treatment of Pulmonary Disease. Statement by the Committee of the American Thoracic Society. Amer. Rev. Resp. Dis., *97*:25, 1968.
24. Pierce, A. K., Taylor, H. F., Archer, R. K., and Miller, W. F.: Responses to exercise training in patients with emphysema. Arch. Int. Med., *113*:28, 1964.
25. Pontoppidan, H., Hedley-Whyte, J., Bendixen, H. H., Laver, M. B., and Radford, E. P.: Ventilation and oxygen requirements during prolonged artificial ventilation in patients with respiratory failure. New Eng. J. Med., *273*:401, 1965.
26. Radford, E. P., Jr., Ferris, B. G., Jr., and Kriete, B. C.: Clinical use of a nomogram to estimate proper ventilation during artificial respiration. New Eng. J. Med., *251*:877, 1954.
27. Refsum, H. E.: Relationship between state of consciousness and arterial hypoxemia and hypercapnia in patients with respiratory insufficiency breathing air. Clin. Sci., *25*:361, 1963.
28. Reid, L.: Measurement of the bronchial mucous gland layer: A diagnostic yardstick in chronic bronchitis. Thorax, *15*:132, 1960.
29. Reinarz, J. A., Pierce, A. K., Mays, B. B., and Sanford, J. R.: The potential role of inhalation therapy equipment in nosocomial pulmonary infections. J. Clin. Invest., *44*:831, 1965.
30. Rotheram, E. B., Jr., Safar, P., and Robin, E. D.: Central nervous system disorders during mechanical ventilation in chronic pulmonary disease. J.A.M.A., *198*:993, 1964.
31. Schwartz, W. B., Hays, R. M., Polack, A., and Hagnie, G. D.: Effects of chronic hypercapnia on electrolyte and acid-base equilibrium: Recovery with special reference to the influence of chloride intake. J. Clin. Invest., *40*:1238, 1961.
32. What you can do about your breathing. National Tuberculosis and Respiratory Disease Association, 1967.
33. Young, W. G., Jr., Sealy, W. C., and Harris, J. S.: The role of intracellular and extracellular electrolytes in cardiac arrhythmias produced by prolonged hypercapnia. Surgery, *36*:636, 1954.

Department of Medicine
University of Miami School of Medicine
P.O. Box 875, Biscayne Annex
Miami, Florida   33152

A Comprehensive Regimen
for Osteoarthritis

David S. Howell, M.D.,* Roy D. Altman, M.D.,**
Harvey E. Brown, Jr., M.D.,† and Norman L. Gottlieb, M.D.‡

The recent information explosion on biochemistry of inflammation and connective tissues, as well as orthopedic materials science, is raising exciting new vistas for future therapeutic approaches to osteoarthritis. However, in this report, only *current* trends in the treatment of osteoarthritis will be reviewed, with special emphasis on personally employed methods of handling of such patients. At present, techniques of treatment are largely operational and empirically based. Unfortunately, there have been too few double-blind, statistically controlled studies to assess quantitatively the relative merits of many of the measures to be recommended. Also, the assessment of objective measures of improvement is difficult enough in respect to overtly inflammatory arthritides, but with osteoarthritis, the intensity of the inflammation may be very slight or questionable, and almost no satisfactory objective handle on the disease is yet available.

Despite these reservations with respect to assessing results, the treatment of osteoarthritis can be a gratifying experience. In few other diseases is it more important to establish a personal interest in the patient and to convey optimism for securing reasonable goals. Cautious and cognizant advantageous use of placebo responses should be taken when they develop in some patients, but not others. In guidance of a therapeutic program, one must adhere, year-in and year-out, to a consistent policy of management with avoidance of therapeutic nihilism on the one hand and over-zealous application of gimmicks on the other.

In order to clarify relationships of treatment to the disease process, a short preliminary description of its nature is included.

---

*Professor of Medicine, University of Miami School of Medicine; Director, Arthritis Training and Research Program, Jackson Memorial Hospital and Veterans Administration Hospital

**Research Associate, University of Miami School of Medicine; Attending Physician, Jackson Memorial Hospital and Veterans Administration Hospital

†Associate Professor of Medicine, University of Miami School of Medicine; Attending Physician, Jackson Memorial Hospital and Veterans Administration Hospital

‡Instructor in Medicine, University of Miami School of Medicine; Attending Physician, Jackson Memorial Hospital and Veterans Administration Hospital

Incidence

Osteoarthritis or degenerative joint disease is probably the common-est form of "rheumatic" disease. The estimated prevalence of osteo-arthritis in the United States was ascertained from x-rays of hands and feet obtained during a health survey from 1960 to 1962.[18] Several con-clusions emerged from that study. It was projected that 40.5 million Americans had an osteoarthritic problem; that by age 75 years, 85 per cent of the population sampled was affected; and that a quarter of them had moderate to severe disease.[18] Although sex incidence overall was roughly equal, under age 45, men were more frequently affected than women, whereas from age 55 on, the prevalence among women was greater.[18] In Finland, by similar x-ray evidence, 13 to 15 per cent of an urban population had osteoarthritis problems.[23] Cobb estimated that one third of those patients with objective evidence of the disease on x-rays examination manifested directly related clinical symptoms.[14]

BRIEF DESCRIPTION OF THE DISEASE

In regard to *primary osteoarthritis,* the disease involves most commonly the knees, hips, bunion joints, proximal and distal inter-phalangeal joints of hands and feet, first carpometacarpal joints, gleno-humeral and acromioclavicular joints, as well as cervical, thoracic, and lumbosacral spine.[14] Early in this disease there is principally periarticu-lar soft-tissue swelling, thickening of the joint capsule, and often syno-vial effusions. Warm erythematous subcutaneous cysts may develop, particularly over the distal interphalangeal joints of the hands.

Osteoarthritis may follow a relentless low-grade, subacute course, or one of remissions and exacerbations. The extent to which cartilage degradation occurs is variable, and this finding does not correlate well with presence of inflammatory signs. Similarly, there is considerable variation in intensity and distribution of marginal bony hypertrophic changes or soft tissue capsular thickening in respect to local pain.

In some patients, the marginal bony overgrowth predominates, whereas in others, the picture is almost entirely one of cartilage degen-eration. In the vast majority of patients, features of both degeneration and repair are observed. The disease is nonfatal and self-limited. Irre-versible crippling effects are minor in comparison to that of many pa-tients with rheumatoid arthritis. In particular, ankylosis or permanent contractures are rarely encountered; bed or wheelchair confinement, except in unusually severe cases of knee, hip, or back disease is uncom-monly required for osteoarthritic patients.

Secondary osteoarthritis describes a clinical syndrome which is not distinguishable from the primary type, except for related causative factors in respect to initiating the local joint damage. The term has been used when osteoarthritis follows fractures, severe sprains, chronic local infections, clear-cut heritable diseases with biomechanical derange-ments of articular function, as well as metabolic disorders, such as ochronosis and chondrocalcinosis involving articular cartilage. Also, rheumatoid arthritis and its variants in an advanced stage often are accompanied by the joint tissue changes of secondary osteoarthritis, the so-called "mixed arthritis." Clinicians confronted with such rheumatic diseases must recognize and delineate the osteoarthritic component of the clinical syndrome at hand before rational treatment can be instituted.

Pathological Findings

These, for present purposes, are best described briefly in terms of the gross and light microscopic findings.

Early in the course of the disease there is noted a patchy superficial loss of staining properties of the articular cartilage of involved joints for normal matrix constituent proteinpolysaccharides (PPC), increased number of cells per basal chondrone ("cloning,"[15, 25, 35]), and evidence of increased PPC synthesis.[25] Also, accelerated matrix degradation of PPC and other constituents develops.[6, 7] Shallow erosions and fissuring of the cartilage gradually extend to form ragged enlarging ulcerations.[35] The loss of cartilage is accompanied or followed by subchondral trabecular bone thickening (eburnation) and formation of subchondral bone cysts. In the process of these changes, coronal capillaries from the marrow space penetrate the subchondral bone table and new cartilage calcification occurs;[22] resorption of the calcified cartilage by chondroclasts, and new bone formation at the joint margins ensue.[22] These cartilaginous and bony disturbances are accompanied by villous hyperplasia of synovial membranes and by scattered infiltration of membranes by mononuclear cells.

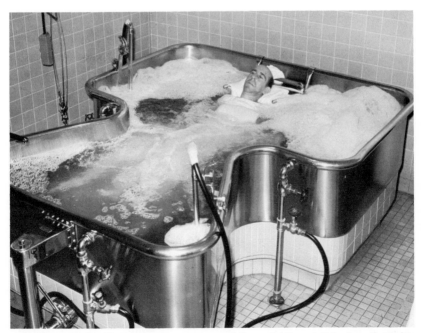

Figure 1.   Hubbard tank treatments are especially useful for painful osteoarthritic hips with associated muscle spasm.

Laboratory Findings

In major joints, the synovial fluid is usually increased in volume, and usually shows a modest leukocytosis (2000 to 3000 cells per cu. mm.) without an increased proportion of polymorphonuclear leukocytes. The fluid is clear or slightly cloudy. Inasmuch as the mucin content and viscous quality are usually within normal limits, the Ropes (acetic acid) test is correspondingly normal. Fluid stained with saffranin O shows, often, evidence of cartilage fibers rich in glycosaminoglycans. Sedimentation rate, serum enzymes, etc., are within normal limits, as are all biochemical profiles studied to date.

Etiology

The causative factors of *primary osteoarthritis* remain disputed, despite several decades of intensive research. Some progress has been made in more clearly defining a profile of contributory factors, of which degeneration from wear-and-tear damage to articular cartilage is particularly prominent. Repeated microtrauma, obesity, and local, ill-defined derangements of bone and cartilage metabolism probably play a role. There are undoubtedly heritable factors and nonspecific effects of aging which remain to be clarified.

It seems likely that altered biomechanical properties of the deteriorated joint, chemical agents released from the deteriorating cartilage,[13] and systemic factors may all contribute to bring about the marginal bony hypertrophy.[6] Much attention by researchers now centers on devising biochemical means of improving cartilage repair at sites of deterioration as well as upon prevention of local enzymic degradation of cartilage matrix. It is conjectured by some investigators that if chemical products of cartilage degradation give rise to the hypertrophic phenomena, as well as the low grade synovial inflammation, these phases of the disease might be curtailed by inhibiting cartilage degradation.

A Philosophy of Management

Our operational perspective of the disease is based upon the histological evidences of low grade local inflammation and upon the fact that many patients follow a course of mild attacks and remissions reminiscent of the acute phase of *rheumatoid arthritis*. By way of exemplification, in the latter disease, treatment is directed toward joint effusions, synovial pouches, acute tenosynovitis, nodules, and muscle spasm, all of which compose the reversible largely inflammatory signs of the disease as opposed to the gradual or rapidly progressing relentless irreversible findings, including ulnar drift, spindling of digits, subluxations and fusion of joints, or nonsoluble contractures of muscle groups (Table 1). The same principal distinctions operate in *osteoarthritis*. Here, the synovial capsular thickening, mild synovitis, synovial effusions, ganglia, soft Heberden's nodes and soluble contractures can be managed as if a component of a *reversible* low-grade inflammation (Table 1) is involved.

In contrast, the firm bony marginal enlargement, articular cartilage loss, bone-on-bone contact, subluxations, subchondral bone table thick-

Table 1. *Comparison of Findings in Two Common Forms of Arthritis with Respect to Reversibility Using Medical Therapy*

OSTEOARTHRITIS		RHEUMATOID ARTHRITIS	
Reversible	Irreversible	Reversible	Irreversible
Joint effusion	Cartilage loss (joint narrowing by x-ray examination and bone-on-bone contact)	Joint effusion	Ulnar deviation of fingers and toes
Synovial thickening	Joint malalignment and subluxations	Joint heat, erythema, edema	Spindling of fingers and toes
Fibromyositic nodules	Ligamentous loosening and joint instability	Synovial pouches	Subluxations
Soft perichondrial and periosteal thickening and edema	Subchondral bony growth and subchondral cysts formation	Bursitis	Bony or fibrous ankylosis
Ganglia	Joint marginal bony and cartilage remodelling	Tenosynovitis	Bone-on-bone contact
Herniated fat pads	"Insoluble" contractures	Early muscle atrophy	"Insoluble" contractures
Bursal inflammation	Advanced muscle atrophy	Nodules	Advanced muscle atrophy
Heberden's nodal cysts		Baker's cysts	Tendon rupture
Muscle spasm			
"Soluble" contractures			
Early muscle atrophy			
Baker's cysts			

ening and remodelled bone, subchondral cysts, as well as aseptic necrosis of cartilage represent *irreversible* changes of this disease, treated by surgical and physical therapeutic means. As in the case of more flagrantly inflammatory arthritides, management is directed to minimize the severity of the subacute attacks and to retard development of the irreversible changes. Thus, after a thorough medical workup, the physician can weigh the relative contribution to the patient's total problems of column I items and column II items (Table 1), and construct an appropriate, comprehensive, therapeutic regimen.

Such a regimen may include (1) reassurance, (2) relief of pain and betterment of joint functions by combined medical and physical therapeutic approaches, (3) correction of the factors which are believed to accelerate deterioration of cartilage, particularly obesity and certain stressful occupational activities, and (4) physical therapy and orthopedic surgical procedures with or without an application of rehabilitative appliances.

TREATMENT MEASURES

Reassurance of the Patient

For primary osteoarthritis, as in other rheumatic disorders, symptoms are magnified and possible inflammatory components worsened by the presence of chronic anxiety. Reassurance that the disease is not fatal and that there need be no worry about crippling is, for a majority of patients, the first order of business. This should be done only following a thorough internal medical and rheumatological workup, because fibromyositic or localized bony symptoms of osteoarthritis may be difficult to separate from those of malignant tumor, multiple myeloma, etc. In many such instances, prognosis is governed by the disease to which the "osteoarthritic" symptoms are secondary. Discussions of prognosis should be couched in understandable terms; statements should always concern the outcome for a similar group of individuals with avoidance of an absolute prediction for the given patient at hand.

Second, the types of treatment available should be discussed in sufficient depth to make it clear to the patient that if the safest, simplest and in most instances, effective regimen tried first gives an inadequate response, that a second or third approach to management can be and usually is applied successively. From each of these approaches a more potent therapeutic action can be anticipated but, pari passu, the chance of unfavorable side effects also increases, so that these approaches are held in reserve. Awareness that there are back-up systems, in case of failure of the primary regimen, is an important emollient to some apprehensive rheumatic patients.

A large percentage of patients with mild osteoarthritis are sufficiently relieved from a discussion of the nature of their disease to pursue their usual daily schedule on no other treatment than intermittent salicylates and exercise programs.

Medical Measures

For osteoarthritic symptoms of weight-bearing joints, more than slight degrees of overweight warrant a weight-losing regimen. Often, partial relief of weight-bearing joint pain accompanies the weight loss.

Sustenance of the weight loss is unfortunately rarely attained without a change of living habits—acquisition of pride in personal appearance, institution of regular exercise, and relief of relevant emotional tensions. In the hip joints, the effective pressures developed during walking between the acetabulum and femoral heads have been found to be about several times greater than the actual body weight carried owing to local biomechanical factors. Damage from shearing forces in extreme limits of motion in knees or hips is probably accentuated by overweight. However, biomechanical evidence of an unfavorable effect of obesity on osteoarthritis is countered to some extent by a negative correlation between osteoarthritis of inbred mice and obesity, noted by Sokoloff,[36] as well as absence of correlation between occurrence of osteoarthritis of the hip in humans and obesity in Saville's report.[32]

Some patients simply cannot or will not muster the effort for sustained weight loss; for such patients efforts in this direction seem futile, so that reliance on other measures to develop symptomatic relief is required.

Rest

The most satisfactory program involves moderate exercise for short periods throughout the day. Patients on a total sanatorium-type regimen can make the exercise period 10 to 30 minutes long, one of formal stretching, postural exercises, and isometric exercises: These may be prescribed for usual performance or may be adapted for Hubbard tank or heated pool usage, where there is added advantage of bouyancy. Increased pain, lasting 1 to 2 hours after the exercises, is an indication for their modification and cut-back. Prolonged exercise or sitting in one position, as before a television screen, should be avoided. Many patients develop a misconception that continuously exercising a stiff painful joint lessens arthritis. Such overactivity of offending joints must be discouraged, as worsening of the process is likely. Persons continuing their daily occupations during treatment should revise their schedule to avoid prolonged over-exercise of an arthritic part, i.e., prolonged uninterrupted typing, standing at a counter, lifting objects, etc. The principal of alternating moderate exercise and rest periods should be applied.

Drugs

The most frequently used and simplest class of agents comprise the salicylates, which have both an analgesic and mild antiphlogistic action. Properly administrated dosages of Aspirin (Ecotrin, Bufferin, Ascriptin, Persistin, choline salicylates) at 2.8 to 4.8 gm. per day, considerably relieve the symptoms of osteoarthritis. Long-acting salicylates, taken at bedtime, are sometimes most effective for night pain.

Sweating, tinnitus, dyspepsia and annoyance at the number of pills required are factors which often lead to abandonment of a simple aspirin regimen. Local irritation of the gastrointestinal tract with erosions, and flareup of peptic ulcer with bleeding occasionally occur; such untoward events are less common than with many oral agents cited below.

Patients on anticoagulants such as heparin or coumadin should not be on salicylates, which affect several aspects of coagulation.[28] In addition, recent finding of the tight chemical binding of acetylsalicylate to certain peptides in albumin raises the question of potential medically important effects of long-term aspirin usage, and is not yet clarified.[29]

The effects of aspirin on cartilage metabolism have been studied. For example, in experimental surgical lesions of rabbit knee cartilage, Chrisman noted improved healing rates in the presence of salicylates.[13, 33] Another agent, comparably safe, is the analgesic acetaminophen (Tylenol); in doses of 0.6 to 0.9 gm. q.i.d., there is less gastrointestinal intolerance, but also slightly less effective pain relief. Caution is advisable in raising acetaminophen dosage above 3.6 gm. per day owing to the possible production of nephropathy.[31]

Propoxyphene (Darvon) alone or with other agents is usually tolerated with minimal side effects, as a moderately potent analgesic agent, but its mechanism of action is not clearly understood.[26]

Indomethacin (Indocin, 25 to 50 mg. t.i.d. or q.i.d.) is usually equally effective or more effective than large dosages of salicylates. This agent is moderately antiphlogistic and should be started at low dosages, e.g., 25 mg. per day.[17] In order to avoid commonly encountered untoward effects of light-headedness, headaches, and gastrointestinal irritation, indomethacin should be given with meals or antacids. For some patients a bedtime dose is all that can be tolerated.

Phenylbutazone (Butazolidin), another effective anti-inflammatory agent, is used over short periods in dosages of 400 to 600 mg. per day. It is not generally recommended for long-term use, and concomitant use with anticoagulants is interdicted. As in the case of indomethacin, gastrointestinal intolerance may be obviated by administration of phenylbutazone with meals and at bedtime, together with skim milk or antacids. Several commonly used antacids must be discontinued during treatment of infections because these antacids interact with certain antibiotics and prevent antibiotic absorption.

Inasmuch as phenylbutazone or phenoxybutazone occasionally cause several other severe untoward events, particular caution must be exerted during the first month of treatment. In the presence of allergic states, hypertension or heart failure, the latter drugs are avoided or used especially carefully because of their propensity to cause dermatitis medicamentosa, elevated blood pressure, and salt and water retention. Bone marrow depression with aplastic anemia or agranulocytosis is an uncommon but serious complication which must be promptly detected. Thus, a complete blood count at 1, 2 and 4 weeks after initiation of treatment is routinely advocated.

Active peptic ulcerations are, of course, a strong contraindication for salicylates, indomethacin, or phenylbutazone. For such patients, local steroid injections, analgesics, and physical therapy are relied upon as

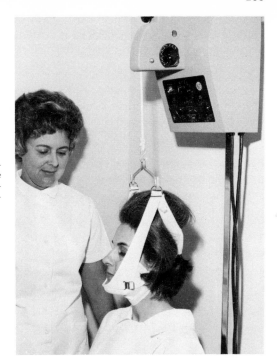

Figure 2. During neck traction, direction of pull should be such that the neck is either partially extended or flexed in a manner to avoid accentuation of pain.

well as occasionally topical counterirritants containing methylsalicylates. Occasionally, degenerative joint pain, particularly of the hip, is sufficiently severe to warrant the use of narcotics such as codeine or percodan, and rarely stronger agents.

New Agents Under Study

Ibuprofen,[10, 40] a recent, moderately potent anti-inflammatory analgesic drug, and such new drugs as mephenamic acid[9] and flufenamic acid,[40] need more study to define their place, if any, in our therapeutic larder.

Agents such as Rumalon,[5, 39] epsilon-amino caproic acid,[16b] and intra-articular silicone[19] have been reported to improve arthritic symptoms, but further documentation of their effectiveness will be needed. Most clinical trials of these agents have been made in Europe.

Local Corticosteroid Injections

The proper role of this form of management in osteoarthritis remains controversial,[3, 4, 11, 20] and, together with techniques, is well discussed by Hollander.[20] In the authors' view, judicious employment of local corticosteroid derivatives, of the long-acting variety,[1, 2] (e.g., Aristospan, Celestone Soluspan, Depomedrol, Hydeltra TBA, Kenalog, etc.), are indicated in the presence of inflammation, however mild, and with failure to respond adequately to the aforementioned programs. A course of as much as 5 or 6 injections separated by 2 to 4 week intervals may be given in any single joint per 6 to 12 month period. Instability or bone-on-contact in a weight-bearing joint is a relative contraindication for intra-articular steroids. Controversy exists whether early cartilage loss is also a contraindication, based on possible acceleration of cartilage destruction.

There are several reports of Charcot-like arthropathy during repeated administration of corticosteroids by the intra-articular route.[4, 11, 37] On the other hand, some patients have shown remarkable tolerance of their joints to large cumulative doses of intra-articular corticosteroids.[8, 20] The stabilization of lysosomes by corticosteroids may block one potential pathway of articular cartilage degradation involving hydrolytic enzymes in chondrocytes.[38] However, concurrent retardation of matrix protein synthesis may theoretically interfere with badly needed repair processes at osteoarthritic sites.[24] In rabbits, cystic degeneration and disintegration of articular cartilage attends repeated corticosteroid injections.[24, 27] The use of injections in humans at sites of a pustule or furuncle may start a septic arthritis; otherwise infection is extremely rare. Occasionally ruptured tendons have been associated with this form of therapy.[21]

Despite these reported ill effects, a follow-up study (unpublished observations of the authors) of 100 patients with osteoarthritis who received multiple corticosteroid injections failed to reveal deleterious effects, except for infrequent transient, local crystal-induced reactions. Excessive frequency of osteochondritis or tabetic type arthropathy, beyond the 2 to 3 per cent expected in 5 year follow-up, was not seen.[20] The controversy concerning the claim that such injections produce chiefly a placebo response is reviewed by Hollander.[20] Eliminating those suspected of being placebo reactors in osteoarthritis, the authors conducted a single-blind study on a group of osteoarthritic patients. Improvement of joint pain for more than 10 days was for injections of lidocaine alone 35 per cent, and for lidocaine mixed with long-acting corticosteroids, 87 per cent (unpublished observations).

All patients should be alerted to the fact that some mild increased joint aching may develop at the site of injection after the lidocaine effects subside, and ends in 6 to 24 hours. In the authors' opinion, incorporation of short-acting steroids such as decadron phosphate in the injection solutions may prevent this effect of irritation. In addition, 1 to 5 per cent of patients develop a more severe reaction, characterized by heat, redness, and swelling of the joint, probably due to the leukotactic effect of steroid crystals.[20] Most crystal-induced reactions respond simply to ice pack and analgesics. Occasionally stronger anti-inflammatory agents are needed such as phenylbutazone.

Physical Therapy

Exposure of the painful joints to hot water in a basin, tub, or shower, 20 to 30 minutes once or twice daily, is easily carried out at home. In more severely afflicted patients, a course of physical therapy may be prescribed for 30 to 60 minute periods, 3 to 5 times weekly for at least a month, subject to renewal. Infrared baker, short-wave diathermy, ultrasound, and hot wet packs are useful modalities, especially for relief of associated fibromyositis in muscle groups surrounding painful joints. After sufficient pain relief from these measures has been obtained, a program of isometric exercise to strengthen involved muscle groups is strongly advised. Regular year-in and year-out recreative swimming seems a most advantageous habit for cultivation by patients afflicted with painful weight-bearing joints. Use of cotton gloves while gardening, rubber gloves in dishwashing, etc., or simply Bandaids to protect involved joints is often recommended for reduction of microtrauma to afflicted parts. If there are bunions or metatarsal prolapse, bars on shoes or arch supports may be helpful. Wrist supports, particularly with Velcro attachments, are useful for carpometacarpal joint pain. Light slings are employed for resting the shoulder or acromioclavicular joints. Unstable knees[34] can be protected temporarily by knee cages or elastic supports containing hinged metal reinforcements. Weight should be shifted away from a degenerated hip, knee, or ankle by use of properly measured canes, crutches,[34] walkers, and rarely wheelchairs.[41]

Indications for Surgical Intervention

Intractable pain, particularly at night, or irreversible hard tissue destruction with joint instability are usually the primary factors in selection of patients for orthopedic surgery. Careful evaluation of the possible benefits is indicated before their recommendation. Certain orthopedic operative procedures consist of resection or fusion, or silastic prostheses of carpometacarpal joints of the thumb, relief of the carpal tunnel syndrome by surgery, osteotomy of the hip or knee joint[30] for pain relief and correction of faulty weight bearing alignments, total hip[12] or knee prostheses, synovectomy and debridement of loose bodies within knee joints and ligamentous repair and tightening for instability of the knee, patellectomy when the cartilage of this bone is severely afflicted, and resection or fusion of metatarsal joint of the great toe for a rigid bunion.

Osteoarthritis of the Spine

Spurs or osteophytes of the spine demonstrable on x-ray films in most patients past middle age are often not the cause of pain. At any age, severe steady pain in all parts of the spine may be of metastatic malignant nature, and work-up to exclude tumor is worthwhile, particularly if conventional medical treatment fails to give at least partial prompt relief.

X-ray films which show spurs encroaching on foramina from which nerve roots emerge, or narrowed intervertebral spaces per se are grounds for suspicion that localized pain may be caused by degenerative disc disease, bony impingement or traction on nerve rootlets at that site. A variable component of slight inflammation and thickening of apophyseal joints, ligaments, and tendons and fibromyositis of the paravertebral muscles contributes to the symptomatology.

Management includes limited trials of the same drugs, and general physical therapeutic measures in the manner already described for peripheral joints. Localized pain, arising from facets and fibromyositic nodules, responds to small injections of lidocaine or corticosteroids, or both, but principal emphasis is placed on physical therapy to release muscle spasm and later to correct postural faults by a long-term exercise program. A firm mattress, bedboard, and small firm pillow are usually important.

In the lumbosacral spine, symptoms from spondylosis may warrant a course of pelvic traction. Eating meals and resting in a contour chair or properly gatched hospital bed, during acute attacks, has often accelerated convalescence.

Acute symptoms in the cervical spine respond to use of a cervical collar and variable periods of vertical or horizontal neck traction. Muscle relaxant drugs, such as metocarbamol, 500 mg. 5 or 6 times daily, or diazepam (Valium), 2 mg. 2 to 4 times daily, are usually prescribed for acute and subacute stages of spondylosis. During acute attacks, patients are kept at bedrest, and during convalescence corsets or belts are worn when the patient is out of bed. In contrast to acute herniation of discs with confined nerve deficits, surgical intervention in spondylosis has been less successful owing to multiple levels of disease involvement and to the complex origin of the pain syndrome.

REFERENCES

1. El Attar, T. M. A.: Study of the metabolism of cortisol. Arth. Rheum., *11*:804, 1968.
2. Bain, L. S., Jacomb, R. G., and Wynn, V.: Parenteral administration of 6 α-methylpredni-solone-21-acetate. Part II: Absorption and duration of effect. Ann. Phys. Med., 9:49, 1967.
3. Baker, D. M.: Intra-articular injections of corticosteroid for degenerative arthritis. Practitioner, 202:431, 1969.
4. Bentley, G., and Goodfellow, J. W.: Disorganizations of the knees following intraarticular hydrocortisone injections. J. Bone Joint Surg., 51(B):498, 1969.
5. Bollet, A. J.: Stimulation of protein-chondroitin sulfate synthesis by normal and osteoarthritic articular cartilage. Arth. Rheum., *11*:663, 1968.
6. Bollet, A. J.: A consideration of the reversibility of osteoarthritis. Trans. Amer. Clin. Climat. Assoc., *80*:212, 1969.
7. Bollet, A. J.: An essay on the biology of osteoarthritis. Arth. Rheum., *12*:152, 1969.
8. Breneman, J. C.: Massive injections of methylprednisolone without harmful side effects. Mich. Med., *68*:135, 1969.
9. Buchmann, E.: Mefamamic acid compared with Indocin and placebo in osteoarthritis. Ann. Phys. Med., 8:119, 1966.
10. Chalmers, T. M.: Clinical experience with Ibuprofen in treatment of rheumatoid arthritis. Ann. Rheum. Dis., 28:513, 1969.
11. Chandler, G. N., and Wright, V.: Deleterious effect of intra-articular hydrocortisone. Lancet, *1*:661, 1958.
12. Charnley, J.: Total prosthetic replacement of the hip. Reconst. Surg. Trauma, *11*:9, 1969.
13. Chrisman, O. D.: Biochemical aspects of degenerative joint disease. Clin. Orthop., *64*:77, 1969.
14. Cobb, S., Merchant, W. R., and Rubin, T.: The relation of symptoms to osteoarthritis. J. Chronic Dis., 5:197, 1957.
15. Collins, D. H.: The Pathology of Articular and Spinal Diseases. London, Arnold, 1960.
16a. Fessel, J. M., and Chrisman, O. D.: Enzymatic degradation of chondromucoprotein by cell-free extracts of human cartilage. Arth. Rheum., 7:398, 1964.
16b. Gaspardy, G., Mituszova, M., and Gaspardy, G.: Results of treatment with Σ-aminocaproic acid of patients suffering from rheumatoid arthritis. Rheumatol. Balneol. Allerg. (Budapest), 9:89, 1968.
17. Golding, D.: General management of osteoarthritis. Brit. Med. J., 3:575, 1969.
18. Health statistics, Series B., No. 36, U.S. Dept of Health, Education and Welfare, 1962. Chronic conditions causing limitation of activities.

19. Helal, B., and Karadi, B. S.: Artificial lubrication of joints; use of silicone oil. Ann. Phys. Med., 9:334, 1968.

20. Hollander, J. L.: Intrasynovial corticosteroid therapy. In Hollander, J. L., ed.: Arthritis and Allied Conditions, A Textbook of Rheumatology. Philadelphia, Lea and Febiger, 1967, ch. 24.

21. Ismail, A. M., Balakrishnan, R., and Rajakumar, M. K.: Rupture of patellar ligament after steroid infiltration. J. Bone Joint Surg., 51(B):503, 1969.

22. Johnson, L. D.: Kinetics of osteoarthritis. Lab. Invest., 8:1223, 1959.

23. Laine, V. A. I.: Rheumatic complaints in an urban population in Finland. Acta Rheumatica Scand., 8:81, 1962.

24. Mankin, H. J., and Conger, K. A.: The acute effects of intra-articular hydrocortisone on articular cartilage in rabbits. J. Bone Joint Surg., 48(A):1383, 1966.

25. Mankin, H. J., and Lippiello, L.: Biochemical and metabolic abnormalities in articular cartilage from osteoarthritic human hips. J. Bone Joint Surg., 52(A):424, 1970.

26. Miller, R. R., Pharm, D., Feingold, A., and Paxinos, J.: Propoxyphene hydrochloride. A critical review. J.A.M.A., 213:996, 1970.

27. Moskowitz, R. W., Davis, W., Sammarca, J., Mast, W., and Chase, S. W.: Experimentally induced corticosteroid arthropathy. Arth. Rheum., 13:236, 1970.

28. O'Brien, J. R.: Effect of salicylates on human platelets. Lancet, 1:779, 1968.

29. Pinckard, R. N., Hawkins, D., and Farr, R. S.: The inhibitory effect of salicylate on the acetylation of human albumin by acetylsalicylic acid. Arth. Rheum., 13:361, 1970.

30. Potter, T. A.: Arthroplasty of the knee with tibial metallic implants of the McKeever and MacIntosh design. Surg. Clin. N. Amer., 49:903, 1969.

31. Prescott, L. F.: Effect of acetylsalicylic acid, phenacetin, paracetamol and caffeine on renal tubular epithelium. Lancet, 2:91, 1965.

32. Saville, P. D., and Dickson, J.: Age and weight in osteoarthritis of the hip. Arth. Rheum., 11:635, 1968.

33. Simmons, D. P., and Chrisman, O. D.: Salicylate inhibition of cartilage degeneration. Arth. Rheum., 8:960, 1965.

34. Smith, E. M.: Bracing the unstable knee. Arch. Phys. Med., 51:22, 1970.

35. Sokoloff, L.: The pathology and pathogenesis of osteoarthritis. In Hollander, J. L., ed.: Arthritis and Allied Conditions, A Textbook of Rheumatology. Philadelphia, Lea and Febiger, 1967, ch. 51.

36. Sokoloff, L., Crittenden, L. B., Yamamoto, R. S., and Jay, G. E., Jr.: The genetics of degenerative joint disease in mice. Arth. Rheum., 5:531, 1962.

37. Steinberg, C. L., Duthie, R. B., and Piva, A. E.: Charcot-like arthropathy following intra-articular hydrocortisone. J.A.M.A., 181:851, 1962.

38. Thomas, L.: The effects of papain, Vitamin A and cortisone on cartilage matrix in vivo. Biophys. J., 4(suppl):207, 1964.

39. Wagenhauser, F. J., Amira, A., and Borrachero, J.: The treatment of arthroses with cartilage-bone marrow extract. Results of multicenter trial. Schweiz. Med. Wschr., 98:904, 1968.

40. Winder, C. V., Lembke, L. A., and Stephens, M. D.: Comparative bioassay of drugs in adjuvant-induced arthritis in rats; flufenamic acid, mephanamic acid, and phenylbutazone. Arth. Rheum., 12:472, 1969.

41. Zinn, W. M.: Reflections on degenerative hip disease. Ann. Phys. Med., 10:209, 1970.

Department of Medicine
University of Miami School of Medicine
P. O. Box 875, Biscayne Annex
Miami, Florida 33152

Microbial Suprainfection

Recognition and Management

Harvey S. Kantor, M.D., and William V. Shaw, M.D.***

The orderliness of man's indigenous microbial flora is striking. Under the usual conditions of exposure, a normal individual's skin and mucous membranes are populated with a varying but nevertheless characteristic range of microorganisms, some of which may be pathogens under special circumstances. The latter are in continual interaction with the host and with other species of the normal flora. The indigenous flora fluctuate within fairly wide limits with respect to number and type of genera, but the dominant species maintain relatively constant proportions to each other.[46] Such examples would be the prominent residence of staphylococci and diphtheroids (Corynebacterium acnes) as the dominant organisms of human skin.[35]

The upper respiratory tract, composed in part of the nose, nasopharynx, mouth, and oropharynx, harbors an extraordinarily varied bacterial flora, numbering no less than 21 genera of bacteria.[46] Although the lower respiratory tract is in direct continuity with the secretions draining the upper respiratory tract, it is, by contrast, normally sterile.[27] That striking alterations in this pattern may occur following the use of antimicrobial agents has been firmly established for almost a quarter of a century.[22, 29, 30] A lack of awareness of this principle has frequently resulted in an erroneous interpretation of positive culture reports and led to the injudicious use of antimicrobial chemotherapy.

The physician's reliance upon antibiotics has increased to a degree which has prompted statements exemplified by that of Finland that their use "has become so thoroughly ingrained in the practice of medicine that the diagnosis or the very suspicion of an infection, or even the mere presence of a fever in a patient, evokes from the great majority of practicing physicians the prescription of an antimicrobial agent – almost as a reflex response."[15]

---

*Instructor in Medicine, University of Miami School of Medicine; Research and Educational Associate, Infectious Disease Section, Veterans Administration Hospital

**Associate Professor of Medicine, University of Miami School of Medicine; Chief, Infectious Disease Section, Veterans Administration Hospital

The importance of the ecology of normal microbial flora in man had not been fully appreciated until evidence was accumulated showing that it can be disorganized by the administration of antimicrobial agents. The indigenous flora play a major role in preventing certain bacterial diseases through effects collectively referred to as bacterial antagonism. The importance of such factors in maintaining proper microbial balance is illustrated by the serious infections that often result from major altera- tions in the bacterial flora of the gastrointestinal tract. When broad- spectrum antibiotics, such as the tetracyclines, are given in large doses for many days, growth of most of the bacteria that thrive in the normal intestinal tract is suppressed. As a result, antibiotic-resistant strains of potentially pathogenic staphylococci, normally held in check by the antagonistic action of coliform and other organisms, may multiply freely in the bowel,[21] and occasionally invade the bowel wall and give rise to the serious and often fatal disease, acute staphylococcal enterocolitis.[1]

A number of mechanisms are probably involved in bacterial antago- nism. At least two have been reasonably well defined: (1) competition for nutrients in the environment[43] and (2) production of inhibitory sub- stances ranging from simple organic acids to highly specific bacterio- cins.[41]

Both cooperative (synergistic) and competitive interactions occur among indigenous microbial species, and between these and either saprophytic or pathogenic intruders. That bacteria with limited synthetic capabilities may acquire essential nutrients from metabolically more competent neighbors is illustrated in vitro by the "satellite phenome- non"[40] frequently exhibited by colonies of Hemophilus influenzae, growing only in the vicinity of staphylococcal colonies which are pro- viding the essential growth-promoting V factor, which has been shown to be the coenzyme diphosphopyridine nucleotide.[33] The antagonism that exists between some microorganisms has occasionally been exploited to man's advantage. Many of the known antibiotics which kill bacteria are produced by fungi (for example, Penicillin G), while certain anti- microbials derived from higher bacteria will kill fungi (Amphotericin B).

Host resistance to sepsis is influenced by the nature of the normal microbial flora. When this normal flora is prevented by the germ-free technique, striking changes take place in susceptibility to certain types of infections. Bacillary dysentery cannot be produced in ordinary guinea pigs, even with large inocula of virulent Shigellae. However, their ad- ministration to germ-free guinea pigs gives rise to fatal ulcerative enteritis.[56]

Although benign changes in the body's microbial population may result from chemotherapy, such alterations may occasionally be followed by overt and even life-threatening disease.[2, 14, 31, 59, 61, 63, 68] The occurrence of this phenomenon was first described in 1947.[61] The superimposition of a new infectious disease on one for which treatment is already being carried out, although well documented, is not often given adequate consideration among the hazards of antimicrobial therapy.

DEFINITION OF TERMS

It may be useful to describe precisely several terms which frequently tend to be confused and, on occasion, used interchangeably. They are: (1) *colonization,* (2) *super*infection, and (3) *supra*infection. These terms and their implications were reviewed in a recent editorial, in which a useful distinction was proposed between superinfection and suprainfection.[65]

Colonization indicates the appearance of or significant increase in numbers of any potential pathogen in the resident microflora after antibiotic therapy is begun. An example would be the emergence of gramnegative bacteria in the course of penicillin G therapy of pneumococcal pneumonia.

Superinfection is a situation in which both microbiological and clinical evidence of a new infection develops, unrelated to antibiotic therapy, but as a secondary complication of an underlying disorder of either an infectious or noninfectious nature. The occurrence of mycotic infections in lymphomas and leukemias is a case in point.

Suprainfection is the appearance of both microbiological and clinical evidence of a new infection developing during the course of antibiotic therapy of a previous one. A necessary prerequisite to suprainfection is colonization by a potential pathogen.

It has been stressed that the differentiation of colonization from suprainfection is of greater significance than the matter of semantics it raises.[59, 65] The magnitude of this issue is sufficiently great to bear quoting the compelling appeal of Weinstein and Musher, that "the difficulty that arises stems from equating change in bacterial numbers, a purely microbiological phenomenon that may be of no importance, with secondary bacterial infection, a clinical event that may have fatal consequences. . . . Failure to distinguish between them may lead, on the one hand, to death from unrecognized or inadequately treated infection and, on the other hand, to treatment of nonexistent disease (colonization). . . . It is clear, therefore, that the best therapy for colonization is not to treat it. Discontinuation of the antibiotic often resolves the problem rapidly."[65]

PATHOGENESIS OF COLONIZATION AND SUPRAINFECTION

It is well known that a consequence of antibiotic therapy is the production of a change which upsets the precarious balance maintained by the normal endogenous or indigenous flora.[22, 29, 30] Little is known, however, of the precise mechanisms which underlie this phenomenon.[5] Born into an environment laden with microbes, the body of an infant, initially sterile prior to his passage through the birth canal, acquires within a few days of birth a flora which is practically identical with that of the adult (called indigenous or autochthonous flora). This flora then establishes a more or less permanent residence according to a remarkable repetitive pattern.[25, 46, 60]

There are obviously mechanisms operating within the first few days of life and continuing throughout life that establish and maintain the microbial status quo. It is not known why certain types of microorganisms have become adapted to specific areas of the body, but it has been suggested that it was probably achieved by competition in a manner analogous to the establishment of a normal flora in soil.[55] With respect to the skin, the predominant organism, C. acnes, has as an absolute growth requirement for the presence of fatty acids[35] and therefore may have an ecological advantage over many other fastidious species because of the availability of fatty acids in the skin. In addition, these organisms appear to exert some restraining influence on the gram-negative bacteria.[53]

Often the type of microbial alteration induced by chemotherapy can be predicted by knowing the spectrum of the antibiotic administered and the duration of therapy. This change is independent of the effect of the antibiotic on the specific organism responsible for the infection.[23] Susceptible bacteria are more or less rapidly eliminated following chemotherapy, resulting in an environment that permits the growth of other resistant microorganisms which, in turn, may eventually attain numbers equal to or greater than those found before the treatment with antibiotics was started.[30] Organisms so few in number that they cannot be detected early in the course increase in number after treatment with most antibiotics. That the secondary infections are not solely the result of the numerical increase of one of the normal microbial inhabitants is suggested by the fact that changes in flora induced by antimicrobial agents are frequently not followed by suprainfection.[63]

Antibiotics may alter the mechanisms responsible for maintaining normal interrelationships among the bacterial populations by selectively removing some organism with "inhibitor" characteristics, thereby permitting an increase in numbers of the organisms subject to such inhibition. The antibiotics having the greatest effect on the "normal flora" result in more striking changes in the bacterial population.[12, 22, 55] The Streptococcus viridans has recently been demonstrated to be a potent inhibitor of gram-negative bacilli that emerge in the sputum following antibiotic therapy, and has been proposed as the inhibitory species responsible for the maintenance of the normal flora of the upper respiratory tract.[55, 57]

Similar mechanisms may be operative during antibiotic therapy in other areas of the body which possess a "normal flora," but they would not account for the increased occurrence of infection in normally sterile organs such as the lung. These infections may arise as a result of increased numbers and virulence of pathogens in contiguous areas which harbor normal flora. Alternatively, antibiotics[11] may actually stimulate the growth of colonizing organisms as has been demonstrated in vitro with certain fungi[7] and bacteria.[19]

It is obvious, therefore, that changes in the microbial population alone probably do not account entirely for the development of suprainfection. Good evidence exists that certain host factors are also significant and these will be described in greater detail below.

FREQUENCY OF SUPRAINFECTION

Accurate data on the incidence of antibiotic-induced suprainfection are not available. The reported frequency of suprainfection has varied markedly and probably reflects the heterogeneity of the patient populations surveyed. In 1954, Weinstein and co-workers[63] reported the prevalence of this complication after antimicrobial therapy and prophylaxis in a wide variety of diseases to be about 2 per cent. A Federal Drug Administration survey of drug reactions carried out between 1953 and 1957 yielded 107 cases of secondary infections.[66] Louria and Kaminski[32] described a frequency of 15 per cent in patients with pulmonary disease who had been exposed to antibiotics. Their findings, however, reflected the appearance of new microorganisms in sputum during treatment and correspond to colonization, not suprainfection as defined above. Tillotson and Finland[59] recently reported their experience in the treatment of pneumonia and found the incidence of colonization and suprainfection to be 59 and 16 per cent respectively.

There have been data to suggest that antibiotics may have some effects predisposing to certain fungal infections,[52] but clear observations on incidence of antibiotic-induced fungal infections are lacking. That patients receiving antibiotics experience proliferation of Candida albicans is no longer a point for dispute.[50] Seelig has summarized the evidence favoring the view that antibiotics enhance the invasiveness of C. albicans.[51]

It has also been suggested that antibiotics may predispose to Candida infections in patients undergoing abdominal surgery.[20] In contrast, the association between antibiotic therapy and failure to survive a fungal infection was not found to be statistically significant.[20] Multiple organ involvement by Candida was also no more common among patients treated with antibiotics.[20] Similarly, studies of patients with acute leukemia and of renal transplant recipients demonstrated that antibiotic therapy was no more frequent in those with fungal infections than in control groups.[4, 45]

Although viral and parasitic infections are rarely considered as fitting the criteria characteristic of suprainfection, there are at least two candidates that warrant consideration for eligibility. They are cytomegalovirus and a protozoan, Pneumocystis carinii. Both of these organisms tend to produce disease under circumstances of altered host resistance. The majority of these patients, in addition to having severe and debilitating underlying diseases such as leukemias, lymphoma, and lupus erythematosus, are often receiving antibiotics as well as corticosteroids and cytotoxic drugs. It is uncertain what role the use of antimicrobial agents may play as a predisposing factor in these diseases. This is particularly so since little is known about their pathogenesis and epidemiology.[10, 48]

Of interest is the frequent observation of coexisting mycotic infections with the above opportunistic pathogens in the same compromised host.[24] The simultaneous association of Pneumocystis, cytomegalovirus, and fungi in a common host may not be particularly unique. Rather, it may represent coincidental infection of highly susceptible hosts with ubiquitous microorganisms.[44] Paradoxically, experience with experimental Pneumocystic carinii infection[17, 54] has shown that immunosuppressed animals will not live to develop pneumocystosis unless otherwise lethal bacterial infections are eradicated by appropriate antibiotics. Studies of patients with acute leukemia, however, demonstrated that antibiotic therapy was no more frequent in those with cytomegalic inclusion disease than in a control group.[5]

SUPRAINFECTION, COLONIZATION, AND THE ORGANISMS INVOLVED

A summary of data relating to suprainfection and the organisms involved, as extracted from two published series, is presented in Table 1. With the exception of the reports cited, the majority of other previous studies,[31, 36, 39] although concerned primarily with factors influencing microbial flora and subsequent superimposed infection, often failed to differentiate or define them adequately.

For the purpose of comparison, the data used were limited to cases of pneumonia that were a consequence of bacterial suprainfection. Separated from each other by approximately two decades, there are expectedly a number of striking differences between these two studies. Not surprising is the predominance of gram-negative bacteria involved in the majority of suprainfections in both series. The relative proportion of gram-positive to gram-negative infections has remained constant. Whereas the most commonly occurring organisms in Weinstein's series

Table 1. *Bacterial Suprainfection Causing Pneumonia*

	NUMBER OF CASES	
	Adapted from Weinstein et al.[63]	Adapted from Tillotson and Finland.[59]
ORGANISM	1946–1953	Feb. to Dec., 1967
Hemophilus influenzae	16	0
Streptococcus pyogenes	8	0
Staphylococcus aureus	5	6
Pseudomonas aeruginosa	3	3
Diplococcus pneumoniae	1	0
Klebsiella pneumoniae	0	2
Escherichia coli	0	2
Proteus mirabilis	0	3
Proteus morganii	0	1
Enterobacter aerogenes	0	1
Total no. of cases	33	18

Table 2.   *Bacteria Causing Colonization of the Respiratory Tract.*
(Adapted from Tillotson and Finland[59])

ORGANISM	NO. OF STRAINS
Klebsiella pneumoniae	37
Staphylococcus aureus	31
Escherichia coli	24
Hemophilus influenzae	23*
Proteus mirabilis	19
Enterobacter cloacae	16*
Serratia marcescens	10*
Pseudomonas aeruginosa	6
Herellea vaginicola	6*
Enterobacter aerogenes	3
Proteus morganii	3
Diplococcus pneumoniae	2*
Streptococcus pyogenes	2*
Total no. of strains	182

*Strains not causing suprainfection.

were Hemophilus influenzae and Streptococcus pyogenes, none of these were found by Tillotson and Finland. They were seemingly replaced by various members of the Enterobacteriaceae and Pseudomonas. It is worth noting, as the authors point out, that the failure to isolate more of the fastidious H. influenzae may have been because special media was not used.

The frequency of bacteria causing colonization was not enumerated in Weinstein's report. Tillotson and Finland found that, although gram-negative bacilli predominated in colonization (Table 2), the Staphylococcus aureus was the single most important species responsible for suprainfection.

Of particular interest was the frequent isolation of Serratia marcescens as a colonizer, although it did not produce a single instance of suprainfection in the experience of Tillotson and Finland. This organism, for many years, had been considered nonpathogenic for man; however, a recent extensive review of this topic[13] should dispel any doubts about its pathogenicity. Patients with S. marcescens bacteremia were studied at the same Boston hospital during the years 1963 through 1967 by independent workers.[67] They found the respiratory tract to be the suspected portal of entry in 13 per cent of cases. Of the various factors that have been associated with the acquisition of S. marcescens, the most prominent has been the prior administration of antimicrobials.[8, 13, 18, 49, 67]

FACTORS INFLUENZING COLONIZATION AND SUPRAINFECTION

Relation to Primary Underlying Disease

It is yet unknown whether suprainfection occurs more often in certain types of treated disease than in others. That a given organ or tissue involved in the primary disease has a much greater chance of being the site of suprainfection has been proposed by some.[63] Others have found this correlation only in permitting colonization to occur, but not in determining whether secondary clinical illness would result from such colonization.[59] Differences in frequency of complicating infection have been related to involvement of different anatomical sites of a specific organ. With respect to the respiratory tract, the lower in the respiratory tract that the primary disease occurred, the greater the risk of suprainfection. In the order of increasing risk, then, are the pharynx, trachea, bronchi, and lungs.[63]

Age and Susceptibility

The age of the patient is frequently correlated with an increased susceptibility to suprainfection, the rates of colonization and fatal suprainfection being significantly higher in elderly patients than in younger ones.[59] What impact the aging process has on host defense mechanisms remains largely unknown. Recently, Burnet has proposed that the process of aging is largely mediated by autoimmune processes, resulting in progressive weakening of immunological surveillance via defects of the thymus-dependent immune system.[6] An obvious accompaniment of increasing longevity has been an increase in the number of patients with chronic and debilitating diseases. The high mortality rate among the aged due to gram-negative bacilli has been substantiated by others.[9, 28, 58] Age itself may be a misleading statistic, however, since it appears that age-associated underlying disease or the preinfection status probably best correlates with the eventual outcome.[9, 16]

Influence of Type of Chemotherapy

The use of antimicrobial agents has been implicated most frequently as the major cause of suprainfection.[32, 68] Of greatest importance is the nature of the drug administered. In general, the narrower the spectrum of bacterial species susceptible to an agent, the lower is the incidence of suprainfection.[62] The use of high doses of penicillin and an aminoglycoside, or broad spectrum antibiotics alone or in combination with penicillin has been well documented as being associated with increased rates of both colonization and suprainfection.[59, 63] It would appear then that broad-spectrum antimicrobials which frequently modify the microbial flora provide a setting in which suprainfection is more likely to occur.

The relationship between penicillin dosage and frequency of suprainfection is of particular interest. Although small dosages of penicillin (less than 3 million units daily) rarely cause suprainfection,[63] the administration of large quantities has been implicated as a common cause of this complication.[31, 32, 59] Large doses of this drug achieve a broad-spectrum effect which includes a variety of gram-negative organisms that, by conventional methods of testing, would be considered to be insensitive.[64] In contrast to these observations, Weinstein and Musher[65] have reported that the administration of 20 to 80 million units of penicillin over a period of as long as 4 weeks resulted in suprainfection infrequently.

Despite this discrepancy over the dose-related infectious complications secondary to penicillin usage, there is agreement that the death rate in patients with suprainfection following large-dose penicillin was significantly lower than in those in whom the superimposed infection was related to the use of other antibiotics.[59]

RECOGNITION AND MANAGEMENT OF SUPRAINFECTION

The diagnostic consideration of suprainfection should be first entertained in a patient who has been given an antimicrobial agent, improves, and then suddenly shows evidence of active infection. Thus, in the case in which chemotherapy abruptly becomes ineffective, the possibility of suprainfection should be carefully searched for. The temperature chart shown in Table 3 illustrates the development of bacterial suprainfection on the sixth hospital day of a patient with bacterial pneumonia, initially of unknown etiology, that subsequently was proven bacteriologically to be pneumococcal in origin. It should be stressed that the continuation of high-dose penicillin and kanamycin in the therapeutic regimen was not warranted when the pneumococcal etiology became known.

Often the apparent progression of an infectious disease is treated more or less empirically by a change of antibiotics without the advantage

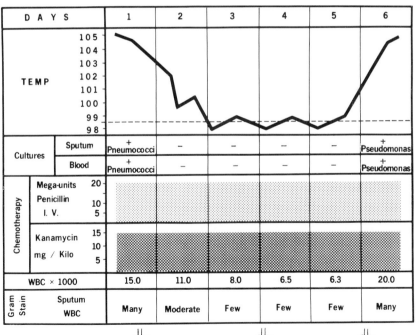

D A Y S			1	2	3	4	5	6
TEMP		105 104 103 102 101 100 99 98						
Cultures	Sputum		+ Pneumococci	–	–	–	–	+ Pseudomonas
	Blood		+ Pneumococci	–	–	–	–	+ Pseudomonas
Chemotherapy	Mega-units Penicillin I. V.	20 10 5						
	Kanamycin mg / Kilo	15 10 5						
WBC × 1000			15.0	11.0	8.0	6.5	6.3	20.0
Gram Stain	Sputum WBC		Many	Moderate	Few	Few	Few	Many

Chest X-Ray

Table 3

of additional information concerning the possibility of a change in etiology. Without specific microbiologic study (both culture and Gram stain of appropriate body fluids), it is impossible to establish specifically the presence of a suprainfection. On the other hand, cultures *alone* fail to differentiate those patients with and without clinical illness caused by the changing flora. In Tillotson and Finland's study,[59] 71 of the 182 potential pathogens colonizing the sputum predominated on culture, but only 24 produced secondary infections. To subject patients to chemotherapy who are colonized with potential pathogens but fail to show objective evidence of new disease (Table 4) not only exposes them to the risks of drug-induced toxic and hypersensitivity reactions but, by further altering the flora, may actually increase the further risk of suprainfection.

It should be mentioned that there are a number of conditions which may simulate suprainfection by meeting all the criteria listed in Table 4. For example, the patient with pneumococcal pneumonia receiving therapy with penicillin may abruptly worsen from a variety of complications of either pneumococcal sepsis (empyema, endocarditis, meningitis) or antibiotic therapy (drug fever, exudative erythema multiforme, or serum-sickness-like reaction). Resolution of such a common clinical dilemma requires an awareness of all the factors involved: (1) knowledge of the chronological sequence of events surrounding the complication, (2) examination of the manner in which the sequelae have begun and progressed, and (3) an understanding of the complications most likely to occur as a consequence of the specific infection or antibiotic involved. Thoughtful appraisal of these factors as well as careful clinical evaluation provides a rational approach which makes possible an etiologic diagnosis that time and laboratory study often prove correct.

Once a diagnosis of secondary infection is made on the basis of clinical and microbiological findings, therapy should be instituted immediately, based on the known antibiotic susceptibilities of the suprainfecting organisms frequently encountered within that particular institution. The choice of drug can be altered if, after sensitivity studies, another antimicrobial agent appears to be more satisfactory.

Table 4.	*Criteria for Diagnosis of Microbial Suprainfection*

Microbiologic Criteria
Demonstration of new organism(s)

Clinical Criteria
History: Antimicrobial administration, recent or current
Physical Signs
    Rise in body temperature
    Evolution of the physical signs, consistent with a disease process not present
        when antimicrobial agents were instituted
Laboratory Values
    Increasing peripheral WBC count
    Increasing erythrocyte sedimentation rate

Interpretation
    Suprainfection: Both microbiologic and clinical criteria present
    Colonization: Only microbiologic criteria present

SUPERINFECTION

The problem of superinfection, namely the development of a secondary infection not primarily related to antibiotic therapy, is a major problem which is being seen with increasing frequency. This increase can be related almost entirely to a growing population of patients with alterations in host resistance.[24] Such individuals owe their susceptibility to the basic disease process such as burns, diabetes mellitus, hematopoietic disorders, renal failure, and liver disease, or to specific therapy including irradiation, the use of antimetabolites and corticosteroids, and the instillation of foreign bodies such as venous and indwelling (Foley) bladder catheters. A review of this problem, often referred to as "opportunistic" infection, is beyond the scope of the present survey. The interested reader is referred to several recent extensive reviews of this subject.[20, 24, 26, 34, 37, 48]

CONCLUDING REMARKS

This review of selected aspects of microbial suprainfection points out again that medical progress has provided physicians with a number of potent agents which under certain circumstances may be deleterious to the host. The most important principle in the prophylaxis of suprainfection is to administer antimicrobial agents only when they are needed. It has been estimated that from 50 to 90 per cent of the time, antibiotics are administered without clear indications.[38, 42, 47] Moreover, it has been shown clearly that the use of antimicrobials to cover so-called "infection-prone" individuals constitutes a leaky umbrella at best and may be distinctly detrimental.[3] The situation cannot be better summarized than in the concluding words of an editorial written almost 20 years ago. "The subtleties of bacterial evasion . . . underscore the need for wisdom in the selection and application of these drugs. The realities of the situation should not escape us in our therapeutic complacency, and should be a warning not to squander our antibiotic fortune at the present prodigal rate. It has been stated often, but it apparently cannot be emphasized enough, that these valuable drugs should not be hurled at the heads of each and every unidentified infection."[11]

REFERENCES

 1. Altemeier, W. A., Hummel, R. P., and Hill, E. O.: Staphylococcal enterocolitis following antibiotic therapy. Ann. Surg., 157:847–858, 1963.
 2. Applebaum, E., and Leff, W. A.: Occurrence of superinfections during antibiotic therapy. J.A.M.A., 138:119–121, 1948.
 3. Beaty, H. N., and Petersdorf, R. G.: Iatrogenic factors in infectious disease. Ann. Intern. Med., 65:641–656, 1966.
 4. Bodey, G. P.: Fungal infections complicating acute leukemia. J. Chronic Dis., 19:667–687, 1966.
 5. Bodey, G. P., Wertlake, P. T., Douglas, G., and Levin, R. H.: Cytomegalic inclusion disease in patients with acute leukemia. Ann. Intern. Med., 62:899–906, 1965.
 6. Burnet, F. M.: An immunological approach to ageing. Lancet, 2:358–360, 1970.
 7. Campbell, C. C., and Saslaw, S.: Enhancement of growth of certain fungi by streptomycin. Proc. Soc. Exper. Biol. Med., 70:562–563, 1949.

8. Dodson, W. H.: Serratia marcescens septicemia. Arch. Intern. Med., *121*:145–150, 1968.
9. DuPont, H. L., and Spink, W. W.: Infections due to gram-negative organisms: An analysis of 860 patients with bacteremia at the University of Minnesota Medical Center 1958–1966. Medicine, *48*:307–332, 1969.
10. Duvall, C. P., Casazza, A. R., Grimley, P. M., Carbone, P. P., and Rowe, W. P.: Recovery of cytomegalovirus from adults with neoplastic disease. Ann. Intern. Med., *64*:531–541, 1966.
11. Editorial. Bacterial versatility. Ann. Intern. Med., *36*:196–202, 1952.
12. Elmes, P. C., Knox, K., and Fletcher, C. M.: Sputum in chronic bronchitis. Effect of antibiotics. Lancet, 2:903–906, 1953.
13. Fields, B. N., Uwaydah, M. M., Kunz, L. J., and Swartz, M.: The so-called "Paracolon" bacteria. Amer. J. Med., *42*:89–106, 1967.
14. Finland, M., and Weinstein, L.: Complications induced by antimicrobial agents. New Eng. J. Med., *248*:220–226, 1953.
15. Finland, M.: The symposium on gentamicin. J. Infect. Dis., *119*:537, 1969.
16. Freid, M. A., and Vosti, K. L.: The importance of underlying disease in patients with gram-negative bacteremia. Arch. Intern. Med., *121*:418–423, 1968.
17. Frenkel, J. K., Good, J. T., and Shultz, J. A.: Latent Pneumocystis infection of rats, relapse and chemotherapy. Lab. Invest., *15*:1559–1577, 1966.
18. Gale, D., and Sonnenwirth, A. C.: Frequent human isolations of Serratia marcescens. Arch. Intern. Med., *109*:414–421, 1962.
19. Garrod, L. P.: The reaction of bacteria to chemotherapeutic agents. Brit. Med. J., *1*:205–210, 1951.
20. Hart, P. D., Russell, E., and Remington, J. S.: The compromised host and infection. II. Deep fungal infection. J. Infect. Dis., *120*:169–191, 1969.
21. Hewitt, W. L., Finegold, S. M., and Sutter, V. L.: Incidence of side effects and changes in fecal microflora following administration of tetracycline and tetracycline-nystatin. Antibiotics Annual 1955–1956. New York, Medical Encyclopedia, Inc., pp. 856–861.
22. Julianelle, L. A., and Siegel, M.: The epidemiology of acute respiratory infections conditioned by sulfonamides. II. Gross alterations in the nasopharyngeal flora associated with treatment. Ann. Intern. Med., 22:10–20, 1945.
23. Keefer, C. S.: Alterations in normal bacterial flora of man and secondary infections during antibiotic therapy (Editorial). Amer. J. Med., *11*:665, 1951.
24. Klainer, A. S., and Beisel, W. R.: Opportunistic infection: a review. Amer. J. Med. Sci., *258*:431–456, 1969.
25. Kneeland, Y., Jr.: Studies on the common cold. III. The upper respiratory flora of infants. J. Exper. Med., *51*:617–624, 1930.
26. Knight, V.: Instruments and infection. Hospital Practice, 2:82–95, 1967.
27. Laurenzi, G. A., Potter, R. T., and Kass, E. H.: Bacteriologic flora of the lower respiratory tract. New Eng. J. Med., *265*:1273–1278, 1961.
28. Lewis, J., and Fekety, F. R.: Gram-negative bacteremia. John Hopkins Med. J., *124*:106–111, 1969.
29. Lipman, M. O., Coss, J. A., and Boots, K. H.: Changes in the bacterial flora of the throat and intestinal tract during prolonged oral administration of penicillin. J. Bact., *51*: 594, 1946.
30. Long, D. A.: Effect of penicillin on bacterial flora of the mouth. Brit. Med. J., 2:819–821, 1947.
31. Louria, D. B., and Brayton, R. G.: The efficacy of penicillin regimens with observations of their frequency of superinfection. J.A.M.A., *186*:987–990, 1963.
32. Louria, D. B., and Kaminski, T.: The effect of four antimicrobial drug regimens on sputum superinfection in hospitalized patients. Amer. Rev. Resp. Dis., 85:649–665, 1962.
33. Lwoff, A., and Lwoff, M.: Studies on codehydrogenases: Nature of growth factor "V." Proc. Roy. Soc., London, S. B., *122*:352–359, 1937.
34. Mandel, G. L., and Hook, E. W.: Opportunistic infections. Hospital Medicine, 4:40–50, 1968.
35. Marples, M.: The Ecology of Human Skin. Springfield, Illinois, Charles C Thomas, Publisher, 1965, pp. 658–668.
36. McCurdy, R. S., and Neter, E.: Effects of penicillin and broad spectrum antibiotics on the emergence of a gram-negative bacillary flora in the upper respiratory tract of infants. Pediatrics, 9:572–576, 1952.
37. Murray, J. F., Haegelin, H. F., Hewitt, W. L., Latta, H., McVickar, D., Rasmussen, A. F., and Rigler, L. G.: Opportunistic pulmonary infections. Ann. Int. Med., *65*:566–594, 1966.
38. Nolen, W. A., Dille, D. E.: Use and abuse of antibiotics in a small community. New Eng. J. Med., *257*:33–34, 1957.
39. Ory, E., Harris, H. W., Meads, M., Wilcox, C., and Finland, M.: Bacteriologic studies of sputum in patients with pneumococcal pneumonia treated with penicillin. J. Lab. Clin. Med., *31*:409–422, 1946.

40. Pickett, M. J., and Stewart, M. A.: Identification of hemophilic bacilli by means of the satellite phenomenon. Amer. J. Clin. Path., 23:713–715, 1953.
41. Reeves, P.: Bacteriocins. Bact. Rev., 29:24–45, 1965.
42. Reimann, H. A.: The misuse of antimicrobics. Med. Clin. N. Amer., 45:849–856, 1961.
43. Ribble, J. C.: A mechanism of bacterial interference in vitro. J. Immunol., 98:716–723, 1967.
44. Rifkind, D., Faris, T. D., and Hill, R. B.: Pneumocystic carinii pneumonia. Studies on diagnosis and treatment. Ann. Int. Med., 65:943–956, 1966.
45. Rifkind, D., Marchioro, T. L., Schneck, S. A., and Hill, R. B.: Systemic fungal infections complicating renal transplantation and immunosuppressive therapy. Clinical, microbiologic, neurologic and pathologic features. Am. J. Med., 43:28–38, 1967.
46. Rosebury, T.: Microorganisms Indigenous to Man. New York, McGraw-Hill Book Company Inc., 1962.
47. Rosenthal, A.: Follow-up study of fatal penicillin reactions: Special report. J.A.M.A., 167:1118–1126, 1958.
48. Ruskin, J., and Remington, J. S.: The compromised host and infection. I. Pneumocystis carinii pneumonia. J.A.M.A., 202:96–99, 1967.
49. Saito, K.: Infections due to Serratia marcescens. Jap. J. Bact., 20:5–13, 1965.
50. Seelig, M. S.: Mechanisms by which antibiotics increase the incidence and severity of candidiasis and alter the immunological defenses. Bact. Rev., 30:442–459, 1966.
51. Seelig, M. S.: The role of antibiotics in the pathogenesis of candida infections. Amer. J. Med., 40:887–917, 1966.
52. Seligman, E.: Virulence enhancement of Candida albicans by antibiotics and cortisone. Proc. Soc. Exper. Biol. Med., 83:778–781, 1953.
53. Shehadeh, N. H., and Kligman, A. M.: The effect of topical antibacterial agents on the bacterial flora of the axilla. J. Invest. Derm., 40:61–71, 1963.
54. Sheldon, W. H.: Experimental pulmonary Pneumocystis carinii infection in rabbits. J. Exper. Med., 110:147–160, 1959.
55. Smith, D. T.: The disturbance of the normal bacterial ecology by the administration of antibiotics with the development of new clinical syndromes. Ann. Intern. Med., 37: 1135–1143, 1952.
56. Sprinz, H., Kundel, D. W., Dammin, G. J., Horowitz, R. E., Schneider, H., and Formal, S. B.: The response of the germ-free guinea pig to oral bacterial challenge with Escherichia coli and Shigella flexneri; with special reference to lymphatic tissue and intestinal tract. Amer. J. Path., 39:681–695, 1961.
57. Sprunt, K., and Redman, W.: Evidence suggesting importance of role of interbacterial inhibition in maintaining balance of normal flora. Ann. Intern. Med., 68:579–590, 1968.
58. Tillotson, J. R., and Lerner, A. M.: Pneumonias caused by gram-negative bacilli. Medicine, 45:65–76, 1966.
59. Tillotson, J. R., and Finland, M.: Bacterial colonization and clinical superinfection of the respiratory tract complicating antibiotic treatment of pneumonia. J. Infect. Dis., 119: 597–624, 1969.
60. Torrey, J. C., and Reese, M. K.: Initial aerobic flora of newborn infants. Amer. J. Dis. Child., 69:208–214, 1945.
61. Weinstein, L.: The spontaneous occurrence of new bacterial infections during the course of treatment with streptomycin or penicillin. Amer. J. Med. Sci., 214:56–63, 1947.
62. Weinstein, L.: Superinfection: A complication of antimicrobial therapy and prophylaxis. Amer. J. Surg., 107:704–709, 1964.
63. Weinstein, L., Goldfield, M., and Chang, T. W.: Infections occurring during chemotherapy. A study of their frequency, type and predisposing factors. New Eng. J. Med., 251:247–255, 1954.
64. Weinstein, L., Lerner, P. I., and Chew, W. H.: Clinical and bacteriologic studies of the effect of "massive" doses of penicillin G on infections caused by gram-negative bacilli. New Eng. J. Med., 271:525–533, 1964.
65. Weinstein, L., and Musher, D. M.: Antibiotic-induced suprainfection (Editorial). J. Infect. Dis., 119:662–665, 1969.
66. Welch, H., Lewis, C. N., Weinstein, H. I., and Boeckman, B. B.: Severe reactions to antibiotics: a nationwide survey. Antibiotics Annual, 1957–1958, pp. 298–309.
67. Wilfert, J. N., Barrett, F. F., and Kass, E. H.: Bacteremia due to Serratia marcescens. New Eng. J. Med., 279:286–289, 1968.
68. Yow, E. M.: Development of proteus and pseudomonas infections during antibiotic therapy. J.A.M.A., 149:1184–1188, 1952.

1201 N.W. 16th Street
Miami, Florida 33125

Pharmacologic Considerations in the Treatment of Anxiety and Depression in Medical Practice

Burton J. Goldstein, M.D.,* and Benjamin Brauzer, M.D.**

The purpose of this chapter is to bring to the attention of the medical practitioner some of the more cogent considerations influencing the outcome of treatment with ataractic (minor tranquilizer and anti-anxiety) and antidepressant drugs. It is not our purpose to recommend specific drugs or classes of drugs for particular emotional states. For information about specific drugs, their uses and limitations, the reader is referred elsewhere.[10, 11, 15, 16]

An article devoted entirely to treatment considerations and the prescribing of drugs for controlling the symptoms of anxiety and depression may appear to be narrow in scope; however, anecdotal information has indicated that between 40 and 70 per cent of the medical practitioner's patients are treated primarily for the target symptoms of anxiety and depression, or these symptoms as concomitants of organic illness.

The extent of psychotropic drug usage, in particular, ataractic and antidepressant drugs, for a typical year may give the reader some idea of the widespread usage of these drugs. In 1967, a total of 1.1 billion prescriptions for drugs of all types were filled in pharmacies throughout the United States at a retail cost of 3.9 billion dollars.[3] Psychotropic drugs accounted for 17 per cent, or 178 million prescriptions, at a consumer cost of 692 million dollars.

The major classes of psychotropic drugs and their distributions by drug class for this period are shown in Table 1.

Considering only those drugs classified as ataractic (antianxiety, minor tranquilizers) or antidepressant, 74.5 million prescriptions were filled. These figures do not include mixtures in which a drug such as chlordiazepoxide (Librium) is used with an antispasmodic agent, nor do these figures include over the counter drugs (Compoz, Tranquil, etc.).

From the Department of Psychiatry, University of Miami School of Medicine, Miami, Florida

*Associate Professor, and Assistant Chairman, Department of Psychiatry
**Assistant Professor of Psychiatry

Table 1. *Major Classes of Psychotropic Drugs and Their Distribution (1967)*

DRUGS	EXAMPLES	DISTRIBUTION
Major tranquilizers		
Phenothiazine derivatives	chlorpromazine, thioridazine	
Butyrophenones	haloperidol	9.5%
Thioxanthines	thiothixene, chlorprothixene	
Minor tranquilizers		
Substituted diols	meprobamate, tybamate	
Benzodiazepines	chlordiazepoxide, diazepam, oxazepam	34.4%
Miscellaneous	hydroxyzine, buclizine	
Antidepressants		
Tricyclics	imipramine, amitriptyline	
Monoamine-oxidase inhibitors	isocarboxazid, phenelzine	8.6%
Others	combination of amitriptyline and perphenazine	
Stimulants		
Amphetamines	dextroamphetamine, methamphetamine	
Others	methylphenidate	15.4%
Sedatives		
Barbiturates – long-acting and intermediate-acting	phenobarbital, butabarbital	12.9%
Others	bromisovalum	
Hypnotics		
Barbiturate – short-acting	pentobarbital, secobarbital	
Non-barbiturate	glutethimide, ethchlorvynol	19.2%

If we consider new and refilled prescriptions dispensed, the minor tranquilizers have shown the greatest increase of all psychotropic drugs, from a total of 45.1 million in 1964 to 59.7 million in 1967. Prescriptions for antidepressant drugs have risen from 9.4 to 14.8 million during the same time period.

The greatest number of ataractic and antidepressant drugs are prescribed for patients in the age group of 40 to 59 years, while stimulant drugs are primarily prescribed for young adults. Knowledge of the latter group is especially important because many physicians prescribe stimulants such as methylphenidate (Ritalin) or an amphetamine for symptoms of tired, lethargic, or "washed out" feelings, which may in fact be prodromal symptoms of depression.

Seventy per cent of all psychotropic drugs are prescribed by physicians other than psychiatrists. Most of the patients receiving these drugs do not have a specific psychiatric diagnosis.

ANXIETY AND DEPRESSION

There are several schools of thought about the manner in which anxiety and depression develop. These theoretical discussions are available to the reader in any standard textbook of psychiatry.[1, 17] It is our belief, however, that the nonpsychiatric physician, and at times the psychiatrist, intuitively treats anxiety and depression as a syndrome[7] –

a complex of signs and symptoms seen in descriptive terms—rather than from an etiological point of view.

These signs and symptoms of anxiety and depression are multiple, and often elusive and vague, as exemplified by the common use of such terms as "masked depression," "depressive equivalent," or "physiological expression of anxiety."

The symptoms and symptom cues listed in Table 2 are compiled from validated, widely used rating scales[12, 20] used in clinical studies to assess the severity of patients' symptoms of anxiety and depression. The symptoms are those most often found in anxious and depressed patients.

Table 2. *Most Frequently Reported Symptoms of Anxiety and Depression*

SYMPTOM CATEGORIES	SYMPTOM CUES
Intellectual	Difficulty in concentration, poor memory
Anxious mood	Worries, anticipation of the worst, fearful anticipation, irritability
Tension	Feelings of tension, fatiguability, startle response, moved to tears easily, trembling, feelings of restlessness, inability to relax
Fears	Of dark, of strangers, of being left alone, of animals, of traffic, of crowds
Depressed mood	Feelings of sadness, hopelessness. The patient expresses pessimism, discouragement and sadness; the facial expression reflects despair or dejection
Feelings of guilt	Self-reproach, feels he has let people down, criticizes himself to an unrealistic degree
Retardation	Slowness of thought and speech; impaired ability to concentrate, decreased motor activity
Work and activities	Thoughts and feelings of incapacity, fatigue or weakness related to activities, work or hobbies; loss of interest in activity, hobbies, or work—either directly reported by patient, or indirect in listlessness, indecision, and vacillation (feels he has to push self to work or activities); decrease in actual time spent in activities or decrease in productivity
Hypochondriasis	Patient is absorbed in his own physical ailments; preoccupation with health
Insomnia	Difficulty in falling asleep, broken sleep, unsatisfying sleep and fatigue on waking, dreams nightmares, night terrors, early awakening
Somatic	Pains and aches, twitching, stiffness, myoclonic jerks, grinding of teeth, unsteady voice, increased muscular tone
Somatic	Tinnitus, blurring of vision, hot and cold flushes, feelings of weakness, pricking sensation, easily fatigued; heaviness in limbs, back, or head, backaches, headache, muscle aches, loss of energy, and fatiguability
Cardiovascular symptoms	Tachycardia, palpitations, pain in chest, throbbing of vessels, fainting feelings, missing beat
Respiratory symptoms	Pressure or constriction in chest, choking feelings, sighing, dyspnea
Gastrointestinal symptoms	Difficulty in swallowing, wind, abdominal pain, burning sensations, abdominal fullness, nausea, vomiting, borborygmi, looseness of bowels, loss of weight, constipation
Genitourinary symptoms	Frequency of micturition, urgency of micturition, amenorrhea, menorrhagia, frigidity, premature ejaculation, loss of libido, impotence
Autonomic symptoms	Dry mouth, flushing, pallor, tendency to sweat, giddiness, tension headache, raising of hair

The reader could expand the items in Table 2 easily by recalling office dialogues with anxious-depressed patients.

In eliciting a review of organ systems, the physician should be aware of the target symptoms that relate to anxiety and depression. All systems may be involved to some degree. The voluntary motor, respiratory, gastrointestinal, and genitourinary systems are most frequently affected. The patient may complain that his neck muscles are frequently sore on arising, that his legs are weak, and that walking is difficult. Young people frequently describe themselves as "up tight." Gastrointestinal problems such as nausea, vomiting, and diarrhea are common manifestations of anxiety; constipation and poor appetite are symptoms more commonly related to depression. Effects on the genitourinary system include frequency of urination during stress, irregular menses, and impotence of recent origin.

As an objective observer, the physician notes the behavioral manifestations of anxiety and depression during each contact with the patient. Table 3 lists a number of signs observed in the anxious-depressed patient. The behavior observed in the interview situation may serve as a convenient barometer of the patient's level of anxiety-depression.

The physician, having identified the syndrome and being convinced there is minimal organic involvement which could be directly responsible for the presenting signs and symptoms, must next consider the appropriate form of intervention — whether it be consultation, referral, counseling, or medication.

The anxious-depressed patient seen by the practicing physician generally presents a preponderance of symptoms of one state or another. The importance of recognizing the coexistence of anxiety and depression lies in the implications for treatment. Hollister and Overall,[20] applying computer profile techniques in analyzing the severity of target symptoms of depressed patients on the Brief Psychiatric Rating Scale (BPRS),[19] were able to distinguish three depressive subtypes: anxious depression, hostile depression, and retarded depression. The majority of patients were classified in the anxious-depressed group. Comparison of drugs by subtype interaction reveal that tricyclic antidepressants (amitriptylene, imipramine, etc.) were most efficacious in the treatment of retarded depression, while the antianxiety drugs were superior in treating the anxious-depression. Hostile depression responded equally well to both classes of drugs. It would thus appear that the antidepressant agents are the drug of choice in the minority of depressions, and then only in the retarded form.

The following discussion is intended to present a frame of reference

Table 3. *Signs of Anxiety and Depression*

Twitching of muscles	Frequent repetitive movements of hands or legs
Grinding of teeth	Tremor of hands
Unsteady voice	Flushing
Sighing	Strained facies
Irregular breathing	Dilated pupils
Fidgeting in the chair	Excessive perspiration

for drug treatment, and should not be construed in itself as being firm criteria for or against treatment.

1. Should the severity of the patient's symptomatology warrant drug intervention? Anxiety and depression are appropriate responses to certain situations and often are required in maintaining a normal discharge of emotion. Anxiety has been considered a catalyst for productivity in some individuals. Comments from everyday life such as, "I work better under stress," "I can never get to work unless I have a deadline to meet," or the student who finds that he must maintain a certain level of anxiety in order to prepare for an examination, exemplify the necessity for "optimal" amounts of anxiety. Grief following the death of a loved one is necessary in working through the loss and allows the mourner to psychologically cope with the tragic event and eventually redistribute his emotional stores. The physician who would interfere with such appropriate feelings by using drugs may be doing the patient a great disservice.

2. The intensity of symptoms will vary from patient to patient. Anxiety and depression experienced by patients exposed to identical stressful situations varies, and must be assessed in terms of the discomfort the patient experiences and not in the expectations of the physician based upon his own personal value system.

3. In assessing the patient's need for pharmacologic intervention, the physician must attempt to use some objective criteria. We would suggest that decrease in productivity be clearly established prior to starting treatment. The decrease in a patient's ability to function in his role (as housewife, parent, spouse, breadwinner) can be determined by history. If it is ascertained that there is a recent onset of diminished level of performance in interpersonal, intrapsychic, social, or economic functioning, medication may be of assistance. Physicians often find themselves treating patients who appear to be clinically anxious and depressed, only to find such patients unimproved or even worsened after a reasonable treatment period with drugs. Often such disappointments can be avoided by a careful assessment of the clinical course, and history of symptoms, as well as responses to previous drug treatment.

The chronically anxious patient is frequently refractory to treatment with minor tranquilizers and presents problems when treated with major tranquilizers.[8] Certain patients appear to have a life-long history of the symptoms of anxiety. These patients generally have received numerous drugs, usually with poor results. With such a patient, one can usually predict equally disappointing results with a "new drug" and it would be to the best interest of the patient to obtain a psychiatric consultation.

The clinical syndrome of depression must, therefore, be differentiated from a life style of depression.[4,5] Certain individuals' personalities are basically gloomy, and their outlook on life is one of sadness, dejection and despair. Such patients are generally refractory to drug treatment. In general, patients who have a history of chronic depression and have received multiple drug treatment warrant psychiatric consultation, in order for the physician to be in a better position to render realistic treatment, rather than make continued haphazard attempts at pharmacologic intervention.

4. Prior to prescribing medication, the physician must decide what changes he expects to effect in his patient. The question of establishing realistic treatment goals is central.

All too often physicians have a tacit expectation that a drug which will reduce anxiety or lift depression will also alleviate social, interpersonal, or intrapsychic problems.[18]

Anxiety and depression are often observed in the middle-aged man who feels that he has reached the highest peak of his career, which is at a lower level than he has strived for, in the woman who feels that her marriage is failing, or in the parents who have difficulty in dealing with the adolescent rebellion of their teenage children. These individuals seek help for relief of their symptoms. At best, drugs may assist these individuals in better coping with their discomfort by altering their physiologic distress, anxiety, and depression; but the basic problems still exist. Drugs cannot be expected to remedy the social, cultural, and interpersonal sources of anxiety. The physician must recognize that reducing the severity of the patient's discomfort may permit the patient to better deal with the sources of the anxiety and depression even though they are not altered. This should be considered a realistic goal and a major achievement.

5. Are anti-anxiety and antidepressant drugs effective? The results of controlled clinical trials have supported the thesis that this is generally the case.[13, 16]

The physician is frequently faced with the dilemma that a particular drug reported to be safe and effective lacks efficacy or produces untoward effects in a particular patient. The variability of responses observed cannot be fully attributed to any single factor.

The relevance of nonspecific factors in drug response has been studied by several investigators during the past five years.[21–25] The influence of patient, doctor, and environmental variables on every aspect of treatment has been demonstrated.

The patient variables consist of the following:

Personality structure
Sociodemographic factors
Duration and intensity of symptoms
Previous drug treatment
Attitudes and expectations of treatment
Symptoms orientation (psychological vs. physiological, whether the patient's major complaint is in the area of emotional feelings of somatically focused)

The personality of the doctor, his expectations and attitudes toward treatment, and those of the patients, as well as the doctor's social class and professional orientation, are all factors influencing results of treatment.

The interaction of sociodemographic factors and presenting symptoms, drug-placebo differences, and side effects will serve as an example.

Rickels[26, 27] in several studies conducted in the medical clinics of public hospitals, and in collaboration with general practitioners in their private practices, using rating instruments to dichotomize presenting symptoms into emotional or somatic clusters. He found that the lower socioeconomic group of patients (clinic) most often present with somatic complaints. The reverse was true with middle-class private patients. The latter group most often complained of worry, apprehension, fear, despair, and sadness (emotional cluster).

In studies in which effects of drugs vs. placeboes were compared, the greatest differences between drug and placebo was observed in private patients; drug-placebo differences were smallest in the clinic patients.[28]

The sedative side-effects of anti-anxiety drugs were best tolerated by clinic patients, and were poorly tolerated by private patients; anti-cholinergic side-effects (nasal stuffiness, constipation, blurred vision) were acceptable to private patients.

The implications of these differences are important in the day to day practice of physicians who prescribe ataractic or antidepressant drugs.

1. Extrapolation of the results of treatment from one population to another is hazardous because marked differences exist, and the results of clinical trials of a drug carried out in a public clinic population may not be applicable to the middle-class private patient.

2. Patients who present with predominantly somatic complaints and have little insight into their emotional feelings are often less responsive to treatment with ataractic or antidepressant drugs. Conversely, the patient who is able to verbalize his anxiety and depression generally responds more satisfactorily.

3. The sedative side-effects encountered with all the ataractic drugs may be a source of difficulty to middle-class patients, while they are acceptable to clinic patients.

The influence of non-drug factors in effecting the outcome of treatment has been well demonstrated. However, at this time the specific interactions of non-drug factors and treatment outcome has not reached the stage of sophistication where the physician in practice can predict their effects in a specific patient. Non-drug factors are always operative, although not always predictable or consistent. It is important for the physician to recognize the existence of these factors and be cognizant of their influence upon the results of treatment.

The physician who is aware of the existence of the nonspecific factors and is willing to accept their influence upon treatment will find himself less frustrated, less likely to change medication frequently, and less likely to prescribe combinations of drugs.

TREATMENT SUGGESTIONS

1. The sedative effects of the benzediazepenes (chlordiazepoxide, diazepam, oxazepam) and the glycerol alcohol derivatives (meprobamate, tybamate) may be utilized to advantage.[13] Most patients who exhibit anxiety and depression suffer from varying degrees of insomnia, which may be successfully treated by giving a larger portion of the daily dose of drug at bedtime. The relatively long half-life of the benzediazepenes makes it possible to reduce the traditional three to four times a day divided dose to two daily doses. This provides added convenience for the

patient who may be reluctant to take medication at work.

2. If treatment with an antidepressant drug is warranted, the tricyclic antidepressant drugs (imipramine, amitriptylene) are the drugs of first choice; the monoamine oxidase inhibitors should be used sparingly and only with extreme caution. The major concern, in spite of its relatively rare occurrence, is the possible hypertensive crisis and death due to cerebral vascular accident. Ingestion of foods containing pressor amines in patients receiving monoamine oxidase inhibitors increases the quantity of circulating biogenic amines and, if levels are sufficiently high, may lead to severe hypertensive sequelae.[2, 8, 29]

Drugs such as methylphenidate (Ritalin) or pipradol (Meratran) have been used with some success in treating symptoms of lethargy and fatigue related to mild or prodromal depression.[9]

We strongly discourage the use of amphetamines in the treatment of depressive symptoms. While we recognize the ability of amphetamines to lessen overt symptoms of depression, the stimulant activity of these drugs is short lived, tolerance develops rapidly, depression follows their discontinuance, and the potential of abuse is always present. A further danger is this drug's ability to precipitate rather bizarre paranoid behavior in a certain percentage of patients, without advanced warning.[32] The geriatric patient whose psychological controls are beginning to wane may develop overt paranoid psychosis and severe agitation with even small doses of amphetamines.

3. The use of combinations of drugs, whether they are two drugs of the same class, or drugs with two different desired actions, (i.e., two antianxiety drugs or an anti-anxiety and an antidepressant drug) have little to offer over agents used alone.[14] The disadvantage of this type of combination is frequency of occurrence of side-effects commonly associated with the administration of two strongly anticholinergic agents. Patients complain of dryness of mouth, thirst, blurred vision, constipation, and other symptoms which override any beneficial effects that might be obtained. Iatrogenic creation of intestinal ileus and urinary retention must always be considered in the elderly patient. The physician who uses these drugs, especially in geriatric patients, should do so with caution with regard to the dose administered and side-effects which may occur.

The combination of a tricyclic antidepressant and a monoamine oxidase inhibitor is potentially dangerous and should be discouraged.

The combination of a major tranquilizer and a tricyclic antidepressant such as perphenazine and amitriptylene (Trival or Etrafon) has been demonstrated to be effective in the depressed patient with agitation, tension, and moderately severe anxiety.[6] The physician should carefully assess the patient for signs and symptoms of at least moderate severity. We would suggest using the combination only after a reasonable trial with minor tranquilizers or antidepressants.

Our opinion as to the use of combination drugs is negative. They generally offer little over the individual ingredients alone.

4. The use of major tranquilizers in low doses for the treatment of anxiety and depression has limited usefulness. For the majority of nonpsychotic patients, major tranquilizers produce uncomfortable subjective feelings.[31] Patients tend to describe these feelings as "dopey, de-

tached, sleepy but unable to sleep, etc." The use of the piperazine pheno-
thiazines (Stelazine, Trilafon, etc.) in small doses, especially in younger
patients, has resulted in severe dystonic reactions[33] which have occurred
following only one or two doses of these drugs.

5. The question of treatment duration is a common problem. Physicians recognize that some patients take medication for exceedingly
long periods of time; however, it has been our observation that many
patients discontinue treatment too quickly. It is important for the practitioner to stress the necessity of taking medication for at least 3 to 4 weeks
on a regular schedule. This becomes especially important with tricyclic
antidepressants where there is a latency of therapeutic effects of 7 to 14
days. In our experience, patients require 3 to 4 weeks of treatment for
their symptoms to subside; but, more important, time is required for the
patient to develop coping mechanisms to handle the stresses that brought
them to the physician's office.

A second factor is that the placebo response tends to last for about 2
weeks, and if the patent discontinues medication prior to this point in
time,[30] it becomes difficult to assess the efficacy of the drug treatment.

One should carefully explain to the patient the possible discomforts
that may be experienced with any new medication. The patients should
be forewarned regarding sedation, dryness of mouth, constipation,
blurred vision, etc., which can be predicted from the pharmacologic
profiles of the drug being given. Patients should be reassured that if
side-effects occur the physician will be available by phone to discuss the
problem. In fact, one might state that some of the side-effects should be
expected. Patients forewarned in this manner are less likely to become
frightened and prematurely discontinue medication should such side
effects occur.

6. The final area that we will consider is the question of consultation.
The figures given in the first portion of the chapter attest to the fact that
nonpsychiatric physicians treat the majority of patients suffering from
the symptom complex of anxiety and depression. It is our desire to enhance the physician's effectiveness in his treatment of such a patient.
In keeping with good medical practice, consultations should be obtained
not as a court of last resort, but as a constructive educational experience
for both patient and physician. The patient may be hesitant because of
the "stigma" (that still exists) of seeing a psychiatrist, or the belief that
the physician no longer wishes to undertake his treatment. Forming a
brief or long-term alliance among patient, physician, and consultant can
be a rewarding experience.

Not all patients who suffer from anxiety-depression are candidates
for drug therapy or psychotherapy. Early consultation may prevent therapeutic failures, as well as unnecessary exposure of patients to multiple
drug therapy.

REFERENCES

1. Arieti, S., ed.: American Handbook of Psychiatry. New York, Basic Books Inc., 1966.
2. Backwell, B.: Hypertensive crisis due to monoamine-oxidase inhibitors. Lancet, 2:849–
   851, 1963.

3. Balter, M. B., and Leviene, J.: The nature and extent of psychotrophic drug usage in the United States. Psychopharm. Bull. 5:3–13, 1969.
4. Beck, A. T.: Depression. New York, Hoeber Medical Division, 1967.
5. Bibring, E.: The mechanism of depression. In Greenacre, P., ed.: Affective Disorders. New York, International Universities Press, 1953.
6. Chacon, C., and Downham, E. T.: Amitriptyline and amitriptyline with perphenazine in depression. A retrospective study. Brit. J. Psychiat., 113:201–207, 1967.
7. Claghorn, J. L., and Johnstone, E. E.: A quantitative relationship of anxiety with depression—A unitary concept. Scientific Exhibit, Section on Psychiatry, American Medical Association Meeting, June, 1970.
8. Davies, D. B.: A pilot study of nialamide at Cambridge. J. Soc. Genet. Med., 123:163–172, 1959.
9. Drug Treatment in Psychiatry. Veterans Administration Medical Bulletin, 1B-11-2, 1970.
10. Ephron, D. E., ed.: Psychopharmacology, A Review of Progress. Public Health Service Publication No. 1836, U.S. Government Printing Office, Washington, D.C., 1968.
11. Goldstein, B. J., and Slater, V.: Comparison of Mesoridazine and chlordiazepoxide in psychoneurotic patients. Current Therapeutic Research, Vol. II, No. 2, November, 1969.
12. Hamilton, M.: A rating scale for depression. J. Neurol. Neurosurg. Psychiat., 23:56, 1960.
13. Hollister, L. E.: Clinical use of psychotherapeutic drugs. Clin. Pharmacol. Therap., 10: 170, 1969.
14. Hollister, L. E.: Combinations of psychotherapeutic drugs. Presented at the tenth meeting of Collegium Internationale Neuropsychopharmacologium, August, 1970, Prague, CSSR.
15. International Psychiatry Clinics. Vol. 2, No. 4, October, 1965.
16. Klein, O. F., and Davis, J. M.: Diagnosis and Drug Treatment of Psychiatric Disorders. Baltimore, Williams and Wilkins, 1969.
17. Kolb, L. C., ed.: Noyes' Modern Clinical Psychiatry. Philadelphia. W. B. Saunders, 1968, 7th ed.
18. Lennard, H. L., Epstein, L., and Bernstein, A.: Hazards implicit in prescribing psychoactive drugs. Science, 169:438–441, 1970.
19. Overall, J. E., and Gorham, D. R.: Brief psychiatric rating scale. Psychol. Rep., 10:799–812, 1962.
20. Overall, J. E., et al.: Imipramine and thoridazine in depressed and schizophrenic patients. J.A.M.A., 189:605–608, 1964.
21. Rickels, K.: Developments in psychopharmacology. Psychosomat., 7:274–277, 1966.
22. Rickels, K.: Drug use in outpatient treatment. Amer. J. Psychiat., 124(Suppl.):20–31, 1968.
23. Rickels, K.: Important and relevant aspects of tranquilizer therapy. J. Neuropsychiat., 5:442–447, 1964.
24. Rickels, K.: Some comments on non-drug factors in psychiatric drug therapy. Psychosomat., 6:303–309, 1965.
25. Rickels, K., and Anderson, F. L.: Attrited and completed lower socioeconomic class clinic patients in psychiatric drug therapy. Comp. Psychiat., 8:90–99, 1967.
26. Rickels, K., Baumm, C., Raab, E., Taylor, W., and Moore, E.: A psychopharmacological evaluation of chlordiazepoxide, LA-1, and placebo carried out with anxious, neurotic medical clinic patients. Medical Times, March, 1965.
27. Rickels, K., Boren, R., and Stuart, H. M.: Controlled psychopharmacological research in general practice. J. New Drugs, 4:138–147, 1964.
28. Rickels, K., and Downing, R. W.: Drug and placebo-treated neurotic outpatients. Pretreatment levels of manifest anxiety, clinical improvement, and side reactions. Arch. Gen. Psychiat., 16:369–372, 1967.
29. Rickels, K., Downing, R. W., and Downing, M. H.: Personality differences between somatically and psychologically oriented neurotic patients. J. Nerv. Ment. Dis., 142: 10–18, 1966.
30. Rickels, K., Jenkins, B. W., Zamostien, B., Raab, E., and Kanther, M.: Pharmacotherapy in neurotic depression. Differential population responses. J. Nerv. Ment. Dis., 145:475–485, 1967.
31. Rickels, K., Raab, E., Gordon, P. E., Laquer, K. G., DeSilverio, R. V., and Hesbacher, P.: Differential effects of chlordiazepoxide and fluphenazine in two anxious patient populations. Psychopharmacologia (Berlin), 12:181–192, 1968.
32. Sjoqvist, F., and Tottie, M., eds.: Abuse of Central Nervous System Drugs. New York, Raven Press, 1969.
33. Stelazine in Psychiatry. Philadelphia, Smith, Kline and French Laboratories, 1966.

University of Miami School of Medicine
P. O. Box 875, Biscayne Annex
Miami, Florida   33152

Drug Interactions

Roger F. Palmer, M.D.[*]

Explosive interest has occurred in the area of adverse reactions to drugs. Patients receiving multiple drugs (the usual situation) appear to have a greater propensity for adverse reactions, reflecting in a crude sense a conclusion drawn from basic pharmacological data that drugs may interact with one another to alter each other's effects. It is somewhat surprising that many of these interactions of drugs, although well known to pharmacologists, have only recently been recognized to be of clinical importance. This is more a commentary on the general lack of communication between basic scientists and clinicians, rather than on neglect on the part of the latter.

The truism "the harder you look, the more you find" is never better exemplified than by the area of drug interactions. In the course of a patient's illness, many bizarre or at least atypical symptoms may appear which, because of a lack of an adequate explanation, are discarded or attributed to an unusual manifestation of the underlying disorder. Armed with the knowledge of how drugs interact, one can explain these symptoms and make appropriate adjustments to alleviate them. How frequently this occurs is a matter of conjecture, but from the vast array of potential drug interactions, it would seem that any patient receiving four to seven drugs simultaneously ought to have an interaction, some overtly manifest by symptoms.

It will be the attempt of this review to organize what may appear to be a great list of complicated facts into a cohesiveness that lends itself to clinical implementation.

Drugs as chemicals can interact with each other outside the organism. However, when two drugs are ingested, many possibilities for interactions occur. It seems appropriate to categorize potential and existing areas of drug interactions.

1. Interactions outside the patient; for example, in intravenous solutions, syringes, etc.
2. Interference with absorption or distribution: plasma binding, membrane transport blockade

---

[*]Professor and Chairman, Department of Pharmacology and Professor of Medicine, University of Miami School of Medicine, Miami, Florida

3. Interference with metabolism of drugs: inhibition or enhancement of one compound's metabolism of the other
4. Inteference with renal or biliary eliminations
5. Alteration of adrenergic mechanisms: inhibition of catecholamine uptake, precipitation of catecholamine release, false neurohumor production, inhibition of drug uptake
6. Indirect modification of a drug's action by electrolyte balance.

Interactions Outside the Patient

Many reactions occur in bottles used for intravenous infusion. Certain drugs, because of acid or alkaline lability, cannot be mixed with acidic or basic compounds unless the solution is buffered. For example, methicillin is acid labile, so the pH of dextrose, saline, or other solutions must be adjusted to the alkaline range.

Levarterenol (Levophed) should be given in acid solutions (e.g., dextrose) to prevent its oxidation.

Some solutions, such as amphotericin and nitroprusside, are light sensitive.

Regular insulin binds to glass. Tetracycline can be photo-oxidized by the riboflavin in vitamin B complex.[8]

Any questions regarding possible interactions of drugs in I.V. bottles can be referred to a competent hospital pharmacist for advice. Indeed, it would be ideal to have such an individual perform the actual mixing of the solutions.

Interference with Absorption

Many drugs have anticholinergic properties which, by decreasing intestinal movements, delay or reduce absorption of drugs. Most of the tricyclic antidepressants and many of the major tranquilizers have this property.[9]

Another device whereby drug absorption is affected is by complexation of drugs by various substances in the gut. For example, calcium and tetracycline, in an alkaline environment such as is achieved when alkaline calcium salts are used as antacids, will complex and the absorption of tetracycline will be reduced.[11] Cholestyramine, a non-absorbable resin, will reduce the amount of thyroxin absorbed.[4]

Dilantin, by inhibiting an intestinal conjugase, inhibits the absorption of folic acid, particularly in susceptible individuals.[6] Natural folate occurs as a polyglutamate and must be broken down to the monoglutamate form in the intestinal wall by conjugase. Dilantin has the ability to inhibit this enzyme, thus preventing the absorption of folic acid. Nitrofurantoin[18] appears to inhibit folic acid conjugase in man and therefore may be associated with megaloblastic anemia. Recently, oral contraceptives and triampterine, a pteridine like diuretic, have been reported to inhibit absorption of folic acid.[18]

A second mechanism whereby drugs may interact is by displacement of each other's binding to plasma proteins. As is well known, drugs bind to amino groups of plasma albumin. A drug thus bound is considered inactive, since it is no longer free to diffuse to the active receptor site. However, it is in equilibrium with a free form. The binding capacity of human plasma albumin for a drug of molecular weight of 200 or so is about 200 micrograms per ml.[15] Obviously, when the binding capacity of albumin is exceeded, more free drug will be present in the system.

Figure 1 depicts what happens when drug A is bound to plasma albumin. For example, suppose 98 per cent of the orally administered drug is bound to albumin and 2 per cent is free. If another drug that also binds to plasma albumin is given in sufficient doses, it will cause displacement of drug A. When the two drugs are given together, 96 per cent of drug A is bound and 4 per cent is free, the additional 2 per cent having been displaced by drug B. Since the free concentration is that concentration which determines the pharmacologic activity of a drug,[2] then the free concentration in this case has doubled, a situation tantamount to giving twice the dose of the drug.

An example of such an interaction is the interaction between warfarin sodium (Coumadin) and phenylbutazone. When given together, both of these highly acidic, highly bound drugs can induce a release of warfarin sodium from plasma albumin and will precipitate bleeding.[16] Other drugs known to displace warfarin sodium from binding sites are indomethacin, oxyphenbutazone, and clofibrate.[17] Aspirin can displace protein-bound penicillin analogs, long-acting sulphonamides, or chlorpropamide.[12] In the case of chlorpropamide, displacement by aspirin can result in a hypoglycemic episode even though the dose of chlorpropamide has not been altered. Methotrexate, a competitive inhibitor of folate reductase is bound to plasma albumin and can be displaced by various acidic drugs, including sulfonamides and salicylates,[7] thereby enhancing the toxicity of methotrexate.

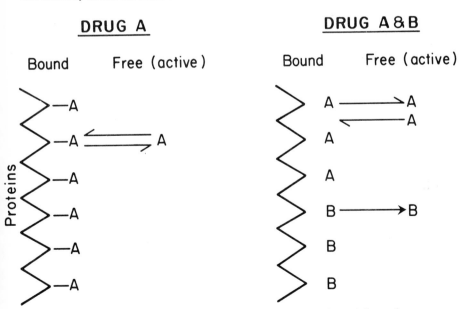

Figure 1. Diagrammatic representation of displacement of Drug A from plasma protein-binding sites by Drug B. Note that when A and B are combined, the free active concentration of A increases.

Many of these drug interactions of a plasma protein binding basis are not completely known; therefore, *as a general rule it may be said that any acidic highly bound drug, when given simultaneously with another acidic highly bound drug, sets up a potential interaction by mutual displacement.* Certainly, one should be able to ascertain from the package insert or, indeed, a recent textbook of pharmacology, the degree of plasma protein binding of the compound as well as its pKa.

It is also possible for drugs to displace each other from nonspecific binding sites and tissues. Pamaquine, an anti-malarial that localizes in the liver, can displace quinacrine, another antimalarial, to increase plasma levels of pamaquine, thus reducing the rate of disappearance of this drug from plasma.[20] Therefore, quinacrine increases the toxicity of pamaquine.

Interference with Metabolism

The third category whereby drugs can interact is through interference with metabolism, either augmenting or inhibiting each other's breakdown. It has been well known for at least a decade that certain drugs, particularly phenobarbital, have the ability to increase liver size and increase the amount of endoplasmic reticulum in animal liver. The increase in liver weight and amount of subcellular structure is correlated with an increase in enzyme activity that is of a nonspecific variety. That is, not only is the metabolism of the inducing drug increased, but the metabolism of other drugs as well.

This process, known as enzyme induction, requires about 48 hours for onset and offset of action after exposure to the inducing substance. For example, phenobarbital enhances the metabolism of warfarin sodium (Coumadin). If a patient is receiving phenobarbital at the time that his warfarin sodium dosage is adjusted and then he spontaneously stops taking the phenobarbital, his effective dose of warfarin sodium will be increased, since the rate of degradation is no longer as rapid in the absence of the inducer.[4] Conversely, if a patient is taking warfarin sodium and then phenobarbital is prescribed, the effective concentration of the warfarin sodium will be reduced and the patient's prothrombin time may come out of the therapeutic range.

Chloral hydrate, in addition to phenobarbital, is a potent inducer of enzymes in man. Cucinell et al.[5] reported fatal hemorrhage in a patient who was treated with chloral hydrate as well as with bishydroxycoumarin. The hemorrhage occurred shortly after secobarbital was substituted for chloral hydrate. Secobarbital is a weak inducer and chloral hydrate is very potent. With the dosage of secobarbital employed, there was no increase in the activity of the drug-metabolizing enzyme. Table 1 lists drugs known to induce hepatic enzymes in man.

In addition to causing the stimulation of hepatic microsomal enzymes, drugs can inhibit the metabolism of each other. Chloramphenicol has the ability to inhibit the metabolism both of phenytoin (Dilantin) and tolbutamide, in one case producing hypoglycemia and in the other phenytoin toxicity manifested by nystagmus and confusion.[3] Obviously, it is impossible to document all cases of drug interactions resulting from

Table 1. *Drugs Known to Increase Hepatic Microsomal Enzyme Activity in Man*

Phenobarbital	Chloral hydrate
Butabarbital	Ethchlorovynol
Heptabarbital	Meprobamate
Amobarbital	Griseofulvin
Secobarbital	Phenytoin
Glutethimide	

this mechanism. *However, as a general rule, if a drug is primarily metabolized and is combined with another drug that is primarily metabolized, either inhibition or enhancement of the other drug's metabolism is possible.* Again the information concerning whether a drug is metabolized or not should be available from the package insert or from standard textbooks.

Inhibition of Renal Secretory Mechanism

Drugs can affect each other's rate of elimination by virtue of their competition for weak-acid-secreting sites. In this regard the weak acids such as the thiazide diuretics, penicillin, and some sulfonamides will compete for uric acid-secreting sites, thereby elevating the plasma level of uric acid.[19] Salicylates are notorious in this regard, since at low doses they act as competitors for weak acid-secreting sites in the kidneys and elevate the concentration of other acidic drugs. *As a general rule any drug that is acidic, and is not metabolized, will be secreted by the kidney and will have the capacity to interact with any other nonmetabolized acidic drug by competing for the same secretory site.*

The excretion of a drug can be affected by affecting the pH of the urine. For example: acetazolamide, by virtue of its ability to alkalinize the urine, will enhance the excretion of any acidic compound. Thus, acetazolamide enhances the secretion of salicylates, the reason being that once a drug is secreted in the proximal tubule it has the capacity to back-diffuse in the lower nephron.[14] The capacity to back-diffuse is determined by the un-ionized species. That is, the un-ionized species can readily pass through membrane barriers into the renal venous blood. In the presence of an alkaline milieu there is a greater proportion of ionized drug, thereby decreasing back diffusion. So any maneuver that influences urinary pH can influence the secretion of a drug with a pKâ between 4 and 8. For example: ammonium chloride, potassium citrate, vomiting, metabolic acidosis, and other diuretics alter the excretion of drugs.

This mechanism is perhaps the most complicated and requires a basic understanding of adrenergic pharmacology. In summary, catecholamines, principally norepinephrine, are stored at postganglionic nerve terminals and in presynaptic and postsynaptic neurons in the central nervous system. With an appropriate stimulus, usually a nerve action potential, norepinephrine is released from the mobile pool where it interacts with a receptor, either alpha or beta. Norepinephrine is synthesized within these sites from tyrosine. Norepinephrine is also broken down in these granules through the participation of monoamine oxidase. In the extracellular fluid norepinephrine is then broken down by an enzyme, catacholorthomethyl-transferase. These important steps are depicted in Figure 2.

These steps become clinically important in the following areas: When norepinephrine is released, the majority of it is taken back up by the nerve terminal and is thereby inactivated. Certain chemical substances have a capacity to inhibit this re-uptake. Common ones are reserpine and the tricyclic antidepressants.[9] Cocaine and toxic concentrations of digitalis also inhibit norepinephrine uptake.[9] Not only are the naturally occurring amines taken up by the nerve terminal, but other exogenously administered amines may be as well. For example, phenyl-

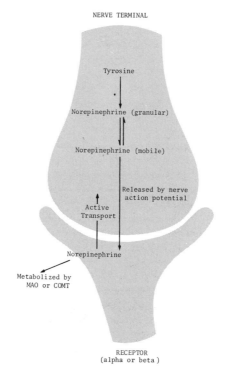

Figure 2. Representation of a postganglionic adrenergic nerve terminal indicating synthesis, storage and release of norepinephrine. Norepinephrine is synthesized from tyrosine, to be stored in a granular pool which is in equilibrium with a mobile pool. Norepinephrine is released from the mobile pool by a nerve action potential to interact with the alpha or beta receptor. Most of the norepinephrine is taken up again by active transport. That which is not taken up again is metabolized by monamine oxidase (MAO) or catechol-ortho-methyl transferase (COMT).

Certain chemical substances can interfere at different points in this process. Synthesis of norepinephrine from tyrosine can be blocked by alpha-methyl-p-tyrosine. Norepinephrine can be released from the mobile pool by tyramine or ephedrine. The nerve action potential can be blocked by local anesthetics. Receptors are blocked by propranolol dibenzyline. The uptake of norepinephrine can be blocked by reserpine, tricyclic antidepressants, or cocaine. Inhibition of monamine oxidase, which metabolizes circulating norepinephrine in the liver, can produce norepinephrine-like effects.

ephrine and metaraminol are also taken up by the nerve ending and stored; and it is here that this relationship has important clinical implications.

A recent patient was referred to me because of paroxysms of hypertension. These paroxysms occurred whenever he used a nasal inhaler containing phenylephrine. The patient had been taking reserpine for a number of years for mild diastolic hypertension. Recall now that reserpine has the ability to block the uptake of phenylephrine at the nerve ending. So when the phenylephrine, some of which was absorbed through the nasal mucosa, reached the nerve terminal, reserpine inhibited its inactivation, leaving more remaining to interact with the alpha receptor, producing hypertension. It is interesting to note that this man underwent a diagnostic work up for pheochromocytoma because of this rather simple pharmacologic maneuver.

Certain drugs, such as guanethidine, that must be taken up by the nerve terminal for their action can be less effective in the presence of a blocking agent. For example, the tricyclic antidepressant desiprimine can block the uptake of guanethidine, negating its action.[13] Incidentally, the tricyclic antidepressants, by their ability to inhibit norepinephrine uptake, may produce symptoms related to increased circulating catecholamines, such as nervousness and insomnia.

Certain compounds present in food, such as tyramine, have the ability to precipitate a release of catecholamines. Under ordinary circumstances this is virtually without effect. However, if a patient is taking a monoamine oxidase inhibitor such as pargyline, the precipitous release of catecholamines can be hazardous, since monoamine-oxidase would ordinarily degrade the released catecholamines under conditions of inhibition. Severe hypertensive crisis can result, and subarachnoid hemorrhage has resulted.[10] Patients on monoamine-oxidase inhibitors should be warned of the hazards of eating foods containing tyramine.

False neurohumor production can be used for therapeutic benefit. Probably the mechanism of action of alpha-methyldopa is at least partially through this mechanism. This compound is metabolized to alpha-methylnorepinephrine and stored in the nerve terminal, displacing the more potent norepinephrine.[9] The nerve terminal becomes filled with alpha-methylnorepinephrine. Thus when a nerve action potential stimulates the release of this catecholamine, it is less effective than the ordinary norepinephrine, and hypotension results. Metaraminol causes a release of catacholamines resulting in a hypertensive effect. Yet, metaraminol itself can replace norepinephrine in the nerve terminal. After prolonged usage of metaraminol, it becomes less effective; little norepinephrine remains, since the nerve terminal is filled with the less potent metaraminol. This mechanism may explain the difficulty in "weaning a patient off aramine."

As a general rule, any drug that is reported to exert its effect by influencing the adrenergic nervous system has the potential for interacting with any other drug working through the same system by the mechanisms listed above.

The last category of drug interactions involves alterations of acid-base metabolism, thus indirectly influencing the action of another drug.

The most classic example of course is the use of thiazide diuretics with digitalis. Thiazide diuretics produce potassium loss, which potentiates the toxic effects of digitalis but not the therapeutic effect.[9] Other examples can be sited. For example, tubocurarine is much more potent in the presence of low potassium levels, as are some of the depolarizing blocking agents, the neuromuscular blocking agents. Any diuretic that alters the urinary pH can alter the excretion of a compound that is handled principally by the kidney.

REFERENCES

1. Bressler, R.: Combined drug therapy. Amer. J. Med. Sci., 255:89, 1968.
2. Brodie, B. B.: Displacement of one drug by another from carrier or receptor sites. Proc. Roy. Soc. Med., 58:946, 1965.
3. Christensen, K. L., and Skovsted, L.: Inhibition of drug metabolism by chloramphenicol. Lancet, 2:1397, 1969.
4. Cucinell, S. A., et al.: Drug interactions in man. 1. Lowering effect of phenobarbital on plasma levels of bishydroxycoumarin (Dicumarol) and diphenylhydantoin (Dilantin). Clin. Pharmacol. Therap., 6:420, 1965.
5. Cucinell, S. A., et al.: The effect of chloral hydrate of bishydroxycoumarin metabolism. J.A.M.A., 197:366, 1966.
6. Dahlke, M. B., and Mertens-Roesler, E.: Malabsorption of folic acid due to diphenylhydantoin. Blood, 30:341, 1967.
7. Dixon, R. L., Henderson, E. S., and Rall, D. P.: Plasma protein binding of methotrexate and its displacement by various drugs, Fed. Proc., 24:454, 1965.
8. Fowler, T. J.: Some incompatibilities of intravenous admixtures. Amer. J. Hosp. Pharm., 24:450, 1967.
9. Goodman, L. S., and Gilman, A.: The Pharmacologic Basis of Therapeutics. New York, MacMillan Co., 1970, 4th ed.
10. Horwitz, D., et al.: Monamine oxidase inhibitors, tyramine, and cheese. J.A.M.A., 188:1108, 1964.
11. Kunin, C. M., and Finland, M.: Clinical pharmacology of the tetracycline antibiotics. Clin. Pharmacol. Therap., 2:51, 1961.
12. McDougal, M. R.: Interaction of drugs with aspirin. J. Amer. Pharm. Assoc., Vol. NS10:85, 1970.
13. Mitchell, J. R., Arias, L., and Oates, J. A.: Antagonism of the antihypertensive action of guanethidine sulfate by desipramine hydrochloride. J.A.M.A., 202:973, 1967.
14. Schanker, L. S.: Passage of drugs across body membranes. Pharmacol. Rev., 14:501, 1962.
15. Solomon, H. M.: Displacement of drugs from plasma binding sites as a factor in drug toxicity. In Goldstein, S. W., ed.: Development of Safer and More Effective Drugs. Washington, D.C., American Pharmaceutical Association, 1968.
16. Solomon, H. M., and Schrogie, J. J.: The effect of various drugs on the binding of warfarin-^{14}C to human albumin. Biochem. Pharmacol., 16:1219, 1967.
17. Solomon, H. M., Schrogie, J. J., and Williams, D.: The displacement of phenylbutazone-^{14}C and warfarin-^{14}C from human albumin by various drugs and fatty acids. Biochem. Pharmacol., 17:143, 1968.
18. Toole, J. F., et al.: Neural effects of nitrofurantoin. Arch. Neurol., 18:680, 1968.
19. Yu, T. F., Dayton, P. G., and Gutman, A. B.: Mutual suppression of the uricosuric effects of sulfinpyrazone and salicylate: A study in interactions between drugs. J. Clin. Invest., 42:1330, 1963.
20. Zubrod, C. G., Kennedy, T. J., and Shannon, J. A.: Studies on the chemotherapy of the human malarias. VIII. The physiological disposition of pamaquine. J. Clin. Invest., 27:114, 1948.

Department of Pharmacology
University of Miami School of Medicine
P.O. Box 875, Biscayne Annex
Miami, Florida 33152

Disorders of Potassium Metabolism

James L. Katsikas, M.D., and*
*Carl Goldsmith, M.D., F.A.C.P.***

NORMAL POTASSIUM METABOLISM

The major cation of the extracellular fluid is sodium, and its main function is to maintain the tonicity and, therefore, the volume of body fluids. By contrast the major cation of the intracellular fluid is potassium. Potassium is important not so much because it maintains the tonicity of intracellular fluid, for there may be many other substances within the cell that are capable of doing this, but because the metabolism of potassium is intimately concerned with cellular function. In the extracellular fluid, the normal potassium concentration is 3.5 to 5 mEq. per liter. (In the intracellular fluid the potassium concentration is around 150 mEq. per liter.) The average total body potassium is approximately 3200 mEq. in men, and 2300 mEq. in women. Only about 2 per cent is extracellular. It is, therefore, not surprising that the serum potassium level is often not indicative of total body potassium.

Potassium Balance

In the normal person on an average diet, intake of potassium is equal to the output, which is usually 50 to 100 mEq. per day. Potassium intake consists of ingested and administered potassium as well as potassium which is released from cells during tissue breakdown and from red cells during hemolysis. Formed stools contain approximately 5 to 10 mEq. of potassium per day. The amount of potassium lost in sweat or by desquamation of the skin is not clinically significant. The kidney, therefore, is the main route of excretion. In contrast to the renal mechanisms for conservation of sodium, which are highly developed and very efficient, the kidney responds to diminished intake of potassium quite slowly. When a subject receives no salt intake, within a 4 day period of time, urinary sodium as well as stool sodium will fall to nil. However, even in severe potassium depletion urinary potassium rarely falls below 5 to 10

---

*Senior Fellow in Nephrology, University of Miami School of Medicine
**Associate Professor of Medicine, University of Miami School of Medicine; Chief, Renal Section, Jackson Memorial Hospital, Miami, Florida

mEq. per day. On the other hand, increased intake promotes a very rapid response in the normal kidney, and the excess is rapidly excreted. Virtually all the potassium which is filtered at the glomerulus is reabsorbed in the proximal tubule.

Potassium that appears in the urine is derived from secretion into the distal tubule. Thus, the ability of the kidney to excrete potassium is critically dependent on those factors which influence distal tubular function. The initiating event in potassium secretion is the active extrusion of sodium from the cell into the peritubular fluid. This results in a fall in the sodium concentration within the cell.

Sodium in the tubular urine then diffuses into the cell along concentration gradients. To the extent that chloride is not reabsorbed with sodium, increased electronegativity develops in the tubular urine, promoting the secretion of both potassium and hydrogen ion. Therefore, the secretion of potassium in the distal tubule depends on the ability of the tubular cell to reabsorb sodium. Furthermore, it appears that potassium and hydrogen ion are in competition for secretion in exchange for sodium. Therefore, the ability of the tubular cell to secrete potassium depends on the availability of both potassium and hydrogen ions.

It is apparent that certain other factors are required for potassium elimination. Among these are the functional integrity of the distal tubular cell, the presence or absence of mineralocorticoid, which appears to enhance the reabsorption of sodium at the site of potassium and hydrogen secretion, and those factors which determine the relative availability of potassium and hydrogen ions within the cell.

Function

The main physiological function of potassium is the maintenance of excitability of certain cells. It is the derangements in excitable tissue which usually offer the acute clinical problems. There is frequently confusion when one speaks of potassium deficiency and potassium excess, because under certain circumstances the serum level of potassium may be an inadequate reflection of total body potassium. Furthermore, since the functional integrity of excitable tissues depends on certain aspects of the cell membrane, potassium affects the activity of the cell membrane by alterations in its relative distribution inside and outside the cell. Therefore, the critical factor to take into account when evaluating the status of body potassium is the relationship of intracellular to extracellular potassium concentrations.

The extracellular fluid potassium is easily measured as serum potassium. Intracellular potassium concentration is not at present a clinically feasible determination. How then does one determine the status of potassium metabolism?

First of all the serum potassium is measured. Generally in potassium deficiency the serum potassium is low. Most people regard the normal range to be between 3.5 and 5.0 mEq. per liter. An elevated serum potassium is frequently a sign of potassium excess. However, other factors must be taken into consideration. For example, if the serum potassium is elevated, but at the same time intracellular potassium is likewise elevated, there could conceivably be a normal ratio of intracellular to extracellular potassium and no clinical symptoms would result. On the other hand, in the presence of a diminished concentration within the cell, clinical signs and symptoms of potassium intoxication may occur at modestly elevated levels of serum potassium.

The history is quite important and is a good method of evaluating the status of intracellular potassium. If a patient is hypokalemic and historically one finds that this patient's potassium deficiency is most likely on the basis of inadequate intake over prolonged periods of time, perhaps coupled with low-grade diarrhea and resulting gastrointestinal losses, one may expect that intracellular potassium stores are low. On the other hand, the patient who comes in with a brief history of severe intractable vomiting, hypokalemia, and alkalosis could be suspected of having normal intracellular stores of potassium. The same holds true for potassium excess.

The status of acid-base balance is a critical part of the evaluation of potassium metabolism. Hydrogen ion excess is to a large extent buffered within cells. Thus, in the presence of acidosis with excess hydrogen ion present in the extracellular fluid, hydrogen ions move into the cell and are buffered there, and potassium ions are displaced into the extracellular fluid. Under these circumstances, the relationship between intracellular and extracellular potassium is moving in an undesirable direction, with an elevation of serum potassium and a simultaneous fall in intracellular fluid potassium concentration.

Conversely, in the presence of metabolic alkalosis, hydrogen ions leave the cell and move into the extracellular fluid. Potassium ions then move from the extracellular fluid into the intracellular fluid. The relationship between the pH of the extracellular fluid and the corrected serum potassium value is crudely approximated by changing the measured serum potassium value 30 per cent for each 0.1 of a pH unit change from normal.

Consider a patient with a blood pH of 7.1 and a serum potassium of 5.6 mEq. per liter. This patient's blood is 0.3 pH units more acid than the normal of 7.4; therefore, as his acidosis is corrected, serum potassium will decline in the following manner: pH 7.2, K 3.7; pH 7.3, K 2.5; pH 7.4, K 1.6. Thus, this degree of acidosis masked severe potassium deficiency by slightly elevating serum potassium above normal. Furthermore, while such a patient is acidotic, he is in danger from the effects of high serum potassium coupled with low intracellular potassium. When the acidosis is corrected, he is endangered by the effects of hypokalemia. The finding of a normal or elevated serum potassium in the face of severe potassium depletion is commonly seen in diabetic ketoacidosis.

The ECG is an extremely useful guide to the status of body potassium. The important results of alternations in potassium metabolism are those which affect neuromuscular excitability. The best clinical guides to the status of potassium metabolism are those which directly reflect this. Since the most critical organ affected by a disordered potassium metabolism is the heart, the ECG is the most sensitive guide to diagnosis of alternations in potassium metabolism. It can be done at the bedside, the answer is immediate, and the changes seen reflect the relative changes in the intracellular and extracellular levels. The ECG is useful and often mandatory in monitoring the patient during therapy.

HYPERKALEMIA

Manifestations

With an elevated serum potassium concentration, there is muscular weakness and loss of deep tendon reflexes. Paralysis of skeletal muscle is rare except in very severe hyperkalemia or in hyperkalemic paralysis[5] (adynamia episodica hereditaria), which is thought to be due to a defect in the potassium transport system of skeletal muscle. There may be mental symptoms and the patient may complain of paresthesias. Cardiac abnormalities are the most important, manifested by bradycardia, ventricular fibrillation, hypotension, or cardiac standstill.

Diagnosis

Diagnosis may be suggested by the clinical setting, but almost always is made on the basis of serum levels or ECG changes, or both. In managing a patient with hyperkalemia, one should keep in mind causes of erroneous elevations of serum potassium levels: (1) hemolysis of the blood specimen due to trauma to the blood in the syringe or when placing it in the tube, or delay in separation of the red cells from the serum; (2) thrombocytosis of any etiology;[10] (3) excess muscular contraction of the forearm prior to drawing blood. The later has shown to result in elevations of serum potassium by as much as 2.7 mEq. per liter.[8] The ECG manifestations of hyperkalemia consist of elevation and peaking of the T waves, depression of the ST segment and some diminution of R wave amplitude, prolongation of the QRS and PR intervals, diminished P wave amplitude with ultimate disappearance or inversion of P wave, diminished T wave amplitude as the QRS widens, and finally a sine wave ECG (Fig. 1.) Arrhythmias may appear at any time.

Causes of Hyperkalemia

Increased serum potassium can result from the administration of excessive potassium, from decreased renal excretion of potassium, or from release of potassium from the cells. Ingestion of excessive potassium is an uncommon cause of hyperkalemia except in the clinical setting of associated renal dysfunction. Decreased renal excretion is frequently seen in acute renal failure, and if the patient is markedly oliguric or anuric, severe hyperkalemia may result even in the absence of potassium intake because of tissue catabolism. In chronic renal failure, significant hyperkalemia is uncommon unless the patient is terminally oliguric or severely acidotic, and in the end stage of chronic renal failure.[9] Adrenal insufficiency may be associated with decreased excretion and

HYPERKALEMIA

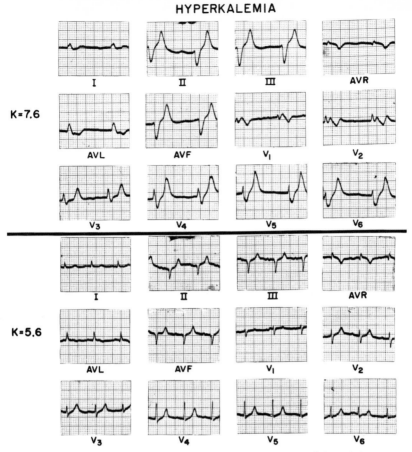

Figure 1. Electrocardiographic manifestations in a patient with hyperkalemia.

Table 1. *Causes of Hyperkalemia*

Administration of excessive potassium

Release of potassium from cells
Hemolysis
Acidosis
Ketoacidosis
Lactic acidosis
Intoxication with salicylates or methanol
Catabolic states
Infection
Trauma
Surgery

Decreased renal excretion
Acute renal failure
Chronic renal failure
Adrenal insufficiency
Certain diuretics

result in hyperkalemia. When this occurs, it is usually associated with an elevated BUN. Rapid release of potassium from cells may result from severe acidosis of any cause such as diabetic ketoacidosis, lactic acidosis, or salicylate or methanol intoxication.

Catabolic states with increased tissue breakdown may result in the release of large amounts of potassium into the extracellular fluid. This may be seen with severe infection, marked hemolysis, and extensive tissue trauma, such as may be seen with crush injury or some major surgical procedures. In the presence of associated decreased glomerular filtration rate, hyperkalemia resulting from any of the above will be accentuated.

Treatment

The best treatment of hyperkalemia is preventive therapy. One must be aware that the patient has renal insufficiency or oliguria, or both. One must check for overlooked sources of exogenous potassium. For example, penicillin G contains 1.7 mEq. of potassium per each million units. If necessary, one can use sodium penicillin G. Bank blood, after one week of storage, can contain up to 30 mEq. of potassium per liter in the plasma. Low-salt milk can contain 60 mEq. per liter. Finally, most salt substitutes are potassium salts.

From the therapeutic point of view, it may be useful to divide hyperkalemia into categories of minimal, moderate, and severe.[7] Assuming no disorder of acid-base status, in *minimal hyperkalemia* the serum potassium is less than 6.5 mEq. per liter and there are only minimal ECG changes. In *moderate hyperkalemia* the plasma potassium is 6.5 to 8 mEq. per liter and the ECG changes are limited to peaking of the T waves. *Severe hyperkalemia* exists if the serum potassium is above 8.0 mEq. per liter, or at any plasma level where ECG abnormalities such as widened QRS, heart block, or ventricular rhythms are seen.

Hyperkalemia is treated by measures that result in a decreased intake of potassium, antagonism of the effects of potassium, moving of potassium into the cells, or actually removing potassium from the body. In minimal hyperkalemia often all that is necessary is to restrict potassium and, if possible, liberalize sodium ingestion. Moderate to severe

Table 2.   *Treatment of Hyperkalemia*

Stop ingestion or administration of potassium

Shift potassium into cells
  Alkalinization
  Glucose and insulin

Antagonism of the effects of potassium
  Calcium

Removal of potassium from the body
  Cation exchange resins
  Peritoneal dialysis
  Hemodialysis

hyperkalemia necessitates immediate therapeutic measures. Calcium directly antagonizes the cardiac effects of hyperkalemia and should be used first if severe cardiac toxicity is present. Ten to 30 ml. of a 10 per cent calcium gluconate solution is given intravenously with continuous ECG monitoring over a 5 minute period. If this is not effective, it is unlikely that additional calcium will be of any benefit. The effect is usually transient if the hyperkalemia is not decreased by other measures. If the patient is digitalized, calcium administration is quite hazardous, and should be used only as a "last resort."

Alkalinization of the extracellular fluid with sodium bicarbonate causes potassium to shift into cells. Depending on the urgency of the situation, 1 ampule (44 mEq.) can be given intravenously over 5 minutes, and the dose repeated in 10 to 15 minutes if needed. Also, one can add 2 or 3 ampules of sodium bicarbonate (44 mEq. per ampule) to 1 liter of 5 per cent dextrose in water administered by slow intravenous drip. Alkalinization is especially effective if acidosis is present, but is useful even when acid-base balance is normal.

Glucose, in the presence of insulin, also causes potassium to shift into cells. Two hundred to 500 ml. of a 10 per cent glucose solution can be given in the first half hour, then maintained at a slower rate. Ten to 15 units of regular insulin may be added to the solution, but this frequently is not necessary unless the patient is diabetic. Some observers[3, 7] recommend a "therapeutic cocktail" that consists of 2 ampules of sodium bicarbonate added to either 1 liter of 5 per cent dextrose in water and normal saline, or 10 per cent dextrose in water with insulin if the patient is diabetic. The first third can be given in 30 minutes, and the remainder in 2 to 3 hours.

Potassium can actually be removed from the body by the use of either cation exchange resins or dialysis. The most commonly used cation exchange resin is polystyrene sulfonate (Kayexalate), which is a sodium cycle resin. Approximately 1 mEq. of potassium is removed for each gram of the resin, by exchange with 1 mEq. of sodium. If the patient is able to cooperate, the Kayexalate should be given orally, because it is more effective by this route. It is desirable to institute diarrhea for two reasons: to counteract the constipating effect of the resin and prevent bowel obstruction, and to decrease the amount of sodium absorbed from the gut. In the presence of renal failure or congestive heart failure, up to 200 mEq. of sodium a day can be exchanged in the gut, and if a significant amount is absorbed, this may result in pulmonary edema or even death.[1]

Kayexalate is given orally in a dose of 20 to 50 gm. 3 or 4 times a day (two heaping teaspoons is equivalent to 15 gm.). To produce a diarrhea, 15 to 20 ml. of a 70 per cent sorbital solution is given with each dose of the resin. This can be increased until several loose stools are produced each day.

If a more rapid effect is desired, or if the patient cannot tolerate the oral resin, the resin can be given by retention enema (a Foley catheter with a 30 ml. bag inserted into the rectum and blown up will promote retention for the desired time). The enema is prepared by dissolving 50 gm. of Kayexalate in a mixture of 50 ml. of a 70 per cent sorbital solution and 150 ml. of tap water. An alternative is to dissolve the resin in 150 ml. of a 1 per cent methyl cellulose solution. If the enema is retained for 30 to 60 minutes, a single enema may reduce the serum potassium level by 0.5 to 1.0 mEq. per liter. This form of therapy can be repeated every 4 to 6 hours if necessary.

Hemodialysis is an effective method of removing potassium, but is usually not practical because necessary equipment and personnel are usually limited to large medical centers, and even if available, significant delay is often necessary before the patient is prepared for hemodialysis. Peritoneal dialysis can remove potassium from the body, but usually more slowly. Even if no potassium is present in the dialysate, assuming an exchange volume of two liters each hour and assuming complete equilibration, only twice the serum potassium in mEq. per liter can be removed each hour.

In patients who, in addition, are also acidotic, dialysis would correct the acidosis rather rapidly with a resulting shift of potassium into cells. Peritoneal dialysis should especially be considered in those patients in whom sodium administration is contraindicated. In patients who have a combination of hyperkalemia and acidosis, and are salt and water overloaded and in renal failure, peritoneal dialysis is desirable because it can control all these abnormalities simultaneously.

HYPOKALEMIA

Manifestations

When hypokalemia is present, there may be weakness and loss of deep tendon reflexes, which may progress to complete paralysis. This may be life-threatening if it progresses to involve the muscles of respiration. Smooth muscle involvement is usually indicated by the presence of paralytic ileus. Mental symptoms and somnolence have been attributed at times to hypokalemia.

The most life-threatening manifestation of hypokalemia is its cardiovascular effects. There may be a wide pulse pressure due primarily to decreased diastolic pressure. There may be arrythmias, and finally cardiac arrest.

Although cases of acute renal failure associated with hypokalemia and apparently cured by the administration of potassium[4] have been reported, this is probably quite rare and in most cases is due to coexistent factors. Moderate elevations in BUN, however, can be seen in apparently uncomplicated potassium deficiency states. The most prominent renal functional abnormality in potassium depletion is a defect in the tubular reabsorption of water with resultant isosthenuria which is resistant to vasopresin. Hypokalemia also affects renal acid-base handling by diminishing the ability to acidify the urine.

Diagnosis

Although it may be suspected on clinical grounds, the diagnosis must be confirmed by serum determinations and the electrocardiogram.

The ECG manifestations are disappearance of the T wave with prominence of the U wave appearing like prolongation of the Q-T interval, inversion of the T wave, and ST depression.

Causes

Causes are listed in Table 3. (1) Potassium depletion from the gastrointestinal tract. This includes any cause of diarrhea, vomiting, ureteroenterostomy, chronic use of laxatives (a history of diarrhea may not be obtained), biliary or intestinal fistulas, and villous adenomas of the rectosigmoid. (2) Renal losses, via renal tubular disorders, such as renal tubular acidosis, Fanconi's syndrome, the recovery phase of acute tubular necrosis, and perhaps chronic pyelonephritis. Renal losses are also seen in Cushing's syndrome, aldosteronism, the use of diuretics, and osmotic diuresis (i.e., mannitol infusion or glycosuria). (3) Poor intake is an unusual cause except in patients on potassium-free parenteral fluids, or in elderly people living alone who eat little more than toast and tea. (4) Shift of potassium into cells as in some forms of periodic paralysis.

Treatment

In most situations, hypokalemia is not an emergency and oral therapy is adequate. At times, the ingestion of the natural foods high in potassium will suffice. If this is inadequate, oral therapy is indicated. If there is no associated alkalosis and dietary chloride is adequate, and there is no tendency to sodium retention, any of the proprietory potassium-containing compounds are satisfactory (Kaon, K-Triplex, Kaylyte). If any

Table 3. *Causes of Hypokalemia*

Potassium depletion from gastrointestinal tract
Diarrhea
Vomiting
Ureteroenterostomy
Chronic laxative use
Fistulas
  Biliary
  Intestinal
Villous adenoma of rectosigmoid

Renal losses
Renal tubular disorders
  Renal tubular acidosis
  Fanconi's syndrome
Recovery phase acute tubular necrosis
Chronic Pyelonephritis (?)
Cushing's syndrome
Aldosteronism
Diuretics

Poor intake
Parenteral fluids
"Tea and toast" syndrome

Shift of potassium into cells
Alkalosis

of the above complications are present, potassium must be given as the chloride salt, because neither the alkalosis nor the potassium ion deficiency can be corrected without the administration of chloride.[6] It should be given in a liquid form, diluted in juice or water, and given after meals to minimize gastric irritation. Enteric-coated tablets should not be used because of the possibility of small bowel perforation and because absorption is variable. If the patient cannot take potassium orally or if there is a severe deficit, it can be administered in concentrations up to 80 mEq. per liter or 20 mEq. per hour without producing hyperkalemia. In the presence of severe potassium deficiency, with constant ECG monitoring and frequent blood determinations, up to 40 mEq. per hr. can be given.

Initially, potassium should be given with saline rather than glucose solution because glucose will tend to shift potassium into the cells, resulting in even further lowering of the serum potassium. Eventually, the increase in sodium excretion produced will enhance urinary potassium losses, rendering replacement therapy less effective. In replacing potassium, it is well to remember that the potassium must cross a relatively small extracellular pool (50 to 70 mEq. per liter) in order to replace the intracellular stores of approximately 3000 mEq.

REFERENCES

1. Berlyne, G. M., Janabi, K., Shaw, A. B.: Dangers of resonium A in the treatment of hyperkalemia in renal failure. Lancet, 1:167–169, 1966.
2. Bland, J. H., ed.: Clinical Metabolism of Body Water and Electrolytes. Philadelphia, W. B. Saunders, 1963.
3. Chamberlain, M. J.: Emergency treatment of hyperkalemia. Lancet, 1:464, 1964.
4. Gropper, A. J.: Acute renal failure responding to potassium replacement therapy. Amer. J. Med., 24:153, 1958.
5. Herman, R. H., and McDowell, M. K.: Hyperkalemic paralysis (adynamica episodica hereditaria). Amer. J. Med., 35:749, 1963.
6. Kassirer, J. P., Berkman, P. M., Lawrenz, D. R., and Schwartz, W. B.: The critical role of chloride in the correction of hypokalemic alkalosis in man. Amer. J. Med., 38:172, 1965.
7. Levinsky, N. G.: Management of emergencies. VI. Hyperkalemia. New Eng. J. Med., 274:1076, 1966.
8. Myerson, R. M., and Frumin, A. M.: Hyperkalemia associated with the myeloproliferative disorders. Arch. Int. Med., 106:479, 1960.
9. Schwartz, W. B.: Potassium and the kidney. New Eng. J. Med., 253:601, 1955.
10. Skinner, S. L.: A cause of erroneous potassium levels. Lancet, 1:418, 1961.

Department of Medicine
University of Miami School of Medicine
P.O. Box 875, Biscayne Annex
Miami, Florida   33152
(Dr. Goldsmith)

Nutritional Management of Kidney Disorders

*Kurt Lange, M.D., F.A.C.P.**

BASIC PRINCIPLES OF PROTEIN METABOLISM

While the National Research Council considers the intake of 1 gm. of protein per kg. of body weight per day as desirable, this figure can be varied with impunity within wide ranges, especially when the biological value of the ingested proteins is taken into consideration. We know from the studies of Rose,[14] Giordano,[4] and Giovannetti and Maggiore[5] that a positive nitrogen balance can be maintained with nitrogen intakes of as little as 3 gm. per day, corresponding to approximately 18 gm. of protein, provided that the ingested protein contains all eight indispensable essential amino acids, leucin, isoleucin, lysine, phenylalanine, threonine, tryptophan, valine, and methionine. Thus the value of an ingested protein will depend not only on the amount ingested, but also its content of essential amino acids. The lack of a sufficient amount of even one of these proteins will prevent positive nitrogen balance, and body-owned muscle and liver protein will be broken down in an attempt to restore nitrogen balance.

While approximately 20 gm. of egg protein per day will cover the vital nitrogen need for positive balance, only 33 gm. of high class meat protein will serve the same purpose.[8] Thus the mere statement of a given amount of protein intake is of relatively little value in critical situations in which protein intake must be reduced to a minimum to reduce the amount of nitrogenous waste products which a functionally severely damaged kidney may not be able to eliminate. The caloric need must be amply covered to avoid the mobilization of body-owned nitrogen for energy needs with the subsequent increase in nitrogenous wastes.

It has also been suggested that a diet rich in carbohydrates may have

From the Renal Service and Laboratory, Departments of Medicine and Pediatrics, New York Medical College, New York, New York

*Professor of Medicine, Professor of Clinical Pediatrics; Chief, Renal Service and Laboratory; Attending Physician, Flower and Fifth Avenue Hospitals, Metropolitan Hospital, and Bird S. Coler Hospital; Consultant, Horton Memorial Hospital, Middletown, New York, and Chenango Hospital, Norwich, New York

Supported by Contract PH43-67-654, National Institutes of Health, and research grants from the Kidney Foundation of New York

a nitrogen-sparing effect.[13] The end-products of carbohydrate metabolism, carbon dioxide and water, do not require renal work since the small amount of metabolic water can readily be eliminated through sweat, lungs, and feces. In contrast, undue exposure to cold leads to increased nitrogen use and breakdown of body-owned protein, with the undesirable side-effects of overloading of the insufficient kidney.

ACUTE GLOMERULONEPHRITIS

In the first few days of acute glomerulonephritis we are dealing with an acute glomerulotubular imbalance produced by diffuse endothelial and mesangial proliferation in the glomeruli, leading to markedly reduced renal blood flow and diminished glomerular filtration rate; at the same time, tubular reabsorption of sodium is maintained at near normal levels, thus leading to salt and water retention and edema formation with expansion of the circulating blood volume.

Vollhard[17] has suggested that complete fluid and food abstention during the first days of the disease may be of decisive value. Animal experiments by Smadel and Farr,[15] using marked protein restriction in acute experimental glomerulonephritis, seemed to prove the value of such a dietary regimen, inasmuch as it markedly reduced animal mortality in uremia. These types of therapy have, however, been abandoned, since they did not seem to be of clinical value.

We have modified such an approach by giving our patients with acute glomerulonephritis a completely protein-free diet, consisting only of fruit juices, fortified with sugar or dextrose for the first 2 to 3 weeks of the disease. Since acute glomerulonephritis is based on an antigen-antibody reaction[9, 12] wherein the streptococcus contributes the antigens[16] and the body forms antibodies to these antigens and fixes complement in this reaction, as the mediator of cellular damage, it was felt that a diet which depresses antibody formation might be useful in alleviating and possibly shortening the course of the disease.

Cannon's classical experiments[3] seemed to indicate that complete withholding of essential amino acids from the diet markedly reduce the possibility of antibody formation. We are not sure as yet whether such a dietary regimen reduces length of morbidity or influences the final outcome; it appears very apparent to us, however, that with this therapy the occurrence of severe (although short-lasting) hypertension is avoided, that convulsive episodes are not seen, and that a rapid diuresis occurs. In general the patients feel subjectively better than the paired controls treated with a regular diet. The blood urea nitrogen values remain very low even in the presence of markedly depressed clearance values, whereas the serum creatinine values differ but little from those of the controls. It is important, however, that the caloric intake represented mostly by carbohydrates is sufficient to avoid excessive endogenous protein breakdown. Sodium intake must be restricted even in patients on regular diet to depress glomerular tubular imbalance as much as possible.

CHRONIC GLOMERULONEPHRITIS WITH MODERATE RENAL INSUFFICIENCY

If kidney function begins to decline, restriction of protein intake seems advisable. This, however, is frequently overdone, especially under the influence of the good results obtained with the Giordano-Giovannetti diet in uremia as described below. Figure 1 illustrates the fact that until clearance values have receded to approximately 50 per cent, a restriction of protein intake, except for reduction of real excesses, does not appear indicated. With clearance values between 50 and 10% of normal, gradual restriction of protein intake appears advisable. As long as the protein intake can be reasonably kept at more than 30 gm. per day without leading to marked elevations in blood urea nitrogen, good quality meat can represent the main source of proteins. Vegetable protein should not be used as the major source of proteins at this stage because of their low

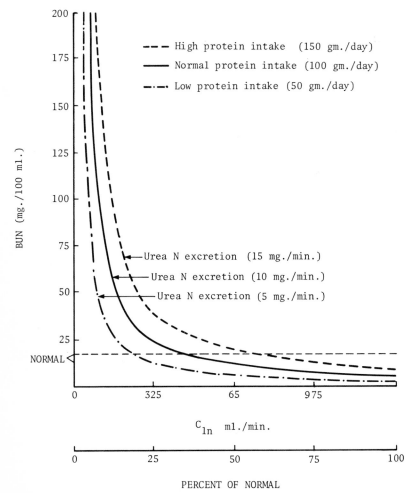

Figure 1.   Relation between protein intake clearance and blood urea nitrogen level. (Courtesy of Dr. John Maher.)

percentage of essential amino acids. When the glomerular filtration rate (GFR) falls to 10 ml. per min. or below, usually accompanied by serum creatinine values above 6 mg. per 100 ml., much more stringent dietary measures are indicated.

UREMIA

The patient with a glomerular filtration rate below 10 ml. per min., caused by chronic renal insufficiency, begins to show symptoms of uremia: severe anorexia, nausea, vomiting, and frequently diarrhea. With this vicious cycle of dehydration, acidosis, and further diminution of food intake, endogenous protein breakdown is initiated. While hemodialytic therapy and transplantation may be unavoidable in the long run, considerable alleviation and frequently complete abolishment of subjective complaints can be achieved by strict dietary measures.

Based on Rose's experimental observation[14] that only very small amounts of protein intake are needed to establish a nitrogen balance provided the proteins contain the essential amino acids, Giordano[4] composed such a synthetic diet for uremics and observed the astonishing fact that within 2 to 3 weeks the blood urea nitrogen values receded very significantly. In our own observation of 66 patients, these values receded by an average of 55 per cent and remained so as long as patients followed the diet conscientiously and the glomerular filtration rate did not decrease further. Appetite returned promptly, nausea, vomiting, and diarrhea disappeared, and a reasonable degree of well-being was re-established.

The synthetic diet was soon replaced by diets containing the essential amino acids in the minimally necessary quantities in natural proteins, and such highly restricted selected protein diets known as G-G diets (Giordano-Giovannetti) were adapted to the tastes of the population of different countries by several investigators.[1, 5, 7, 10] A diet scheme for American taste developed by our group is shown in Table 1. The need for a special bread using wheat starch as a source of carbohydrates is indispensable to reduce the supply of nonessential amino acids and at the same time to serve as a good and well-accepted source of calories.

With such a diet, the urea in the intestinal tract is transformed into ammonia by gastric and bacterial urease and is thus made available as building blocks for nonessential amino acids which the body seems to produce avidly. With the decreasing blood urea levels, formation of ammonia in the stomach and intestinal tract is markedly reduced and the gastrointestinal symptoms disappear rapidly, and the patient feels markedly improved. Serum creatinine values remain unaltered or recede only slightly, since endogenous creatinine production is independent of protein intake. Depending on the rapidity with which the kidney function dwindles, the effectiveness of the diet decreases. When the glomerular filtration rate goes below 3 ml. per min. and the creatinine value above 12 mg. per 100 ml., the diet becomes usually ineffective and dialytic therapy is indicated.

With the G-G diet, marked increases in potassium levels are ob-

Table 1. *Renal Diet*

BREAKFAST
> Fruit or juice and dextrose or grapefruit
> Bacon rinds and fat (crisply grilled NO LEAN) on fried gluten-free bread
> *or* Tomato or fried apple rings
> Gluten-free bread, toast
> Butter (from day's allowance)
> Marmalade, honey or jam

MID-MORNING
> Fruit juice and dextrose or tea (with milk from allowance)
> Special biscuits or cup cakes

LUNCH
> Vegetables (not peas, beans, or lentils) as a pie with wheat starch and vegetable margarine pastry
> *or* as a pie with 5 oz. potato topping
> *or* as a curry + 3 oz. (cooked weight) boiled rice
> *or* 3 oz. boiled rice + savoury fried vegetables

PUDDINGS
> 1. Fruit crumble + wheat starch + vegetable margarine + sugar, topping
> *or* 2. Fruit pie + wheat starch and vegetable margarine pastry
> *or* 3. Fruit or fruit mold (wheat starch or cornstarch thickening). (+ 1 oz. cream once or twice weekly only)
> *or* 4. Fruit puree + wheat starch or cornstarch sauce
> *or* 5. Boiled rice + ½ egg yolk, spread with jam, and meringue topping (½ egg white)
> *or* 6. Fruit + ½ egg yolk, with meringue topping (½ egg white)
> *or* 7. Sponge pudding (wheat starch + ½ egg) + syrup

MID-AFTERNOON
> Fruit juice + dextrose or tea (with milk from allowance)
> Gluten-free bread + butter + jam or honey
> *or* Special biscuits (wheat starch) or cake

EVENING MEAL
> Clear broth + rice or vegetables
> Vegetable salad or vegetable stew
> Gluten-free bread
> Fruit, if desired + dextrose or sugar

IMPORTANT
> During the day, one to two whole eggs *must* be taken
> If ½ egg is used in pudding, you can still take ½ egg with salad or ½ egg scrambled at another meal or in less advanced cases one additional egg
> *or* Take one egg — boiled, fried, poached, as omelette, or hard boiled in salad.

N.B. Methionine 0.5 gm. (two tablets) and iron tablets must be taken daily, as prescribed.

Notes on Renal Diet

DAILY ALLOWANCE
> 1½ oz. butter
> 1 to 2 eggs
> 6½ oz. milk (measured carefully) for tea or coffee

MARGARINE
> Use only vegetable margarine (Tomor, Crisco, Fleischman's)

FRYING
> Any vegetable oil may be used

SUGAR AND DEXTROSE
> Should be used liberally

FOODS FORBIDDEN
> Ordinary flour in any form, meat, fish, cheese

(Table continues on following page.)

Table 1. *Renal Diet* (Continued)

RECIPE FOR GLUTEN-FREE BREAD

    1   lb. wheat starch
    10½ ozs. water
    1   oz. yeast
    1   oz. sugar
    2   ozs. margarine/veg. oil
        Mix yeast with sugar. Warm special flour, rub in fat, add warm water. Mix to a
        soft batter consistency. Beat well. Pour into greased tins. Allow to stand in a
        warm place until it has risen to fill the tin. Bake at 450–500° F

Note: Bread, cupcakes, and cookies suitable for the G-G diet may be obtained from
Wuest Diet Bakeries, 176 Sherman Avenue, Jersey City, New Jersey.

served in approximately 50 per cent of the patients, probably because of
the copious intake of fruit in the diet. With oral sulfonic resins (Kayexalate) this difficulty can usually be overcome with ease.

It was interesting to note that a uremic patient who underwent
nephrectomy prior to transplantation was fairly well stabilized on the
G-G diet. When the daily allowance of essential amino acids was with-
drawn in favor of a more liberal diet, but deficient in one essential amino
acid, the blood urea nitrogen rose in significant daily increments. Restoration of the full complement of essential amino acids promptly reduced
the blood urea nitrogen values again.

In the period during which the patients were on the G-G diet, we observed that motor nerve conduction velocity frequently decreased, as
it would without the benefit of the diet. Similarly, when already present
at the onset of dietary therapy, such a significant decrease did not
vanish, in spite of the subjective improvement of the patient. EEG
changes in the form of slow wave activity, present at onset of dietary
therapy, did not disappear and occasionally appeared while the patient
was on "the diet." This is in contrast to dialytic therapy which, when
carried out properly, will reduce or normalize the neurologic abnormalities. It is thus evident that the dietary therapy does not remove some
very important uremic toxins in contrast to chronic peritoneal or hemodialysis.[11]

We consider the appearance of significantly reduced nerve conduction time an indication to abandon pure dietetic therapy and to replace
it either by mixed dietetic and dialytic therapy, or by complete transfer
to hemodialysis treatment. Since chronic dialysis therapy, however,
represents a major intervention into the patient's life, and is cumber-
some, very expensive, and available for only a small percentage of
chronic uremics, dietary therapy of uremics should be used exclusively
until the hand of the treating physician is forced by the above-mentioned
circumstances. The value of the diet can hardly be overestimated, since
it may prolong the patient's well-being for months or years, especially
in cases with very slow progression of the functional defect, e.g., in
polycystic kidneys.

While protein restriction is helpful in chronic hemodialysis to avoid
rapid rises in uremic toxins between the individual sessions, attention
should be paid to the fact that considerable amounts of amino acids are
lost with each hemodialysis; still greater amounts are lost with peritoneal
dialysis. The loss of folic acid during dialysis, as a contributing factor in
the anemia of the uremic,[17] is still under discussion, but the addition of

15 mg. of folic acid to the diet often seems to improve the hematologic situation somewhat.

Since most patients in uremia suffer from hypertension, the temptation is great to restrict their sodium intake extremely, as one would probably do in hypertension without uremia. Such management can be disastrous. Certain patients, for reasons poorly understood, become salt-wasters in the advanced stages of the disease, probably owing to damaged nephrons and disturbed interstitial transport in the counter-current apparatus. Another explanation is the intact nephron theory of Bricker,[2] wherein the still functioning nephrons have shown increased filtration but relative suppression of proximal tubular reabsorption leading to salt loss. By markedly diminished salt intake in uremia, salt-losing can be diminished, but at the expense of extracellular fluid depletion, resulting in further deterioration of the patient's condition. The hypertension of advanced uremia should be treated by suitable antihypertensive medication, but not by salt restriction. On the other hand, if the patient is in a chronic hemodialysis program, having no or only minimal urine excretion, these rules do not apply and strict sodium restriction may be useful in combating the hypertension.

DIET IN THE NEPHROTIC SYNDROME

In all forms of the nephrotic syndrome, the marked proteinuria, which may vary from 3 to 30 gm. per 24 hours, has led to an indiscriminate "forcing" of protein intake. It is a well-established fact, however, that any increase in plasma proteins by forced protein feeding, or still more clearly by the intravenous infusion of salt-poor albumin, leads to a prompt increase in urinary protein loss. Intravenously infused albumin can usually be recovered quantitatively from the urine within 48 to 72 hours, above and beyond the amount of proteinuria which the patient excretes regularly before the infusion. While a somewhat increased protein intake may be advisable, the frequently encountered massive protein feeding has no value whatsoever. Unless the permeability of the glomerular basement membrane for proteins can be reduced, improvement of the hypoproteinemia by intravenous or increased oral protein intake cannot be expected to occur, nor can a positive nitrogen balance be re-established by such measures. Similarly, restriction of salt intake does not seem to influence the edema since it is mostly, if not completely, caused by the lowered oncotic pressure. For that same reason, even massive doses of diuretics are usually ineffective and, if very rarely effective, may lead to shock by further reduction of the already markedly reduced circulating blood volume.

DIETARY TREATMENT OF ACUTE RENAL FAILURE

The early and frequent use of peritoneal or hemodialysis in acute renal failure has recently been common practice in some institutions. It is thus forgotten that probably the majority of cases of acute renal failure can be treated by proper medical management alone. The rise in

KURT LANGE

nitrogenous waste products should not be the indication for dialytic therapy unless it is excessively fast (BUN by more than 30 mg. per 100 ml. per day). Fluid restriction remains the backbone of therapy: 500 ml. per 24 hours, to which the amount of fluid lost by urine, diarrhea, or vomitus may be added, should represent the only fluid given to the patient. Five to 10 per cent dextrose in water administered intravenously with 1 unit of insulin added per 10 gm. of dextrose is the method of choice. The life-threatening rise in potassium level can be combated with Kayexalate, with careful blood electrolyte determinations carried out every 12 hours.

Most recently, the introduction of the G-G diet with careful estimation of its water content (which must be included in the fluid balance mentioned above) seems to yield promising results, especially in patients with markedly prolonged oliguria where provision of an adequate caloric intake may be of importance. The available high carbohydrate additives to the ingested fluids can make this task easier. It should be understood, however, that dialysis therapy should be instituted early when an ingested or inhaled dialyzable and not yet tissue-fixed poison plays the major role in the acute renal failure.

REFERENCES

1. Berlyne, G. M., Shaw, A. B., and Nilwarangkur, S.: Dietary treatment of chronic renal failure. Experiences with a modified Giovannetti diet. Nephron, 2:129, 1965.
2. Bricker, N. S., Klahr, S., Lubowitz, H., and Rieselbach, R. E.: Renal function in chronic renal disease. Medicine, 44:263, 1965.
3. Cannon, P. R.: Antibodies and the protein-reserves. J. Immunol., 44:107, 1942.
4. Giordano, C.: Use of exogenous and endogenous urea for protein synthesis in normal and uremic subjects. J. Lab. and Clin. Med., 62:231, 1963.
5. Giovannetti, S., and Maggiore, Q.: A low-nitrogen diet with proteins of high biological value for severe chronic uraemia. Lancet, 1:1000, 1964.
6. Hampers, C. L., Steriff, D., and Nathan, R.: Megaloblastic hematopoiesis in chronic renal failure. Clin. Res., 14:379, 1966.
7. Kluthe, R., and Quirin, H.: Diätbuch für Nieren Kranke. Stuttgart, Georg Thieme Verlag, 1968.
8. Lang, K., and Ranke, O. F.: Stoffwechsel und Ernährung. Berlin, Springer, 1950.
9. Lange, K., Slobody, L., Graig, F., Ogur, G., Oberman, J., and LoCasto, F.: Changes in serum complement during the course and treatment of glomerulonephritis. Arch. Int. Med., 88:433, 1951.
10. Lonergan, E. T., and Lange, K.: Use of a special protein-restricted diet in uremia. Amer. J. Clin. Nutr., 21:595, 1968.
11. Lonergan, E. T., Semar, M., and Lange, K.: Transketolase activity in uremia. Arch. Int. Med. (in press).
12. Mellors, R. C., and Ortega, L. G.: Analytical pathology. III New observations on the pathogenesis of glomerulonephritis, lipid nephrosis, periarteritis nodosa, and secondary amyloidosis in man. J. Path., 32:455, 1956.
13. Munro, H. N.: Carbohydrate and fat as factors in protein utilization and metabolism. Physiol. Rev., 31:449, 1951.
14. Rose, W. C.: The amino acid requirements of adult man. Nutr. Abstr. Reviews, 27:631, 1957.
15. Smadel, I. E., and Farr, L. E.: The effect of diet on the pathologic change in rats with nephritotoxic nephritis. Amer. J. Path., 15:199, 1939.
16. Treser, G., Semar, M., Ty, A., Sagel, I., Franklin, M. A., and Lange, K.: Partial characterization of antigenic streptococcal plasma membrane. J. Clin. Invest., 49:762, 1970.
17. Vollhard, F.: Die doppelseitigen Nierenerkrankungen. In Handbuch innerische Medizin. 2nd ed. Berlin, Springer Verlag, 1931, vol. 6, p. 1.

New York Medical College
Flower and Fifth Avenue Hospitals
New York, New York   10029

Index

Note: Page numbers of symposium and article titles are in **boldface** type.

ACIDOSIS, renal tubular, in chronic renal failure, 347
  cirrhosis and, 369
  treatment, 339
Adrenergic receptors, blockers of, cardiac arrhythmias and, 289
  for angina pectoris, 428
Airway, artificial, 451
  obstruction, **445–456**
Alcoholism, hepatitis and, 386
Alkalosis, diuretic-induced, 365
Aminophylline, as bronchodilator, 450
Amylopectin sulfate, in peptic ulcer disease, 312
Anemia, chronic renal failure and, 348
Angina pectoris, stable, diagnosis and treatment, **420–433**
Antacids, in peptic ulcer disease, 310
Anti-anxiety drugs, in medical practice, **485–494**
Antibiotic drugs, microbial suprainfection and, **471–483**
Anticholinergic drugs, in peptic ulcer disease, 311
Antidepressant drugs, in medical practice, **485–494**
Antigens, hepatitis-associated, chronic hepatitis and, 383
Antihypertensive drugs, 320–324
Antimicrobial agents, as cause of suprainfection, **472–483**
Anxiety, depression and, drug therapy in medical practice, **485–494**
Arrhythmias, cardiac, adrenergic blocking agents and, 289
  after acute myocardial infarction, treatment, **273–293**
    treatment, basic considerations, **435–444**
Ascites, tense, treatment of, 370

Asthma, bronchial, airway obstruction in, 446
Ataractic drugs, in medical practice, **485–494**
Atropine, for cardiac arrhythmia, 277

BIGUANIDES, in diabetes mellitus, 300
Biopsy, muscle, in diagnosis of diabetes mellitus, 297
Blocking agents. See *Adrenergic receptors, blockers of.*
Blood, glucose, in diabetes mellitus, control of, 298
  pressure, high. See also *Hypertension.*
    reduction of, hazards in, 317
  urea nitrogen, glomerular filtration rate and, 343
Body weight. See also *Obesity.*
  in diabetes mellitus, management, 299
Bone lesions, chronic renal failure and, 349
Bretylium tosylate, for cardiac arrhythmias, 442
Bronchitis, chronic, airway obstruction in, 445
Bronchospasm, management, 447
Bricker hypothesis, 343

CALCIUM insufficiency. See *Hypocalcemia.*
Caloric balance, positive. See *Obesity.*
Caloric intake, in acute renal tubular insufficiency, 338
Carbenoxolone, for peptic ulcer disease, 312
Carbohydrate intolerance, causes, 296
Cardiac fiber conduction, electrophysiology of, 435–438

Cardiopulmonary system, uremic manifestations in, 351
Carotid sinus nerve stimulation for angina pectoris, 429
Cell function, potassium and, 503
Cholestyramine, for pruritus of biliary cirrhosis, 374
Cirrhosis, biliary, pruritus and, treatment, 373
    renal tubular acidosis with, 369
Colonization, in microbial suprainfection, 473
Coma, hepatic, treatment, 373
Contraceptives, oral, hyperlipemia and, 407
Cor pulmonale, chronic bronchitis and, 451
Coronary care unit, intermediate, 290
Corticosteroids, for bronchospasm, 450
    for osteoarthritis, 465
Creatinine, serum, glomerular filtration rate and, 343

DEPRESSION, anxiety and, drug therapy in medical practice, **485–494**
Diabetes, hyperlipemia and, 414
    mellitus, insulin-independent, complications, 302
        diagnosis and treatment, **295–304**
Dialysis, chronic intermittent, in end-stage renal disease, 353
    in acute renal tubular insufficiency, 340
Diet, Giordano-Giovannetti, 516
    low-protein, for uremic symptoms, 352
    therapy, in edema, 366
        in kidney disorders, **513–520**
        in obesity, 396
        in peptic ulcer disease, 309
Digitalis, for cardiac arrhythmia, 286
Diphenylhydantoin, for cardiac arrhythmias, 440
Diuresis, effects of, 361
Diuretics, clinical use, 365–371
    for chronic hypertension, 320
    for edema, **359–371**
    outpatient use, 371
Drugs, dosage, renal failure, and, 341
    interactions in multiple drug therapy, **495–502**

EDEMA, diuretic drug therapy for, **359–371**
    pulmonary, acute, treatment, 370
    refractory, treatment, 367
Emphysema, airway obstruction in, 445
Encephalopathy, hypertensive, 329
Epinephrine, for bronchospasm, 447
Ethacrynic acid, toxic effects, 366
Extracellular fluid. See under *Fluids*.

FATS, malabsorption, with cirrhosis, treatment, 374

Fluids, and electrolytes, abnormalities, in chronic renal failure, 345
    therapy, in acute renal tubular insufficiency, 338
    urinary concentration, diuretics and, 363
    extracellular, overload syndromes, symptomatic treatment, **359–371**
    volume maintenance, in chronic renal failure, 346
Furosemide, toxic effects, 366

GASTRIC acid secretion, peptic ulcer and, 305
Gastrointestinal tract, abnormalities, in uremic syndrome, 351
Gastroscopy, in peptic ulcer disease, 308
Giordano-Giovannetti diet, 516
Glomerular filtration rate, blood urea nitrogen and, 343
Glomerulonephritis, dietary management, 514, 515
Glucose tolerance test, in diabetes mellitus, 295
Guanethidine, for hypertension, 323

HAA. See *Hepatitis-associated antigen*.
Halothane, fulminant hepatic failure and, 377
Heart, arrhythmias. See *Arrhythmias*.
    block, after myocardial infarction, treatment, 278–285
    electrophysiology of, 435–438
Hepatic coma, treatment, 373
Hepatic failure, fulminant, treatment, 377
Hepatitis, alcoholic, treatment, 386
    chronic, treatment, 380
    viral, acute uncomplicated, treatment, 374
Hepatitis-associated antigen (HAA), chronic hepatitis and, 383
Hepatoma, hypercholesterolemia and, 404
Hydralazine, for hypertension, 322
Hypercholesterolemia, diagnosis and treatment, 404
Hyperglycemia, hyperlipemia and, 414
    in diabetes mellitus, management, 298
Hyperkalemia, diagnosis and management, 506–510
    in chronic renal failure, 347
    in oliguric patient, management, 339
Hyperlipemias, causes, 407
    diabetes mellitus and, 303
    primary, 408–414
Hyperlipidemias, carbohydrate-induced, 296
    clinical approach to, **403–419**
    plasma lactescence and, 404
Hypertension, chronic, treatment, **317–324**
    crises, **325–332**
    encephalopathy (crisis) in, 329
    malignant, 325–329
    renal failure and, chronic, 349
Hypertriglyceridemias, diabetes mellitus and, 303
Hypocalcemia, in chronic renal failure, 348
Hypokalemia, diagnosis and management, 510–512

Hyponatremia, diuretic therapy and, 364
Hypoxemia, in acute respiratory failure and obstructive airway disease, management, 446

INFECTION, antibiotics and suprainfection, **471–483**
Intact nephron hypothesis, 343

JOINT disease, degenerative. See *Osteoarthritis.*

KIDNEY. See also *Renal.*
disorders, nutritional management, **513–520**

LACTULOSE, for hepatic coma, 373
Lidocaine, for cardiac arrhythmias, 275, 440
Liver. See also *Hepatic.*
Liver disease. See also *Hepatitis.*
obstructive, hypercholesterolemia and, 404
therapeutic considerations in, **373–390**

MALABSORPTION, fat, cirrhosis and, treatment, 374
Medical disorders, common, treatment of, symposium on, **273–520**
Methyldopa, for hypertension, 322
Microbial suprainfection, recognition and management, **471–483**
Muscle biopsy, in diagnosis of diabetes mellitus, 297
Myocardium, infarction, arrhythmias after, treatment, **273–293**
heart block after, 278–285
Myxedema, hypercholesterolemia in, 404

NATRIURETIC drugs, 359
Nephrotic syndrome, diet in, 519
hyperlipemia and, 407
Nervous system abnormalities, in uremia, 351
Nitrites, for angina pectoris, 426
Nitrogen balance, protein metabolism and, 513

OBESITY, carbohydrate intolerance and, 296
causes of, 392
management, **391–401**
Oliguria, in acute renal tubular insufficiency, treatment, 337
Osteitis fibrosis, chronic renal failure and, 350

Osteoarthritis, comprehensive regimen for, **457–469**
Osteodystrophy, renal, treatment, 349
Osteomalacia, treatment, 349

PACEMAKER, cardiac, in heart block with acute myocardial infarction, 281, 284
Pargyline, for hypertension, 323
Peptic ulcer, uncomplicated, treatment, **305–315**
Pericarditis, fibrinous, uremia and, 351
Phenformin, in diabetes mellitus, 301
Plasma, lactescence, hyperlipidemias and, 404
triglycerides, in diagnosis of hyperlipidemias, 403
volume, diuretics and, 362
Pneumonia, bacterial suprainfection and, 476
Potassium, cell function and, 503
excess. See *Hyperkalemia.*
metabolism, disorders, diagnosis and treatment, **503–512**
Procainamide, for cardiac arrhythmias, 439
Propranolol, for angina pectoris, 428
for cardiac arrhythmia, 275, 287, 441
for hypertension, 323
Protein metabolism, nitrogen balance and, 513
Pruritus of biliary cirrhosis, treatment, 373
Pulmonary edema, acute, treatment, 370

QUINIDINE, for cardiac arrhythmias, 438

RENAL failure, acute, diagnosis and treatment, **335–342**
dietary management, 519
chronic, diagnosis and treatment, **342–357**
metabolic consequences, 344
drug diseases and, 341
Renal osteodystrophy, 349
Renal tubular acidosis. See *Acidosis, renal tubular.*
Renal tubular insufficiency, acute, diagnosis and treatment, 335
Reserpine, for hypertension, 321
Respiration, assisted, in obstructive airway disease, 452–455
Respiratory failure, acute, in obstructive airway disease, 446
Rickets, chronic renal failure and, 349
Roentgen treatment, for peptic ulcer disease, 314

SALICYLATES, for osteoarthritis, 463
Sodium, renal excretion, diuretics and, 359–361
in chronic renal failure, 345
Spine, osteoarthritis of, 467

Sulfonylureas, in diabetes mellitus, 300

Superinfection, microbial, 473

Suprainfection, microbial, recognition and management, **471–483**

Surgery, for peptic ulcer disease, 313

TOTAL body water, diuretics and, 362

Tranquilizers, in medical practice, **485–494**

Triglycerides, plasma, in diagnosis of hyperlipidemia, 403

Trimethaphan, for hypertensive emergencies, 331

ULCER, peptic. See *Peptic ulcer.*

Urea nitrogen, blood, glomerular filtration rate and, 343

Uremia, dietary management, 516

manifestations and treatment, 350–355

VENTILATION, mechanical, 451

Virus, hepatitis from, uncomplicated acute, treatment, 374

WATER, deficiency, in chronic renal failure, management, 346

total body, diuretics and, 362

ZIEVE'S syndrome, hyperlipemia and, 407

FIRST CLASS
PERMIT NO. 101
PHILADELPHIA, PA.

BUSINESS REPLY MAIL
NO POSTAGE STAMP NECESSARY IF MAILED IN UNITED STATES

POSTAGE WILL BE PAID BY

W. B. Saunders Company

West Washington Square
Philadelphia, Pa. 19105

...cal checkup!

On the move?